Advances in Diabetes

Novel Insights

Advances in Diabetes

Novel Insights

Second Edition

Editor

GR Sridhar MD DM FACE FRCP
Director
Endocrine and Diabetes Centre
Visakhapatnam, Andhra Pradesh, India

Foreword

PV Rao MD PhD FRCP (Lond)

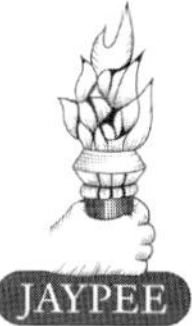

JAYPEE BROTHERS MEDICAL PUBLISHERS
The Health Sciences Publisher
New Delhi | London

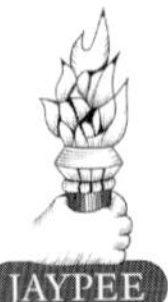

Jaypee Brothers Medical Publishers (P) Ltd

Headquarters
EMCA House
23/23-B, Ansari Road, Daryaganj
New Delhi 110 002, India
Landline: +91-11-23272143, +91-11-23272703
+91-11-23282021, +91-11-23245672
E-mail: jaypee@jaypeebrothers.com

Corporate Office
Jaypee Brothers Medical Publishers (P) Ltd.
4838/24, Ansari Road, Daryaganj
New Delhi 110 002, India
Phone: +91-11-43574357
Fax: +91-11-43574314
E-mail: jaypee@jaypeebrothers.com

Overseas Office
JP Medical Ltd.
83, Victoria Street, London
SW1H 0HW (UK)
Phone: +44-20 3170 8910
Fax: +44(0)20 3008 6180
E-mail: info@jpmedpub.com

Website: www.jaypeebrothers.com
Website: www.jaypeedigital.com

Inquiries for bulk sales may be solicited at: jaypee@jaypeebrothers.com

Advances in Diabetes: Novel Insights / *GR Sridhar*

First Edition: 2016

Second Edition: **2024**

ISBN: 978-81-947090-3-9

Printed at: Sterling Graphics Pvt. Ltd. India

To
Nagamani

Contributors

EDITOR

GR Sridhar MD DM FACE FRCP
Director
Endocrine and Diabetes Centre
Visakhapatnam, Andhra Pradesh, India

CONTRIBUTING AUTHORS

Ajay Raj Mallela MD DM
Consultant Endocrinologist
Department of Endocrinology
Arka Multispeciality Hospital
Gudivada, Andhra Pradesh, India

Anton B Tonchev MD DSc
Department of Anatomy and
Cell Biology
Medical University
Varna, Bulgaria

Aravind Ramachandra Sosale DNB
FRCP (Glasg and Edin)
Director, DIACON Hospital
Bengaluru, Karnataka, India

Arun Shankar MBBS FDIAB (RSSDI)
PG Dip Diab CCEBDM (PHFI)
Medical Director
Jothydev's Diabetes and
Research Center
Thiruvananthapuram, Kerala, India

Bhavana Sosale MD MRCP (Glasg)
FRCP (Edin)
Consultant Diabetologist and Physician
DIACON Hospital
Bengaluru, Karnataka, India

Chitra Selvan MBBS MD DM MRCP
Associate Professor
Department of Endocrinology
MS Ramaiah Medical College
Bengaluru, Karnataka, India

Deepak K Jumani ACS (USA) FIAMS
FCSEPI MBBS (Bom) PhD (USA) MRCPS
(Glasg) FRCP (Glasg)
Consultant Senior Sexual Health
Physician and Counselor
Honorary Assistant Professor
Department of Medicine (Sexual
Health)
Sir JJ Group of Hospitals and Grant
Government Medical College
Mumbai, Maharashtra, India

Dwaipayan Bharadwaj PhD
Professor
Systems Genomics Laboratory
School of Biotechnology
Jawaharlal Nehru University
New Delhi, India

Ganesh Chauhan PhD
Associate Professor
Department of Genetics and Genomics
Rajendra Institute of Medical Sciences
Ranchi, Jharkhand, India

George N Chaldakov MD PhD DHC FIACS
Department of Anatomy and
Cell Biology and Translational Stem
Cell Biology
Research Institute, Medical University
Varna, Bulgaria

G Lakshmi MD
Assistant Professor
Department of Medicine
Gayatri Vidya Parishad Institute of
Healthcare and Medical Technology
Visakhapatnam, Andhra Pradesh, India

G Nagamani MD DGO
Professor and Head
Department of Obstetrics and
Gynecology, Andhra Medical College
Visakhapatnam, Andhra Pradesh, India

Gopika Krishnan BPharm MBA
Academic Head
Jothydev's Diabetes and Research
Center
Thiruvananthapuram, Kerala, India

GR Sridhar MD DM FACE FRCP
Director
Endocrine and Diabetes Centre
Visakhapatnam, Andhra Pradesh, India

Jothydev Kesavadev MD FRCP (Lond, Glasg, Edin) FACE FACP
Chairman
Jothydev's Diabetes and
Research Center
Thiruvananthapuram, Kerala, India

K Madhu MD
Former Professor and Head
Department of Psychology
Andhra University
Visakhapatnam, Andhra Pradesh, India

Kudugunti Neelaveni MD DM
Professor
Department of Endocrinology
Osmania Medical College
Osmania General Hospital
Hyderabad, Telangana, India

Levent Özturk MD DSc
Faculty of Medicine
Department of Physiology
Trakya University
Edirne, Turkey

Luigi Aloe PhD DHC
Fondazione Iret Tecnopolo R
Levi-Montalcini
Rome, Italy

Marco Fiore PhD
Institute of Biochemistry and
Cell Biology
Section of Neurobiology
National Research Council (CNR)
Rome, Italy

Mythili Ayyagari MD DM FACE
Professor
Department of Endocrinology
Andhra Medical College
Visakhapatnam, Andhra Pradesh, India

Nitya SN Malladi MD DNB MNAMS
Speciality Registrar in Dermatology
University Hospital of Wales
Cardiff, United Kingdom

Prasanna Kumar KM MD DM
Director and Consultant
Endocrinologist
Department of Endocrinology
Center for Diabetes and Endocrine Care
Bengaluru, Karnataka, India

Rao Tatavarti MS (IIT Madras) PhD (Dalhousie, Canada) DRDS FOSI FAPAS
Director and Distinguished Professor
Gayatri Parishad Scientific and Industrial Research Centre (GVP-SIRC) and Gayatri Vidya Parishad College of Engineering
Visakhapatnam, Andhra Pradesh, India

Rouzha Z Pancheva MD DSc
Faculty of Public Health
Department of Hygiene and Epidemiology
Medical University
Varna, Bulgaria

S Aruna Sri MA (PhD)
Assistant Professor
Department of Psychology
Dr LB College (Affiliated with Andhra University)
Consultant Psychologist
Wellness Hub India Private Limited
Visakhapatnam, Andhra Pradesh, India

Sanjana Narasimhadevara SN MD
Resident Physician
Department of Internal Medicine
BronxCare Health System
Affiliated with Icahn School of Medicine at Mount Sinai, Bronx
Bronx, New York, United States

Sreelakshmi R PhD
Research Scientist
Jothydev's Diabetes and Research Center
Thiruvananthapuram, Kerala, India

Stanislav Yanev MD
Department of Drug Toxicology
Institute of Neurobiology
Bulgarian Academy of Sciences
Sofia, Bulgaria

Sujatha RL Malladi MD DPD (Cardiff)
Senior Consultant in Dermatology
Gagangiri Complex, Chembur
Mumbai, Maharashtra, India

Venkateswarlu Kolichana MD DM FIAN
Emeritus Professor
Faculty of Neurology
Andhra Medical College
Visakhapatnam, Andhra Pradesh, India

Vidya D Kharkar MD DVD
Professor and Head
Department of Dermatology
Seth GS Medical College and KEM Hospital
Mumbai, Maharashtra, India

Rama Kumar MBBS DipDiab (Croatia) FIDF (Sweden) FDI
Certified Laughter Yoga Leader
SVR Diabetes Care and Research Centre
Guntur, Andhra Pradesh, India

Foreword

Knowledge about diabetes is exploding. It threatens to overwhelm, rather than inform and educate. Attending any of the many conferences entails a careful choice of sessions of interest. The editor and contributors of this monograph have done a wonderful job in making some of the choices for its readers, who wish to read, rather than listen. From the topics and the expertise of the authors, these are choices well made; a synthesis of clinical and basic science and other topics that both educate and amuse.

This is an intriguing addition to the literature on diabetes.

PV Rao MD PhD FRCP (Lond)
Professor and Head
Department of Endocrinology and Metabolism
Nizam's Institute of Medical Sciences
Hyderabad, Telangana, India

Preface to the Second Edition

While a week could be a long time in politics, 6 years certainly is in diabetes—the time elapsed since the previous volume of "Advances in Diabetes."

There were advances in areas long thought of as being "established", with little to add: Newer ways to classify diabetes based on emerging pathogenic mechanisms which allow more rational treatment. Attempts were made to develop drugs modulating secretions from adipose tissue and skeletal muscles.

Twenty years of genomics is time enough to see where the promise of the Human Genomic Project has led and what the future holds. Air pollution is traditionally thought to cause respiratory disease. It is now shown to have a role in obesity and diabetes mellitus. Professor Rao Tatavarti et al. describe simpler methods to measure air pollutants.

Advances have been made in the pathogenesis, identification, and management of diabetes-related vascular disease. They are highlighted in chapters on cerebrovascular disease, peripheral artery disease, and nephropathy. Professor Vidya et al. present the skin vasculature as an accessible window to diabetic microangiopathy. Professor Jumani updates therapeutic approaches in male sexual dysfunction in diabetes, a frequent gray zone. Not just a proximate complication in pregnancy, high blood pressure has long-term implications for the woman even later. Professor Nagamani et al. present an account of this important aspect.

With the deluge of available data, artificial intelligence (AI) has been in the forefront of diabetes management. Professor Aravind et al. share their experience on using AI in identifying diabetic retinopathy, the first robust application in clinical care. Prevention of hypoglycemia utilizing AI is reviewed in another chapter.

Two years of the pandemic compromised access to medical clinical care, thereby highlighting the need for teleconsultation. Professor Jyothydev et al. share their decades-long experience in this area. Similarly, the use of corticosteroids in the management of COVID-19, with its attendant risks and benefits, has been addressed.

No matter what the technical advances and potential drug targets, managing "self" is a crucial and often difficult part in diabetes treatment. An account of mindful meditation by Professor K Madhu et al. is timely. Similarly, humor plays a part in patient–physician relation. Rather than employ it in an ad hoc manner, Dr Ram Kumar et al. formalized the role of humor ("Geletology") as an adjunctive management of diabetes.

There have been fascinating advances in unusual areas targeting obesity and diabetes mellitus: Timing of food rather than just the quality or quantity, and potential use of drugs to regulate nerves to adipocytes in managing metabolic syndrome. Finally, the Renaissance group of drugs, the SGLT-2 inhibitors, find extended use beyond diabetes mellitus.

All in all, the second volume of "Advances in Diabetes: Novel Insights" has a mix of updating concepts, advances in vascular involvement, self-care, remote delivery of treatment, and a clutch of potential applications—the science fiction of diabetes mellitus.

GR Sridhar

Preface to the First Edition

Does diabetes need yet another publication? Ever since the 'Progress in Medicine' series edited by Professor MMS Ahuja, there have been similar efforts in various specialties of medicine. Diabetes seems to be relatively untouched by such efforts, and hence this monograph. Even with the proliferation and access to information, one sometimes wants a crystallized digest of the field, that as described in the Foreword both educates and amuses.

The genetic basis of diabetes, its relation with epigenetics and the limitations of genomics are well brought out, followed by an account of β-cell development, which can be utilized to replicate and replenish lost pancreatic β cells. Insulin signaling pathway is then brought up, as a basis for the use of insulin and the perceived adverse effects that have been recently highlighted. Other molecules and ligands, which have come into mainstream such as incretins and dual peroxisome proliferator-activated receptors (PPAR) agonists are also covered, where basic science leads to newer drug molecules. In the management aspects, the status of bariatric surgery as a potential cure and its current limitations are highlighted.

To put into perspective that science and knowledge alone cannot change behavior, psychological stress, and relaxation response have been delineated; the role of physical exercise, often prescribed to prevent obesity and diabetes, also seems to preserve cognition. Depression, which is in close companionship with obesity and diabetes, finds a place. Scientific advances in society – the electric light have changed the distinction between day and night and its relation to sleep, and to diabetes completes the behavioral aspects.

There are some surprising associations with diabetes which have come to the fore; the close relation of bone and energy metabolism is being increasingly recognized. Oral health seems to be important in the pathogenesis of diabetes and has been highlighted. The field of bioinformatics provides new areas of investigation; sequences related to human insulin were found in plant kingdom, suggesting that plants may be a source of glucose modulating agents. Finally, if a bariatric surgeon can 'cure' diabetes, can hypertension be left off? Ablation of sympathetic nerves in the treatment of resistant hypertension, seen also in diabetes, is an emerging concept.

I thank all the contributors for sparing their time to share their expertise for this volume.

GR Sridhar

Acknowledgments

My appreciation and sincere thanks to the authors and coauthors who have spared their time and effort to share their knowledge: Professors George N Chaldakov, Rao Tatavarti, Dwaipayan Bharadwaj, Venkateswarlu Kolichana, Prasanna Kumar KM, Kudugunti Neelaveni, Vidya D Kharkar, G Nagamani, Deepak K Jumani, Aravind Ramachandra Sosale, Jothydev Kesavadev, K Madhu (since deceased) and Drs Ram Kumar, G Lakshmi, and Sanjana Narasimhadevara SN.

I also want to express my deepest gratitude to M/s Jaypee Brothers Medical Publishers (P) Ltd, New Delhi, India, special thanks to Shri Jitendar P Vij (Group Chairman), Mr Ankit Vij (Managing Director), Mr MS Mani (Group President), Dr Richa Saxena (Associate Director—Professional Publishing), and Ms Himani Pandey (Development Editor) from Jaypee Brothers for their hard work, patience, and understanding.

Contents

PLATE 1

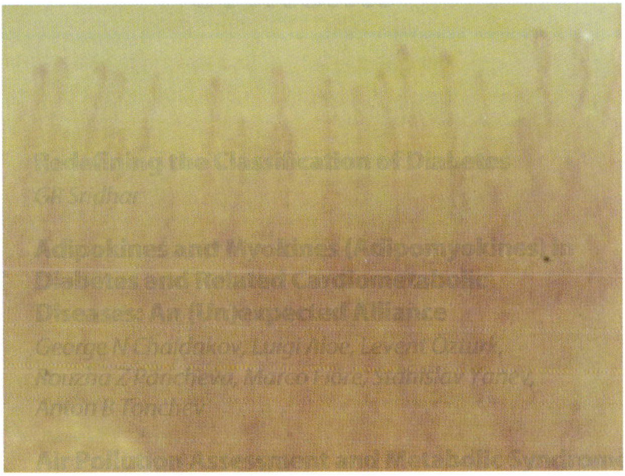

Fig. 1: Normal pattern of capillary vessels. ***(Chapter 8)***

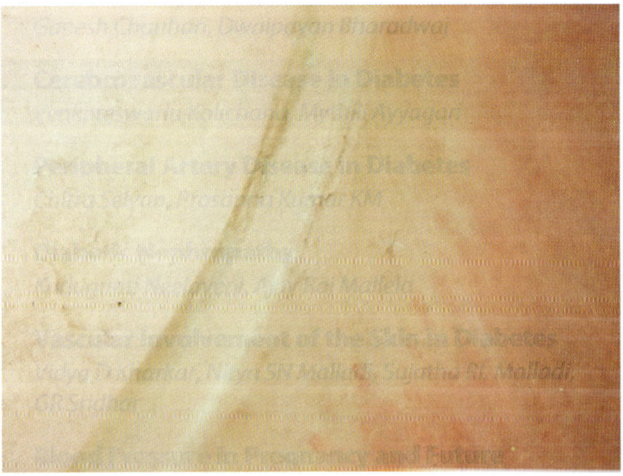

Fig. 2: Tortuous and enlarged capillaries in diabetes. ***(Chapter 8)***

PLATE 2

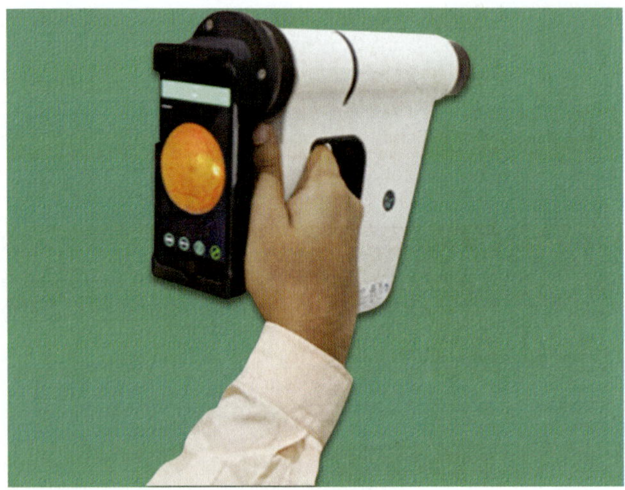

(AI: artificial intelligence; FOP: Fundus on Phone)

Fig. 1: The Remidio FOP with the offline Medios AI. ***(Chapter 11)***

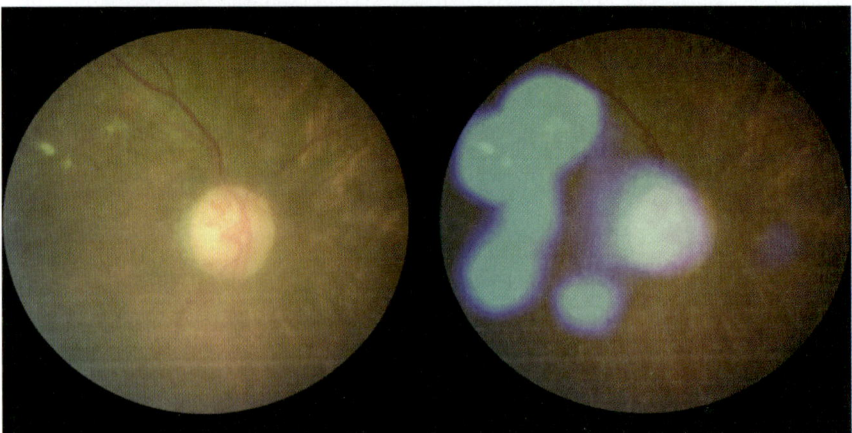

Fig. 2: A report generated by the Medios artificial intelligence (AI) in an individual with diabetic retinopathy. ***(Chapter 11)***

Result: Signs of retinopathy are detected. Examples of lesions are highlighted.

CHAPTER 1

Redefining the Classification of Diabetes

GR Sridhar

ABSTRACT

Identifying diabetes mellitus as a specific entity, unraveling the causes, and finding treatments has occupied nearly 150 years. Hypoglycemia is only one of many manifestations of metabolic abnormalities. Having a more refined diagnostic label is essential for providing individualized and personalized treatment. Clustering models for classification were used with clinical and biochemical variables. To improve the clinical applicability of such clustering tools, addition of genetic scores improves our understanding the pathogenic pathway, leading to refined treatment in individuals.

Keywords: *Glucose, Genetic score, Clustering, Personalized treatment.*

INTRODUCTION

In these times of genomics, proteomics, and metabolomics, it may appear counterintuitive to raise issues about the classification of diabetes. Yet, it is precisely because of advances in these areas that questions are being raised about what we mean by "diabetes mellitus." If one considers a linear progress from physiology to understand the normal followed by pathology to know what is wrong, it is possible to provide treatment for reversion the balance to normalcy. The explosion of knowledge about physiology and pathology of diabetes mellitus calls for a redefinition.

A consensus report from the American Diabetes Association (ADA) and the European Association for the Study of Diabetes published recently summed as a convergence of advances in medical science, human biology, data science, and technology that has enabled the generation of new insights into the phenotype what is called diabetes.[1] The operative word is phenotype because the diagnosis is made on the basis of one phenotype, namely plasma glucose, which is one of many phenotypes. It is increasingly evident that disturbances in glucose are only one of many other metabolic abnormalities.

HISTORICAL ASPECTS OF DIABETES

A disease with the features of what we now called diabetes mellitus was reported in antiquity; it is described in Egyptian manuscripts as early as 1,500 BC and by Indian doctors Sushruta and Charaka, who subclassified them into what are now called type 1 diabetes mellitus (T1DM) and type 2 diabetes mellitus (T2DM).[2] However, it was Aretaeus in the first century AD who coined the term "diabetes" where "no essential part of the drink is absorbed by the body, while great masses of the flesh are liquefied into urine." "Mellitus" was appended to diabetes by the surgeon general of Britain, John Rollo (1798), to distinguish it from diabetes insipidus, which was characterized by tasteless urine;[2,3] diabetes insipidus results from lack of antidiuretic hormone (vasopressin).[4]

A series of events followed: the identification of pancreatic islets of Langerhans, inducing diabetes by removing the pancreas, and finally the pathbreaking extraction of insulin from dog. This established that diabetes mellitus was due related to lack of insulin and that replacing insulin could reverse the manifestations of diabetes.

EVOLUTION OF METHODS TO IDENTIFY DIABETES MELLITUS

Even before diabetes mellitus was recognized as a clinical entity, a British physician in the 17th century described the sweet taste of the urine after evaporation.[5] It was in the 19th century that a qualitative clinical test to identify glucosuria was developed by Trommer.[5] A quantitative test was developed in 1850 by Fehling to measure glucose in the urine. Since then, technological advances took place until Ames Company (1941) introduced a strip test to identify glucose in urine. Rapid progress took place with measurement of glucose in the blood, point-of-care capillary measurements, glycosylated hemoglobin (HbA1c) as a measure of medium-term glycemic control, fructosamine for short-term control, and, recently, continuous tissue glucose monitoring. Diagnosis was based on the blood glucose levels.

CLASSIFICATION OF DIABETES: HISTORICAL CONTEXT

It is now broadly understood that diabetes is a clinically heterogeneous clinical condition resulting from a failure to maintain euglycemia through conversion of food to energy through insulin-dependent mechanisms. It is defined by clinical differences in insulin dependence to maintain euglycemia, the age and suddenness of onset, and the tendency to develop ketosis.[6]

Based on clinical observations, the disease was classified into fat and thin varieties in the 19th century.[7,8] Early in the 20th century, it was categorized depending on age of onset and severity of disease. Himsworth put forward the concept of insulin-resistant and insulin-sensitive diabetes, much before the modern concept of insulin resistance was established.[9] In the mid-50s, diabetes was categorized into juvenile onset and maturity onset; however, overlaps were noticed in clinical presentation, leading to subclassifications such as type 1.5 diabetes mellitus, ketosis-prone diabetes, mild diabetes, and malnutrition-related diabetes.[10] By 1976, the two broad categories were called insulin-dependent diabetes and noninsulin diabetes.[11] Finally, in 1999, the World Health Organization (WHO) classified diabetes into type 1, based on autoimmune destruction of pancreatic β-cells leading to insulinopenia, often seen in youth and T2DM, with a predominant element of insulin resistance, commonly identified in adults.[12]

Overlapping categories of subjects not falling into either T1DM or T2DM were recognized in clinical practice.[13] Similarly, diabetes in childhood and infancy was assumed to be due to autoimmune pancreatic β-cell destruction[14] until monogenic varieties of neonatal diabetes mellitus were identified by genomic studies.

In 2008, Donath compared the defining features that were believed to distinguish T1DM and T2DM; the various parameters tended to overlap between the two groups in differing degrees.[15] Both types can be identified at any age spectrum, although T1DM is more common in the younger age; age per se cannot be used as a differentiating feature. Metabolic stress and genetic predisposition can be found in both. Insulin secretory failure is observed in T2DM, although not as early and as severe as in T1DM, as is β-cell death and reduced β-cell mass. Similarly, circulating islet autoantibodies and insulin resistance are observed in both and cannot be used as to differentiate one from the other.[15]

Identifying the type of diabetes: Does it matter?

The question arises does it really matter whether or not we identify the type of diabetes? In an insightful review on the subject, Hoogwerf describes diabetes as a syndrome covering a number of abnormalities of the genome and epigenome, with differences in pathophysiology and complications.[16] Particularly, the classification of diabetes into type 1 and type 2 has been called as the starting point.[17]

A number of "other" varieties of diabetes are identified other than the major forms referred to above, e.g., maturity-onset diabetes of the young (MODY) or maturity-onset hyperglycemia of youth and latent autoimmune diabetes in adults (LADA).

The human genome project led to anticipation for a quick translation into precision diagnosis and medicine; reality has been different. While a number of genetic markers have been identified,[18] none of them on their own or in combination is really practically useful to subclassify T2DM in a way that helps therapy.[14] Yet, diabetes mellitus is a heterogeneous complex disease that is diagnosed without considering its etiology. Deconvoluting its etiology based on pathophysiological factors aids in management.[19] The current diagnosis of T2DM is by a process of exclusion.

It seems that T2DM is driven by a combination of genetic, lifestyle, and environmental factors. The underlying pathways could involve β-cell mass and function, insulin and glucagon secretion and actions, and fat distribution. Identifying which pathway or combination of pathways is disturbed in an individual allows prediction of progress and outcome of treatment. It might mean that the differently contributing factors in an individual must be plotted in a multidimensional space involving different etiological contributions. Combining them all can then provide an integrative approach.[19]

While monogenic etiology for rare forms of diabetes has been established, the results have not been as clear in the common garden variety of T2DM. Flannick proposed that it could be due to ascertainment bias of genetic studies that were carried in the past rather than due to true differences in the pathophysiological processes.[20] Among common variants for T2DM, a number of signals have been shown to localize within the regulatory pathways involved in monogenic forms of diabetes.

Results from next-generation sequencing methods show that low-frequency alleles that can moderate the effect for T2DM coexist with common alleles of low effect and with rare alleles of high penetrance.[20] Overlapping pathways could comprise genes responsible for glucose-stimulated insulin secretion, insulin signaling in the muscle and fat, and finally transcriptional regulation of pancreatic β-cells. Ultimately, T2DM and monogenic forms of diabetes may be considered as being on either end of a broad spectrum of phenotypes.

RATIONAL AND CURRENT ATTEMPTS AT CLASSIFICATION

Current classification and, thereby, management of diabetes follow a "one-size-fits-all" approach.[21] Insights into the different pathophysiological pathways to diabetes can help in personalized management. Realizing the contributions of genetic and environmental factors leading to progressive β-cell dysfunction and identifying the specific path in an individual helps in individualizing therapy.[21] Treatment depends particularly into understanding the disease trajectory of diabetes as currently defined.

There has been a surge of studies to classify diabetes into different clusters that reflect the possible underlying pathophysiological causes, course of the disease, and, thereby, suggest specific treatment for each group.

Current phenotypic classification into T1DM and T2DM at diagnosis is at best porous.[22,23] Khawandanah proposed that the two forms of diabetes are not separate at all, but lie at two ends of a spectrum, and coined the term *double or hybrid diabetes*.[24] This is based on the *accelerator hypothesis* which proposed that the differences are a result of the tempo of the accelerators, viz., β-cell death, insulin resistance, and β-cell immunity, modified by underlying genetic factors.

GROUPING OF DIABETES INTO CLASSES

Grouping into classes has been suggested based on a combination of clinical, biochemical, immunological, and, sometimes, genetic factors. Recent studies from across the globe are presented.

Type 1 Diabetes Mellitus

A recent study reported a multivariable clinical diagnostic model to differentiate T1DM and T2DM in adults who are aged between 18 and 50 years. Early identification is crucial for appropriate treatment choices. Unfortunately, there is an overlap of clinical factors making differentiation difficult. The authors employed logistic regression method to relate each of the phenotypic features and T1DM, which was defined by severe insulinopenia and early requirement of insulin for glycemic control. Criteria for T1DM: necessity of insulin use at or 3 years forms the diagnosis of diabetes, and a severe degree of insulin deficiency, as defined by a nonfasting C-peptide < 200 pmol/L. T2DM diagnostic criteria were: not requiring insulin for 3 years from the time of identification of diabetes, and when insulin was begun earlier, retained insulin secretory capacity, viz., C-peptide > 600 pmol/L 5 years or more after diagnosis of diabetes.[25]

Subjects with T1DM requiring rapid insulinization were younger, had a lower body mass index (BMI), and a higher rate of autoimmunity [glutamic acid decarboxylase (GAD) antibodies, insulin autoantibodies-2A, or both]. Initially, age at diagnosis and BMI were independent predictors of T1DM; adding autoantibody markers and genetic risk score improved the discriminatory capacity.[25] The authors claimed that it was the first documented clinical developmental model for distinguishing T1DM and T2DM. The generalizability of the results is strengthened because the sample was a population-based cohort from a primary care setting, which more truly reflects reality. However, it was a cross-sectional study that requires replication in longitudinal studies incorporating ethnically diverse group of subjects and across a broader spectrum of age. The current age group was limited between 18 and 50 years.

Diabetes in Adults

Cluster Analysis from Scandinavian Countries

Ahlqvist et al. carried out a data-driven cluster analysis of subjects newly diagnosed with diabetes from Swedish All New Diabetics in Scania (ANDIS) database. The variables chosen were, viz., GAD antibody, age at diagnosis, BMI, HbA1c, and homeostatic model assessment (HOMA) 2 estimates of β-cell function and of insulin resistance.[26] These variables were related to prospective data from patient records on development of complications and prescription of medications. Thereby, they sought to classify subjects with the greatest risk of complications at the time of diagnosis itself before waiting for the complications to manifest, so that treatment regimens can be individualized.

In all, data were obtained from five cohorts: besides ANDIS, the Scania Diabetes Registry (SDR), All New Diabetics in Uppsala (ANDIU), Diabetes Register Vaasa (DIREVA), and Malmö Diet and Cancer Cardiovascular Arm (MDC-CVA). Genotyping was performed for the ANDIS participants. Estimated glomerular filtration rate, macroalbuminuria, diabetic retinopathy, coronary events, and stroke were noted. Subjects with secondary diabetes and extreme outliers [≥5 standard deviations from mean (n = 42)] were not included in analysis. Two-step cluster analysis was performed (k-means and hierarchical clustering).

The following *five clusters* were identified:

1. *Severe autoimmune diabetes* comprised 6.4% of the consort; they had an early onset of diabetes, low BMI, were insulin deficient, and were GAD antibody positive
2. *Severe insulin-deficient diabetes* comprised 17.5%; they also had early-onset disease with a low BMI and were insulinopenic. However, they were GAD antibody negative. Groups 1 and 2 most often presented with ketoacidosis at diagnosis; high HbA1c was the strongest predictor of diabetic ketoacidosis at presentation in the second group. Early diabetic retinopathy was more common compared to the other groups.
3. *Severe insulin-resistant diabetes* had about the same prevalence as the earlier two clusters (15.3%). This group was more insulin resistance and had higher BMI and HOMA-IR index. Nonalcoholic fatty liver disease was most often present. They were also more susceptible to developing chronic kidney disease, including diabetic nephropathy.
4. *Mild obesity-related diabetes* was more common (21.6%) than the earlier three. Subjects in this group were obese, but not insulin resistant.
5. *Mild age-related diabetes,* the last group was the largest (39.1%). Subjects were older than those of other clusters and had modest metabolic derangements (similar to cluster 4).

   However, no genetic variant was associated with all clusters.[26]

Based on these analyses, the authors proposed to develop a web-based tool to slot subjects in specific clusters.

Newer insights obtained from this grouping are: severe insulin-deficient diabetes and severe insulin-resistant diabetes and these are new severe forms of diabetes; they were previously dubbed in T2DM. This group must be targeted with intensified treatment to delay the onset of diabetic complications.

However, clear mechanistic underpinnings cannot be obtained by this analysis; it is possible that subjects may change groups over the course of time and that further refinement can be obtained by employing additional variables such as biomarkers, genotypes, and genetic risk scores. Replication in other ethnic categories is also an issue to be addressed. However, rather than depend only on glucose, merging data from other variables provides a better classification model in diabetes mellitus.[26] In addition, the clustering does not offer personalized therapy.[27]

Clustering in Asian Indians

While similar results were obtained in a smaller sample of adult-onset diabetes from Chinese and US populations,[28] Anjana et al. performed a cluster analysis on a large cohort from the Indian subcontinent.[29] The reasons for studying; South Asians are many: Despite having a lower BMI, have unique features rendering them susceptible to T2DM at a younger age.[30] Among these predisposing factors are a greater amount of abdominal fat, hyperinsulinemia and insulin resistance, higher levels of the inflammatory marker C-reactive protein, lower levels of adiponectin, and dyslipidemia characterized by low levels of high-density lipoprotein (HDL) cholesterol, elevated levels of triglycerides, and higher levels of small dense low-density lipoprotein (LDL) particles. All these increased the susceptibility to T2DM and coronary artery disease.[30]

They performed a data-driven cluster analysis from the INSPIRED study, which[29] was a retrospective analysis of electronic medical records of a tertiary care center for diabetes in India, with 50 branches spread over the country. In all 55,429 subjects aged between 10 and 97 years were studied. The following baseline data for analysis was available viz., age at diagnosis, BMI, waist circumference, HbA1c, serum triglycerides, serum HDL cholesterol, and C-peptide. From these, 20,850 were further subselected who had a reported duration of diabetes <5 years at the first clinic visit. Further exclusion of outliers ($n = 188$) and those with a positive GAD antibody ($n = 66$) left 19,084 subjects for final analysis.

K-means clustering and sensitivity analysis were performed for clustering. To ensure that the clinic-based sample is representative of the general population, clustering was replicated in the dataset obtained from the Indian Council of Medical Research-India Diabetes (ICMR-INDIAB) study, which is a nationally representative sample. Data on HOMA-B and HOMA-IR were not available in the ICMR-INDIAB sample.

Based on this, *four clusters* were identified:

1. *Severe insulin-deficient diabetes* comprising 26.2% of the subjects. They had the lowest BMI and waist circumference, lowest C-peptide levels, low HOMA-B and HOMA-IR, and the highest HbA1c levels. They were more likely to use insulin than those in the other groups.
2. *Insulin-resistant obese diabetes,* is a unique group, comprising a quarter of all subjects (25.9%). They had the highest BMI and waist circumference, the highest C-peptide levels, and highest HOMA-B and HOMA-IR. Metabolic control was intermediate. Subjects in this cluster were likely to be on metformin treatment.
3. *Combined insulin-resistant and insulin-deficient diabetes* cluster comprised 12.1% of all subjects. They had the lowest age of onset, with a BMI and waist circumference that were intermediate between clusters 1 and 2. Their triglyceride levels were the highest and the HDL levels were the lowest. C-peptide levels were intermediate, suggesting a coexistence of both insulin deficiency and insulin resistance. Metabolic control was poor; only 15% were on insulin.
4. *Mild age-related diabetes,* the most frequent cluster of all (35.8%) was characterized by a later age of onset compared to others; they had the highest HDL cholesterol and preserved C-peptide. Subjects in this had the best metabolic control of all clusters and were least likely to be on insulin.

Compared to the clusters identified in the Scandinavian, US, and Chinese subjects, the Asian clusters reflected the three defining features described earlier, viz., younger age at diagnosis, less severe obesity, greater insulin resistance, and potentially early and rapid β-cell dysfunction.[29]

Of the four clusters reported by Ahlqvist et al.,[26] the Indian clusters had a different expression, namely insulin-resistant obese diabetes and combined insulin-resistant and insulin-deficient diabetes.[31] Ethnic-specific clustering helps in subclassifying diabetes to plan treatment based on pathophysiology and to provide prognostic information.

How do clusters compare with simple patient characteristics?

To compare the prognostic information obtained by the clustering methods described above with simple patient characteristics, Dennis et al. used data from clinical trials (ADOPT and RECORD).[32] The main question posed was the clinical utility of subgrouping based on the clustering method. Significant advantages of using clinical trial datasets included the availability of protocol-driven randomized follow-up to assess outcomes and responses to different treatments. Subjects in the ADOPT trial were newly diagnosed subjects with T2DM, who were drug-naïve and on follow-up. The RECORD trial participants were drawn from a cardiovascular outcomes trial in those with established T2DM.

For the ADOPT sample, clustering approach of Ahlqvist was employed; then for RECORD, each individual was placed in their ADOPT-derived cluster based on their Euclidean distance from each cluster center.[32] The aim was to assess whether assigning to clusters was more useful in the selection of a drug compared to simple clinical features.

Essentially, the clusters identified in the earlier study[26] were reproducible in the trial data; clusters were relatively stable over time. However, what was interesting and *clinically relevant was that simple clinical features were as good and even better at predicting disease progression* (viz., age at diagnosis for progression of glycemic levels and baseline renal function for renal deterioration).[32] Treatment response could also be predicted by clinical measures (viz., age, sex, HbA1c at baseline, and BMI). It appeared that models for prediction which combined phenotypes to predict specific outcomes in an individual subject could have more clinical utility than assignment to a subgroup.[32]

Hornbak et al. compared diabetic genetic risk variants to discriminate progression to drug use in freshly identified subjects with T2DM. They found that common phenotypic information was as good as genetic variants; the variables assessed were: HbA1c (higher), fasting triglycerides (high), lower HDL, greater BMI, and younger age.[33]

Despite absence of unequivocal evidence of clinical utility of clustering, subgrouping of persons is useful in integrated health systems; they help in improving population health by more accurately targeting better and more effective services.[34] A merging of data from multiple sources, electronic medical records, and multiple omics sources in biobanks can improve the usability of clustering.

GENETICS IS NOT ALL GENES

It is being increasingly realized that variations in noncoding regions of DNA account for much of the complex diseases such as T2DM. A number of gene regulatory regions exist such as enhancers and promoters.[35] Most genetic loci for T2DM obtained by genome-wide association studies (GWAS) lie in the noncoding regions of DNA. Kyona et al. proposed that rather than studying genetic regions in isolation, context for interpretation is important. The variables include flanking sequences of DNA and environmental factors such as environmental exposure, which have the potential to reveal molecular signatures across different regions, which improve patient care more effectively.[35]

Rather than defined clusters based merely on phenotypes, addition of genetic loci could improve their assessment in terms of being causal, consequential, or coincidental to the pathogenesis of T2DM. Udler et al. identified relevant T2DM genetically anchored and physiological pathways to deconstruct the heterogeneity of T2DM.[36] Employing soft clustering of genetic loci associated with T2DM resulted in mechanistic pathways supported by logical biological regions; it could be the next step toward personalized treatment of diabetes.

CONCLUSION

Diabetes mellitus is a heterogeneous condition with contributions from genes, environment, and lifestyle, manifesting as hyperglycemia and associated metabolic abnormalities. In order to tailor treatment more accurately, better subgroupings of diabetes are necessary. With the availability of large clinical datasets and data from multiple omics repositories, it is possible to refine the diagnosis of diabetes mellitus for better targeted personalized treatment.

REFERENCES

1. Chung WK, Erion K, Florez JC, Hattersley AT, Hivert MF, Lee CG, et al. Precision medicine in diabetes: a Consensus Report from the American Diabetes Association (ADA) and the European Association for the Study of Diabetes (EASD). Diabetologia. 2020;63:1671-93.
2. Lakhtakia R. The history of diabetes mellitus. Sultan Qaboos Univ Med J. 2013;13:368-70.
3. Sanders LJ. From Thebes to Toronto and the 21st century: an incredible journey. Diabetes Spectr. 2002;15:56-60.
4. Sridhar GR. Disorders of the posterior pituitary. In: Kamath SA (Ed). API Textbook of Medicine. Mumbai: Association of Physicians of India; 2019. pp. 749-51.
5. Kirchhof M, Popat N, Malowany J. A historical perspective of the diagnosis of diabetes. UWOMJ. 2008;78:7-11.
6. Grant SFA, Wells AD, Rich SS. Next steps in the identification of gene targets for type 1 diabetes. Diabetologia. 2020;63:2260-9.
7. Apollinaire B. (1875). De la glycosurie, ou, Diabète sucré: son traitement hygiénique: avec notes et documents sur la nature et le traitement de la goutte, la gravelle urique, sur l'oligurie, le diabète insipide avec excès d'urée, l'hippurie, la pimélorrhée, etc. [online] Available from https://archive.org/details/delaglycosurieou00bouc. [Last accessed June, 2021].
8. Taylor R, Barnes AC. Translating aetiological insight into sustainable management of type 2 diabetes. Diabetologia. 2018;61:273-83.
9. Himsworth HP. Diabetes Mellitus: Its Differentiation into Insulin-Sensitive and Insulin-Insensitive Types. Lancet. 1936;227:127-30.
10. Sridhar GR. Malnutrition-related diabetes mellitus. J Assoc Physicians India. 1994;42:561-4.
11. Elbein SC, Hoffman MD, Mayorga RA, Barrett KL, Leppert M, Hasstedt S. Do non-insulin-dependent diabetes mellitus (NIDDM) and insulin-dependent diabetes mellitus (IDDM) share genetic susceptibility loci? An analysis of putative IDDM susceptibility regions in familial NIDDM. Metabolism. 1997;46:48-52.
12. Classification and Diagnosis of Diabetes Mellitus: Standards of Medical Care in Diabetes. Diabetes Care. 2018;41:S13-27.
13. Sridhar GR. Diabetes in India: snapshot of a panorama. Curr Sci. 2002;83:791.
14. Sridhar GR. Diabetes Mellitus in Children below the Age of Five. Indian J Endocrinol Metab. 1997;1:13-5.
15. Donath MY, Ehses JA. Type 1, type 1.5, and type 2 diabetes: NOD the diabetes we thought it was. PNAS. 2006;103:12217-8.
16. Hoogwerf BJ. Type of diabetes mellitus: does it matter to the clinician? Cleve Clin J Med. 2020;87:100-8.
17. American Diabetes Association. 2. Classification and Diagnosis of Diabetes: Standards of Medical Care in Diabetes-2019. Diabetes Care. 2019;42:S13-28.

18. Sridhar GR, Duggirala R, Padmanabhan S. Emerging face of genetics, genomics and diabetes. Int J Diabetes Dev Ctries. 2013;33:183-5.
19. Pearson ER. Type 2 diabetes: a multifaceted disease. Diabetologia. 2019;62:1107-12.
20. Flannick J, Johansson S, Njølstad PR. Common and rare forms of diabetes mellitus: towards a continuum of diabetes subtypes. Nat Rev Endocrinol. 2016;12:394-406.
21. Skyler JS, Bakris GL, Bonifacio E, Darsow T, Eckel RH, Groop L, et al. Differentiation of Diabetes by Pathophysiology, Natural History, and Prognosis. Diabetes. 2017;66:241-55.
22. Sharp PS. Type 1 versus type 2 diabetes: is it time for a change? Pract Diabetes. 2017;34:214-6.
23. Butler AE, Misselbrook D. Distinguishing between type 1 and type 2 diabetes. BMJ. 2020;370:m2998.
24. Khawandanah J. Double or hybrid diabetes: a systematic review on disease prevalence, characteristics and risk factors. Nutr Diabetes. 2019;9:33.
25. Lynam A, McDonald T, Hill A, Dennis J, Oram R, Pearson E, et al. Development and validation of multivariable clinical diagnostic models to identify type 1 diabetes requiring rapid insulin therapy in adults aged 18-50 years. BMJ Open. 2019;9:e031586.
26. Ahlqvist E, Storm P, Käräjämäki A, Martinell M, Dorkhan M, Carlsson A, et al. Novel subgroups of adult-onset diabetes and their association with outcomes: a data-driven cluster analysis of six variables. Lancet Diabetes Endocrinol. 2018;6:361-9.
27. Feher MD, Munro N, Russell-Jones D, de Lusignan S, Khunti K. Novel diabetes subgroups. Lancet Diabetes Endocrinol. 2018;6:439.
28. Zou X, Zhou X, Zhu Z, Ji L. Novel subgroups of patients with adult-onset diabetes in Chinese and US populations. Lancet Diabetes Endocrinol. 2019;7:9-11.
29. Anjana RM, Baskar V, Nair ATN, Jebarani S, Siddiqui MK, Pradeepa R, et al. Novel subgroups of type 2 diabetes and their association with microvascular outcomes in an Asian Indian population: a data-driven cluster analysis: the INSPIRED study. BMJ Open Diabetes Res Care. 2020;8:e001506.
30. Unnikrishnan R, Anjana RM, Mohan V. Diabetes in South Asians: is the phenotype different? Diabetes. 2014;63:53-5.
31. Anjana RM, Pradeepa R, Unnikrishnan R, Tiwaskar M, Aravind SR, Saboo B, et al. New and Unique Clusters of Type 2 Diabetes Identified in Indians. J Assoc Physicians India. 2021;69:58-61.
32. Dennis JM, Shields BM, Henley WE, Jones AG, Hattersley A. The Proposed 5 Subgroups of Diabetes Have Less Clinical Utility Than Models Using Simple Clinical Features: An Evaluation in Randomised Trial Data. Lancet Diabetes Endocrinol. 2019;7:442-51.
33. Hornbak M, Allin KH, Jensen ML, Lau CJ, Witte D, Jørgensen ME, et al. A combined analysis of 48 type 2 diabetes genetic risk variants shows no discriminative value to predict time to first prescription of a glucose lowering drug in Danish patients with screen detected type 2 diabetes. PLoS One. 2014;9:e104837.
34. Ala-Korpela M. Data-driven subgrouping in epidemiology and medicine. Int J Epidemiol. 2019;48:374-6.
35. Kyono Y, Kitzman JO, Parker SCJ. Genomic annotation of disease-associated variants reveals shared functional contexts. Diabetologia. 2019;62:735-43.
36. Udler MS, Kim J, von Grotthuss M, Bonàs-Guarch S, Cole JB, Chiou J, et al. Type 2 diabetes genetic loci informed by multi-trait associations point to disease mechanisms and subtypes: A soft clustering analysis. PLoS Med. 2018;15:e1002654.

CHAPTER 2

Adipokines and Myokines (Adipomyokines) in Diabetes and Related Cardiometabolic Diseases: An (Un)expected Alliance

George N Chaldakov, Luigi Aloe, Levent Özturk, Rouzha Z Pancheva, Marco Fiore, Stanislav Yanev, Anton B Tonchev

ABSTRACT

Today, the most widespread disease around the world is not Coronavirus disease 2019 (COVID-19) or any other communicable disease. Indeed, type 2 diabetes mellitus (T2DM) and obesity (hence, diabesity) have been lionized as the main risks for cardiometabolic diseases (CMD) and their morbidity and mortality signature. Recent studies revealed that the adipose tissue and the skeletal muscles may function as endocrine and paracrine organs secreting multiple proteins termed as adipokines and myokines, respectively. Some of them being produced by both adipose and skeletal tissue, hence dubbed adipomyokines. The contents of this Chapter highlight the following two topics: (1) The progress in knowledge of adipomyokines may lead to better understandings of the pathobiology of T2DM and related CMD; and (2) In-depth studies on Palade–Blobel's general theory of cell protein secretion may allow us to explore its pharmacological potentials for new therapies of these diseases.

Keywords: *Adipomyokines, Irisin, Adiponectin, BDNF, Diabetes, Cardiometabolic diseases.*

INTRODUCTION

In 1962, Thomas S Kuhn published his book *The Structure of Scientific Revolutions* (1st edition, University of Chicago Press, Chicago, USA). Epistemology (Greek epistēmē means "knowledge") is the study of knowledge. Kuhn argued for a model in which periods of "development-by-accumulation" of accepted facts and theories in *normal science* were interrupted by paradigm shifts in *revolutionary science*.

Such a paradigm shift has been Jeffrey Friedman's 1994 discovery of leptin (Greek *leptos* meaning "thin"), a white adipocyte-secreted *Ob* gene-encoded protein.[1] It became a "big bang" for the current explosion of studies on

BOX 1 The paradigm shifts in adipobiology.

From:
Adipose tissue is a lipid and energy storage involved in obesity
To:
- Adipose tissue is an endocrine and paracrine organ
- Adipose tissue is a steroidogenic organ
- Adipose tissue is an immune organ
- Adipose tissue is a source of and target for inflammatory mediators
- Adipose tissue produces all components of renin–angiotensin system
- Adipose tissue is, thus, involved in numerous diseases beyond obesity

adipose-derived secretory proteins designated adipokines.[2,3] Thus, paradigm shifts were emerged (**Box 1**).

In brief, it is an adipose tissue's Renaissance marked by at least two paradigm shifts not listed in **Box 1**: (1) The internal (organ-associated, viewed by imaging technology) adipose depots are even more important in health and disease than the external depots calculated as body mass index (BMI) and other anthropometric criteria; and (2) The brown and beige adipocytes are as important as the white adipocytes in health and disease.

ADIPOBIOLOGY AND MYOBIOLOGY OF CARDIOMETABOLIC DISEASES

One of the biggest recent achievements in studying the pathogenesis of cardiometabolic diseases (CMD) (**Box 2**) is its association with adipomyokines, the secretory proteins released from both adipose tissue and skeletal muscles. There is now increasing evidence that type 2 diabetes mellitus (T2DM, hereinafter, diabetes) is a disease associated with obesity.[1] Thus, diabesity[5-7] has been moving to center stage becoming one of the most challenging medicosocial problems. Moreover, adipomyokines are also involved in the pathogenesis of cognitive disorders.[8-10]

ADIPOKINES AND MYOKINES

There are two major subtypes of adipose tissue: (1) White adipose tissue (WAT), the body's largest endocrine and paracrine organ producing multiple adipokines[2,3,11,12] (**Fig. 1**); and (2) Brown adipose tissue (BAT), the major thermogenic organ. Brite (brown in white) and beige adipose tissues were recognized recently (**Fig. 2**). Also, it was found that some adipomyokines [irisin, brain-derived neurotrophic factor (BDNF), and fibroblast growth factor-21 (FGF-21)] act as browning hormones.[13,14] Accordingly, browning of WAT is considered as a sanogenic phenomenon whereas whitening of BAT—as pathogenic one.

BOX 2 Cardiometabolic diseases (CMD).*

- Atherosclerosis, hypertension, and acute coronary syndromes (coronary heart diseases)
- Congestive heart failure and atrial fibrillation
- Stroke (ischemic and hemorrhagic), the major example of cerebrovascular diseases (CVD)
- Obesity
- *Type 2 diabetes mellitus*:
  - Diabetic neuropathy
  - Diabetic retinopathy
  - Diabetic erectile dysfunction
  - Diabetic nephropathy
- Metabolic syndrome and metabolic-cognitive syndrome
- Type 3 diabetes mellitus (Alzheimer's disease)
- Obstructive sleep apnea

*The term CMD is conceptually more correct than CVD; the latter represents a number of heart and blood vessel diseases and is a conceptually narrow than the list of CMD shown. In the USA, diabetes costs an estimated $174 billion in 2007. In CVD, according to the American Heart Association and the American Stroke Association, the total medical cost moves from $318 billion (2005) to $749 billion (2035)

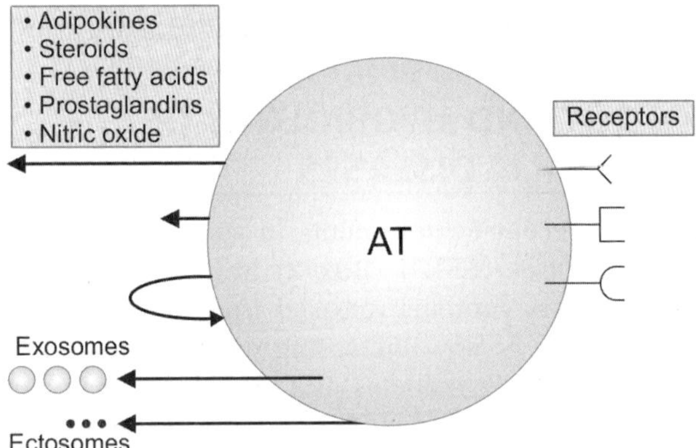

FIG. 1: Schematic illustration of white adipose tissue (AT) as a multicrine organ. Note the AT is consisted of (not shown) adipocytes, fibroblasts, mast cells, macrophages, and other immune cells. All these are *bona fide* secretory cell types, i.e., they synthesize, store, and release >500 different adipokines.[15,16] The arrows, left from up-to-down, indicate endocrine, paracrine, and autocrine pathway; other two arrows show the extracellular vesicles such as exosomes and ectosomes. At the right, depicted are adipose cells receptors for various ligands.

Source: Chaldakov G. Human body as a multicrine system, with special reference to cell protein secretion: from vascular smooth muscles to adipose tissue. Adipobiology. 2017;8:6-17.

Recently, skeletal muscles also "became" an endocrine and paracrine gland in response to contraction. Their secretory products were collectively termed as myokines (**Box 3**). Accumulating findings suggest that myokines may exert anti-inflammatory, antiobesogenic, and insulin-sensitizing effects.[17-20]

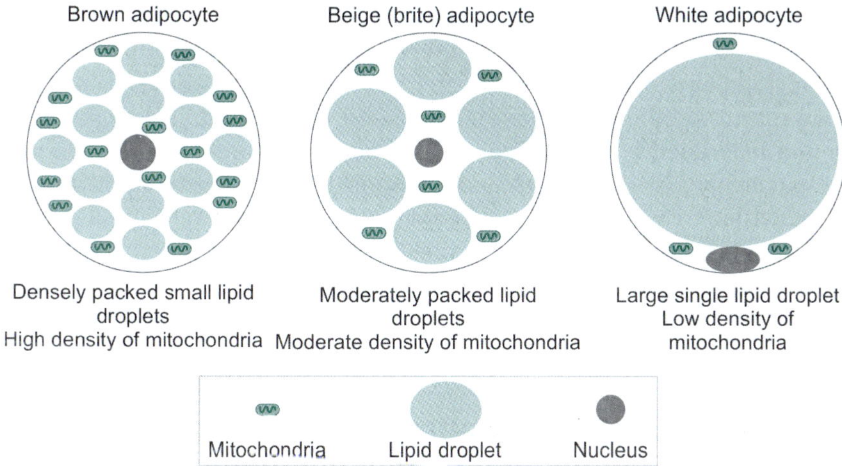

FIG. 2: Schematic presentation of the different types of adipocytes.

Source: Reproduced with permission from Jacob VD, Manoj KM. Are adipocytes and ROS villains, or are they protagonists in the drama of life? The murburn perspective. Adipobiology. 2018;10:1-10.

BOX 3 A selected list of myokines.*

- Irisin—a cleavage protein of fibronectin type III domain 5
- Brain-derived neurotrophic factor
- Interleukins (IL-6, IL-15) and angiopoietin-like 4
- Fibroblast growth factor-21
- Monocyte chemoattractant protein-1 (MCP-1/CCL2)
- Adiponectin and leukemia inhibitory factor
- Myonectin and myostatin [growth differentiation factor-8 (GDF8)]
- Atrial natriuretic peptide (ANP) and B-type natriuretic peptide (BNP)**

*In mice were identified 119 myokines, 79 adipokines and 22 adipomyokines.[21]

**(Un)expectedly, we also include these natriuretic peptides in the list of myokines because the heart muscles cardiomyocytes secrete both ANP and BNP from the cardiac atria and from the ventricles, respectively. ANP decreases blood pressure and cardiac hypertrophy whereas BNP acts locally to reduce ventricular fibrosis.[22]

ADIPOMYOKINES

The adipomyokines are secretory proteins released from both adipose tissue and skeletal muscles for endocrine, paracrine, and autocrine signaling.[13,17,21,23-29] We focus herein on the adipomyokines such as irisin, adiponectin, and BDNF and their relevance to diabetes and associated CMD.

Irisin

Irisin (named after the Greek mythology goddess Iris, a messenger of the gods) is a newly identified adipomyokine. It is a cleavage protein of fibronectin type III domain-containing protein 5 (FNDC5), the latter converted to irisin after exercise. Several recent studies demonstrated an association between irisin and endothelial function. Lower levels of irisin were found to be independently associated with endothelial dysfunction in nonhypertensive, nondiabetic obese subjects.[30] Circulating irisin levels are positively associated with endothelium-dependent arterial dilation in diabetic patients[31] whereas elevated circulating irisin level was suggested to have role in the development of insulin resistance and atherosclerosis in patients with obstructive sleep apnea.[32] Altogether, these data collectively suggest that diabetes and related CMD might, at least in part, be viewed as irisin-mediated disorders.[30-42]

Adiponectin: A "Therapeutical Antikine"

As recently reviewed,[12,43] adiponectin is an adipose tissue-secreted signaling protein and one of the best-characterized adipomyokine[44] with a great potential for developing novel therapeutics for various diseases. Adiponectin is the major endogenous insulin-sensitizing factor, which also exerts anti-inflammatory, antiatherogenic, antidiabetic, antiobesity, antifibrotic, and anticancer effects.[12] Hence, we name it "therapeutical antikine".

There is a strong link between lower adiponectin levels and higher incidence of diabetes and metabolic syndrome.[45] Experimental evidence showed that both aerobic[46] and anaerobic exercise[47] led to significant increase in circulating adiponectin levels.

Brain-derived Neurotrophic Factor

Brain-derived neurotrophic factor belongs to the family of proteins named neurotrophins. It consists of nerve growth factor (NGF),[48] neurotrophin-3 (NT-3), NT-4/-5, and NT-6.[49] These mediate their effects via ligation of receptor tyrosine kinase [tropomyosin-related kinase (Trk)], namely, TrkA (for NGF), TrkB (for BDNF and NT-4), TrkC (for NT-3), and pan-neurotrophin receptor p75NTR and its coreceptor sortilin. Today, BDNF is well-recognized to mediate various trophobiological effects. These latter ranging from neurotrophic to metabotropic effects. For instance, reduced circulating and local NGF and BDNF levels are implicated in the pathogenesis of both neurodegenerative and CMD.[42,50-52] The investigations on TrkB-BDNF agonists, therefore, are critically needed for the therapy of these diseases.[53] For example, (1) polyphenols (in fruit and vegetables, red wine, olives, extra virgin olive oil, green and black tea, coffee, and chocolate) express both cardioprotection and neuroprotection by stimulating the TrkB-BDNF signaling pathway[54] and (2) metformin, a commonly used antidiabetic drug, significantly increased BDNF level.[55] On the contrary, after a brief treatment with metformin in polycystic ovary syndrome women, blood plasma irisin levels and BAT activity were not changed.[56]

Pro-NGF and pro-BDNF are as active as their respective mature forms. These are released extracellularly through the tissue type plasminogen activator (tPA), a serine protease-plasmin pathway. Of note, the cholesterol-lowering drugs statins stimulate tPA, hence releasing pro-BDNF.[57] These "nonaged" NGF and BDNF required further studies in diabetes and its associated cardiometabolic and neurodegenerative diseases. Whether pro-BDNF and pro-NGF may be included in the list of adipomyokines, it remains to be studied.

CELL PROTEIN SECRETION

"-Kines" Sweet "-Kines"

The Human Genome Project was finalized estimating over 20,000 genes encoding >100,000 functionally distinct proteins. "Diabetes has been one of the first major disorders that was studied for its genetic basis, soon after results of the Human Genome Project were published".[58]

In the postgenome time, many other "-ome" projects have emerged including proteome, transcriptome, interactome, metabolome, adipokinome, and connectome, alike. Perhaps, this prompted Jeff Lichtman and Joshua Sanes to entitle one of their connectome articles *Ome sweet ome* (*Curr Opin Neurobiol* 2008;18:346-53)—reminding of the Italian *Casa dolce casa* (Home sweet home).

Discovery of novel secretory proteins, such as cytokines, chemokines, osteokines, hepatokines, adipokines, and myokines, may provide new opportunities for better understanding of the pathogenesis of many diseases. Also for the development of new drug therapies, exported and transmembrane proteins being relevant pharmacological targets. They are accessible to various drug delivery initiatives because they are presented within the extracellular space and the cell surface, respectively.[59] In the same vein, adipomyokines may pharmacologically be targeted by (1) specific antibodies and (2) small molecules boosting or inhibiting their intracellular secretory pathways. Noteworthy, a large-scale effort, termed the Secreted Protein Discovery Initiative (SPDI), was undertaken to identify novel exported and transmembrane proteins.[59]

According to George Palade's classical concept and Günter Blobel's signal hypothesis,[11,12,60] the protein secretory pathway constitutes of several intracellular steps including synthesis, post-translational modifications, sorting, targeting, storage (in case of regulated vs. constitutive secretion), and, finally, exocytosis (**Box 4** and **Figs. 3** and **4**). Each of these steps might be a pharmacotherapeutic target.

Generally, the secretory proteins are four major types: (1) Lysosomal; (2) Plasmalemmal; (3) Recycled; and (4) Exported. Adipomyokines are exported proteins, while glucose transporters (GLUTs) are recycled membrane proteins. Accordingly, we should be focused in-depth on Palade–Blobel's general

BOX 4 The two major protein secretory pathways.

Cell protein secretion:

- *Palade's rough endoplasmic reticulum (RER)-Golgi pathway*: RER-Golgi complex-microtubules-exocytosis/porosomes
- *Günter Blobel*: Signal hypothesis of sorting and targeting of proteins
- *Non-RER-Golgi pathway:*
  - Exosomes [multivesicular body (MVB)-derived microvesicles]
  - Ectosomes (plasmalemma-derived microparticles)

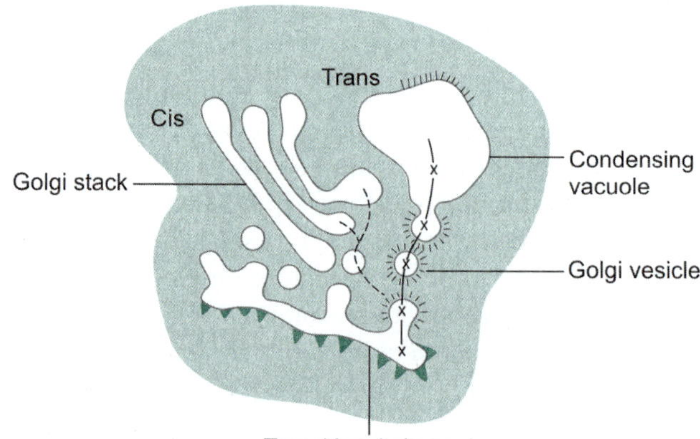

FIG. 3: A diagram illustrating the intracellular secretory pathway in the pancreatic exocrine cell of the guinea pig.

Source: Harvey Cushing/John Hay Whitney Medical Library. (2020). George E. Palade EM Slide Collection. [online] Available from https://library.medicine.yale.edu/find/palade. [Last accessed December, 2020].

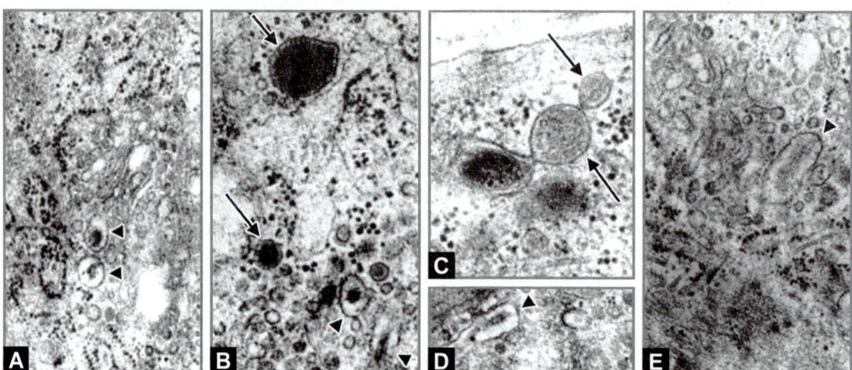

FIGS. 4A TO E: Electron micrographs of secretory-state (secretory phenotype) aortic smooth muscle cells of the rabbit [spherical-shaped (black arrows) and elongated-shaped (black arrowheads) secretion granules] (20,000×).

Source: Chaldakov GN, Vankov VN. Morphological aspects of secretion in the arterial smooth muscle cell, with special reference to the Golgi complex and microtubular cytoskeleton. Atherosclerosis. 1986;61:175-92.

theory of the cell protein secretion to explore its pharmacological potentials for new therapies for diabetes and related CMD. The non-rough endoplasmic reticulum (RER)-Golgi pathway using exosomes and ectosomes (see **Fig. 1**) may also be a target for the discovery of new therapeutics. Likewise, one of the pathways known to be crucial for the function of pancreatic β-cells is the endoplasmic reticulum stress response. Recent study revealed that a group of babies developing diabetes soon after birth had mutations in the *YIPF5* gene involved in the RER-to-Golgi complex trafficking.[61]

Of note, adiponectin inhibits the secretion of the metabolically dangerous tumor necrosis factor-α (TNF-α).[12] Since treatment with the microtubule-disassembling agent colchicine[60,62] also inhibits TNF-α secretion and exerts anti-inflammatory effects, one may wonder as to whether adiponectin may act as microtubule-disassembling agent.[11,12,60] Therefore, dissecting the adiposecretion by (1) the microtubule-disassembling agents such as colchicine and nocodazole, alike, (2) microtubule stabilizers such as taxol (the drug paclitaxel), and (3) brefeldin A, an inhibitor of RER-Golgi complex trafficking, may provide important pharmacotherapeutic information.[11,12]

CONCLUSION

Future studies on adipobiology and myobiology of diabetes and associated CMD might cultivate a more relevant thinking about how we can make adipomyokine secretion that works for the improvement of physical and mental quality of life of our patients. In effect, a hope in understanding and managing diabetes and related CMD might be materialized.[63] Yet, many *food for thoughts* remain to be eaten (**Fig. 5**).

ACKNOWLEDGMENTS

This Chapter expresses our tribute to Albert Claude, Christian de Duve, and George E Palade, the Nobel Prize winners in Physiology or Medicine in 1974 "for their discoveries concerning the structural and functional organization of the cell", including for their conceptual contributions to the knowledge of cell protein secretion. We apologize to the authors of many relevant articles that were not quoted here for reasons of brevity.

Conflict of Interest statement: The authors declare that no conflicts of interest exist.

Authorship note: All the authors contributed equally to this work.

FIG. 5: The dish shown may be viewed as a white adipocyte covered with plasma membrane (dark blue), having marginally located flatten nucleus (dark blue), unilocular lipid droplet (white), and basal (pericellular) lamina (light blue).

REFERENCES

1. Zhang Y, Proenca R, Maffei M, Barone M, Leopold L, Friedman JM. Positional cloning of the mouse obese gene and its human homologue. Nature. 1994;372:425-32.
2. Chaldakov G, Fiore M, Ghenev P, Stankulov IS, Aloe L. Atherosclerotic lesions: possible interactive involvement of intima, adventitia and associated adipose tissue. In Med J. 2000;7:43-9.
3. Chaldakov G, Stankulov I, Hristova M, Ghenev P. Adipobiology of disease: adipokines and adipokine-targeted pharmacology. Curr Pharm Des. 2003;9:1023-31.
4. Chaldakov G, Fiore M, Tonchev A, Dimitrov D, Pancheva R, Rancic G, et al. Homo obesus: a metabotrophin-deficient species. Pharmacology and nutrition insight. Curr Pharm Des. 2007;13:2176-9.
5. Astrup A, Finer N. Redefining type 2 diabetes: 'diabesity' or 'obesity dependent diabetes mellitus'? Obesity Rev. 2000;1:57-9.
6. Farag YM, Gaballa MR. Diabesity: an overview of a rising epidemic. Nephrol Dial Transplant. 2011;26: 28-35.
7. Aloe L, Tonchev AB, Fiore M, Chaldakov GN. Homo diabesus: involvement of metabotrophic factors. Adipobiology. 2013;5:45-9.
8. Naderali EK, Ratcliffe SH, Dale MC. Obesity and Alzheimer's disease: a link between body weight and cognitive function in old age. Am J Alzheimers Dis Other Demen. 2009;24:445-9.
9. Frisardi V, Solfrizzi V, Seripa D, Capurso C, Santamato A, Sancarlo D, et al. Metabolic-cognitive syndrome: a cross-talk between metabolic syndrome and Alzheimer's disease. Ageing Res Rev. 2010;9:399-417.
10. Forny-Germano L, De Felice FG, Vieira MN. The Role of Leptin and Adiponectin in Obesity-Associated Cognitive Decline and Alzheimer's Disease. Front Neurosci. 2018;12:1027.
11. Chaldakov G. Human body as a multicrine system, with special reference to cell protein secretion: from vascular smooth muscles to adipose tissue. Adipobiology. 2017;8:6-17.
12. Töre F, Tonchev A, Fiore M, Tunçel N, Atanassova P, Aloe L, et al. From Adipose Tissue Protein Secretion to Adipopharmacology of Disease. Immunol Endocr Metab Agents Med Chem. 2007;7:149-55.
13. Rodríguez A, Becerril S, Ezquerro S, Méndez-Giménez L, Frühbeck G. Crosstalk between adipokines and myokines in fat browning. Acta Physiol. 2017;219:362-81.
14. Calton EK, Soares MJ, James AP, Woodman RJ. The potential role of irisin in the thermoregulatory responses to mild cold exposure in adults. Am J Hum Biol. 2016;28:699-704.

15. Renes J, Rosenow A, Mariman E. Novel adipocyte features discovered by adipoproteomics. Adipobiology. 2009;1:7-18.
16. Renes J, Mariman E. Application of proteomics technology in adipocyte biology. Mol Biosyst. 2013;9:1076-91.
17. Broholm C, Pedersen BK. Leukaemia inhibitory factor—an exercise-induced myokine. Exerc Immunol Rev. 2010;16:77-85.
18. Matthews VB, Aström MB, Chan MH, Bruce CR, Krabbe KS, Prelovsek O, et al. Brain-derived neurotrophic factor is produced by skeletal muscle cells in response to contraction and enhances fat oxidation via activation of AMP-activated protein kinase. Diabetologia. 2009;52:1409-18.
19. Pedersen BK, Pedersen M, Krabbe KS, Bruunsgaard H, Matthews VB, Febbraio MA. Role of exercise-induced brain-derived neurotrophic factor production in the regulation of energy homeostasis in mammals. Exp Physiol. 2009;94:1153-60.
20. Matsakas A, Foster K, Otto A, Macharia R, Elashry MI, Feist S, et al. Molecular, cellular and physiological investigation of myostatin propeptide-mediated muscle growth in adult mice. Neuromuscul Disord. 2009;19:489-99.
21. Schering L, Hoene M, Kanzleiter T, Jähnert M, Wimmers K, Klaus S, et al. Identification of novel putative adipomyokines by a cross-species annotation of secretomes and expression profiles. Arch Physiol Biochem. 2015;121:194-205.
22. Potter LR, Yoder AR, Flora DR, Antos LK, Dickey DM. Natriuretic peptides: their structures, receptors, physiologic functions and therapeutic applications. Handbook Exp Pharmacol. 2009;191: 341-66.
23. Görgens SW, Eckardt K, Jensen J, Drevon CA, Eckel J. Exercise and Regulation of Adipokine and Myokine Production. Prog Mol Biol Transl Sci. 2015;135:313-36.
24. Li F, Li Y, Duan Y, Hu CA, Tang Y, Yin Y. Myokines and adipokines: Involvement in the crosstalk between skeletal muscle and adipose tissue. Cytokine Growth Factor Rev. 2017;33:73-82.
25. Raschke S, Eckel J. Adipo-myokines: two sides of the same coin—mediators of inflammation and mediators of exercise. Mediators Inflamm. 2013;2013:320724.
26. Trayhurn P, Drevon CA, Eckel J. Secreted proteins from adipose tissue and skeletal muscle—adipokines, myokines and adipose/muscle cross-talk. Arch Physiol Biochem. 2011;117:47-56.
27. Oh KJ, Lee DS, Kim WK, Han BS, Lee SC, Bae KH. Metabolic adaptation in obesity and type II diabetes: Myokines, adipokines and hepatokines. Int J Mol Sci. 2017;18:8.
28. Chung HS, Choi KM. Adipokines and myokines: a pivotal role in metabolic and cardiovascular disorders. Curr Med Chem. 2018;25:2401-15.
29. Kirk B, Feehan J, Lombardi G, Duque G. Muscle, bone, and fat crosstalk: the biological role of myokines, osteokines, and adipokines. Curr Osteopor Rep. 2020;18:388-400.
30. Xiang L, Xiang G, Yue L, Zhang J, Zhao L. Circulating irisin levels are positively associated with endothelium-dependent vasodilation in newly diagnosed type 2 diabetic patients without clinical angiopathy. Atherosclerosis. 2014;235:328-33.
31. Sesti G, Andreozzi F, Fiorentino TV, Mannino GC, Sciacqua A, Marini MA, et al. High circulating irisin levels are associated with insulin resistance and vascular atherosclerosis in a cohort of nondiabetic adult subjects. Acta Diabetol. 2014;51:705-13.
32. Ozturk G, Demirel O, Tekatas A, Celebi C, Avci B, Gurel EF, et al. Circulating irisin levels in newly diagnosed obstructive sleep apnea patients. Scr Sci Med. 2019;51:16-20.
33. Hofmann T, Elbelt U, Stengel A. Irisin as a muscle-derived hormone stimulating thermogenesis: a critical update. Peptides. 2014;54:89-100.
34. Gamas L, Matafome P, Seiça R. Irisin and Myonectin Regulation in the Insulin Resistant Muscle: Implications to Adipose Tissue: Muscle Crosstalk. J Diab Res. 2015;2015:359159.
35. Kurdiova T, Balaz M, Vician M, Maderova D, Vlcek M, Valkovic L, et al. Effects of obesity, diabetes and exercise on Fndc5 gene expression and irisin release in human skeletal muscle and adipose tissue: in vivo and in vitro studies. J Physiol. 2014;592:1091-107.
36. Perakakis N, Triantafyllou GA, Fernández-Real JM, Huh JY, Park KH, Seufert J, et al. Physiology and role of irisin in glucose homeostasis. Nat Rev Endocrinol. 2017;13:324-37.

37. Moreno-Navarrete JM, Ortega F, Serrano M, Guerra E, Pardo G, Tinahones F, et al. Irisin is expressed and produced by human muscle and adipose tissue in association with obesity and insulin resistance. J Clin Endocrinol Metab. 2013;98:E769-78.
38. Aydin S, Aydin S, Kobat MA, Kalayci M, Eren MN, Yilmaz M, et al. Decreased saliva/serum irisin concentrations in the acute myocardial infarction promising for being a new candidate biomarker for diagnosis of this pathology. Peptides. 2014;56:141-5.
39. Zhu D, Wang H, Zhang J, Zhang X, Xin C, Zhang F, et al. Irisin improves endothelial function in type 2 diabetes through reducing oxidative/nitrative stresses. J Mol Cell Cardiol. 2015;87:138-47.
40. Hou N, Han F, Sun X. The relationship between circulating irisin levels and endothelial function in lean and obese subjects. Clin Endocrinol. 2014;83:339-43.
41. Park KH, Zaichenko L, Brinkoetter M, Thakkar B, Sahin-Efe A, Joung KE, et al. Circulating irisin in relation to insulin resistance and the metabolic syndrome. J Clin Endocrinol Metab. 2013;98: 4899-907.
42. More CE, Papp C, Harsanyi S, Gesztelyi R, Mikaczo A, Tajti G, et al. Altered irisin/BDNF axis parallels excessive daytime sleepiness in obstructive sleep apnea patients. Respir Res. 2019;20:67.
43. Yang D, Yang Y, Li Y, Han R. Physical Exercise as Therapy for Type 2 Diabetes Mellitus: From Mechanism to Orientation. Ann Nutr Metab. 2019;74:313-21.
44. Martinez-Huenchullan SF, Tam CS, Ban LA, Ehrenfeld-Slater P, McLennan SV, Twigg SM. Skeletal muscle adiponectin induction in obesity and exercise. Metabolism. 2020;102:154008.
45. Kadowaki T, Yamauchi T, Kubota N, Hara K, Ueki K, Tobe K. Adiponectin and adiponectin receptors in insulin resistance, diabetes, and the metabolic syndrome. J Clin Inves. 2006;116:1784-92.
46. Yu N, Ruan Y, Gao X, Sun J. Systematic Review and Meta-Analysis of Randomized, Controlled Trials on the Effect of Exercise on Serum Leptin and Adiponectin in Overweight and Obese Individuals. Horm Metab Res. 2017;49:164-73.
47. Öztürk G, Kaya O, Gürel EE, Palabiyik O, Kunduracilar H, Süt N, et al. Acute supramaximal exercise-induced adiponectin increase in healthy volunteers: involvement of natriuretic peptides. Adipobiology. 2017;8:9-45.
48. Levi-Montalcini R. The nerve growth factor 35 years later. Science. 1987;237:1154-62.
49. Rocco ML, Soligo M, Manni L, Aloe L. Nerve growth factor: early studies and recent clinical trials. Curr Neuropharmacol. 2018;16:1455-65.
50. Chaldakov GN, Fiore M, Stankulov IS, Manni L, Hristova MG, Antonelli A, et al. Neurotrophin presence in human coronary atherosclerosis and metabolic syndrome: a role for NGF and BDNF in cardiovascular disease? Prog Brain Res. 2004;146:279-89.
51. Sornelli F, Fiore M, Chaldakov GN, Aloe L. Adipose tissue-derived nerve growth factor and brain-derived neurotrophic factor: results from experimental stress and diabetes. Gen Physiol Biophys. 2009;28: 179-83.
52. Yanev S, Aloe L, Fiore M, Chaldakov GN. Neurotrophic and metabotrophic potential of nerve growth factor and brain-derived neurotrophic factor: linking cardiometabolic and neuropsychiatric diseases. World J Pharmacol. 2013;2:92-9.
53. Yanev S, Fiore M, Hinev A, Ghenev P, Hristova M, Panayotov P, et al. From antitubulins to trackins. Biomed Rev. 2016;27:59-67.
54. Carito V, Venditti A, Bianco A, Ceccanti M, Serrilli A, Chaldakov G, et al. Effects of olive leaf polyphenols on male mouse brain NGF, BDNF and their receptors TrkA, TrkB and p75. Nat Prod Res. 2014;28: 1970-84.
55. Fang W, Zhang J, Hong L, Huang W, Dai X, Ye Q, et al. Metformin ameliorates stress-induced depression-like behaviors via enhancing the expression of BDNF by activating AMPK/CREB-mediated histone acetylation. J Affective Disord. 2020;260:302-13.
56. Oliveira F, Mamede M, Bizzi M, Rocha AL, Ferreira C, Gomes K, et al. Effects of Short Term Metformin Treatment on Brown Adipose Tissue Activity and Plasma Irisin Levels in Women with Polycystic Ovary Syndrome: A Randomized Controlled Trial. Horm Metab Res. 2020;52:718-23.
57. Tsai SJ. Statins May Act Through Increasing Tissue Plasminogen Activator/Plasmin Activity to Lower Risk of Alzheimer's Disease. CNS Spectrums. 2009;14:234-5.

58. Sridhar GR. Encode, decode and diabetes. In: Sridhar GR (Ed). Cognitive Science and Health Bioinformatics: Advances and Applications. Singapore: Springer; 2018. pp. 47-55.
59. Clark HF, Gurney AL, Abaya E, Baker K, Baldwin D, Brush J, et al. The secreted protein discovery initiative (SPDI), a large-scale effort to identify novel human secreted and transmembrane proteins: a bioinformatics assessment. Genome Res. 2003;13:2265-70.
60. Chaldakov GN, Vankov VN. Morphological aspects of secretion in the arterial smooth muscle cell, with special reference to the Golgi complex and microtubular cytoskeleton. Atherosclerosis. 1986;61: 175-92.
61. De Franco E, Lytrivi M, Ibrahim H, Montaser H, Wakeling MN, Fantuzzi F, et al. YIPF5 mutations cause neonatal diabetes and microcephaly through endoplasmic reticulum stress. J Clin Invest. 2020;130:6338-53.
62. Chaldakov GN. Colchicine, a microtubule-disassembling drug, in the therapy of cardiovascular diseases. Cell Biol Int. 2018;42:1079-84.
63. Arhire LI, Mihalache L, Covasa M. Irisin: A hope in understanding and managing obesity and metabolic syndrome. Front Endocrinol (Lausanne). 2019;10:524.

CHAPTER 3

Air Pollution Assessment and Metabolic Syndrome

Rao Tatavarti, GR Sridhar

ABSTRACT

Environmental pollution, chiefly air pollution, is recognized to be responsible not for just respiratory illnesses, but for many noncommunicable diseases such as metabolic syndrome, type 2 diabetes mellitus (T2DM), obesity, and coronary artery disease, leading to premature deaths. A number of pathways have been suggested involving both chronic and acute exposure involving chemical mediators, oxidant stress, and impaired vascular function including endothelial dysfunction acting through local and central mechanisms. We present an innovative technique whereby environmental particulate matter (PM) pollutants can be cost-effectively measured in real time from a remote location, to first document the degree of pollution, so that corrective methods can be taken up to prevent or lower the levels of pollutants.

Keywords: *$PM_{2.5}$, NO_2, Ozone, Particulate matter, Detection, Insulin resistance, Oxidative stress, Sensors, Photonic system, "AUM" real time.*

INTRODUCTION

The poor state of air quality all over the world, in general, and across India, in particular, is a cause for extreme concern, as it is directly and indirectly linked to the deterioration of human health and economies of nations.

The many complexities and challenges posed by ambient air quality monitoring prompted the World Health Organization (WHO) to suggest a road map for all nations for the year 2020—to arrive at a consensus for effective air quality monitoring by all stakeholders—nations and governments, regulatory and controlling bodies, nongovernmental organizations (NGOs), scientists and researchers, and private citizens.

As we approach the end of 2021, the multifaceted and multidimensional problems related to effective ambient air quality monitoring still remain herculean and extremely expensive for wider deployment to gather a realistic spatiotemporal information related to ambient air quality, in order to draw up effective plans to curb or mitigate the air pollution.

Air pollution is a relatively young phenomenon in terms of human history. It followed the industrial revolution in the 19th century when manufacturing processes shifted to burning of fuel and the emergence of cities densely populated. The adverse health effects of air pollution were recognized as late as in the 1950s, when dense smog from burning of coal for heating led to dense smog over London.[1] This was associated with about an excess of 12,000 deaths due to the smog and was the first epidemiological evidence linking the two.

Since then a number of large studies were carried out on the risk of death and various diseases—metabolic syndrome, type 2 diabetes mellitus (T2DM), and obesity—with exposure to particulate air pollution. Liu et al. reported the association of inhaled particulate matter (PM) on death among multiple countries (652 cities in 24 countries or regions).[2] Health and environmental data were obtained from the Metropolitan Community College (MCC) database of 652 urban areas from regions where data were available between 1986 and 2015. There was an association between short-term exposure to particulate air pollution and deaths due to cardiovascular and respiratory diseases all across the globe.[2] Although the authors acknowledge the limitations in being limited to only 24 countries from six continents, this is among the largest global studies showing an association of air pollution and death.

Diabetes mellitus has been showing an explosive growth over the world. The causes are both genetic and environmental, the latter including lifestyle factors. Among the modifiable environmental factors are built environment, neighborhood conditions, open spaces, air pollution, and noise pollution.[3,4]

REGIONAL STUDIES

A number of epidemiological reports showed an association of air pollution with prevalence of diabetes, degree of glucose control, insulin resistance, disability, and death due to diabetes.[5,6] Eze et al. performed a meta-analysis on the relation between ambient air pollution and the risk of diabetes mellitus in studies from North America and Europe.[6] Among the 13 studies which were included, eight were on T2DM, two on type 1 diabetes mellitus, and three were on gestational diabetes. The nature of studies was as follows: longitudinal (n = 5), cross-sectional (n = 5), case control (n = 2), and ecologic (n = 1). Essentially, the results showed that the pooled relative risks of T2DM per 10 μg m^{-3} increase in exposure to $PM_{2.5}$ were 1.1 and to NO_2 were 1.08.[6]

A more recent study from a multiethnic cohort by Park et al. showed the effect of long-term exposure to air pollution and T2DM. The authors evaluated the association of prevalent and incident diabetes with exposure to $PM_{2.5}$ and nitrogen oxides. Study population was drawn from a prospective cohort study, the Multiethnic Study of Atherosclerosis (MESA).[7] Out of 6,814 subjects aged 45–84 years without clinical evidence of cardiovascular disease at baseline, follow-up was carried out during four time periods. In all after exclusion, 5,135 individuals were included for analysis.

The ambient $PM_{2.5}$ and NO_2 were estimated over the follow-up period using the hierarchical spatiotemporal model from MESA and air pollution. Taking the 2-week average concentration from each person's home location, annual average concentration was computed.

Other data were obtained related to sociodemographic, behavior, and medical information. At baseline, 11.9% of participants (696/5,839) had diabetes mellitus. Over a median of 9 years follow-up, 12.1% developed diabetes (622/5,135). Those with diabetes at baseline or on follow-up tended to have higher body mass index (BMI), poor built environment, family history of diabetes, and less physically active. There was significant association of diabetes prevalence with $PM_{2.5}$ (odds ratio 1.09) and NO_2 per each interquartile range increase even when adjusted for age, sex, ethnicity, family history of diabetes, and physical activity level.[7] However, neither $PM_{2.5}$ nor NO_2 was associated with diabetes incidence over 9 years of follow-up in the whole population. Earlier studies showed mixed results from West Germany, Los Angeles, Ontario, and the Nurses' Health Study.[7] The reasons for the potential association of air pollution with the prevalence but not incidence of diabetes were speculated: Either those who were susceptible to diabetes had already developed before baseline or that those without diabetes could have been more healthy and less susceptible to the adverse of pollutants. Alternatively, the duration of follow-up may have been insufficient to capture the effects of air pollution or finally the pollution levels on follow-up were not high enough with improved quality of air over time.[7]

Effects of air pollutants on insulin and glucose homeostasis were reported among Mexican Americans in 2016.[8] Insulin sensitivity and secretion were measured using frequently sampled intravenous (IV) glucose tolerance test (GTT) in BetaGene participants, who were Mexican American women with confirmed gestational diabetes within the past 5 years as well as their siblings or cousins with fasting glucose levels <126 mg/dL. Recruitment was done between 2002 and 2008. Ambient air quality information was taken from the US Environmental Protection Agency's Air Quality System. Average air pollution levels were related to 90 days and 12 months before each subjects IV GTT.

Among 1,023 subjects with complete data, there was a robust association with ambient air pollutants and outcomes related to diabetes.[8] Higher daily cumulative average of $PM_{2.5}$ was associated with higher fasting glucose, total cholesterol, and low density lipoprotein cholesterol (LDL-C). The size effect was equivalent to a one unit increased body fat or BMI.

On longer-term association, $PM_{2.5}$ was negatively associated with 2 months period before the IV GTT. Fasting glucose and $PM_{2.5}$ were positive associated from 5 to 12 months. Higher annual average of NO_2 was associated with higher fasting glucose. Dyslipidemia [decreased high-density lipoprotein cholesterol (HDL-C), increased LDL-C, and triglycerides] is associated with exposure to air pollutants.[9] It was concluded that air pollution may be as important as obesity in the development of T2DM in the metabolically susceptible population.[8]

GLOBAL STUDY

Bowe et al. published a global and national study to define and quantify the risk of diabetes, which is attributable to pollution due to $PM_{2.5}$. One group, which was comprised the longitudinal cohort, was obtained from the US Department of Veterans Affairs' database; they were US veterans who did not have previous history of diabetes mellitus. This was linked to the US Environmental Protection Agency's Community Multiscale Air Quality Modeling System of $PM_{2.5}$.[10]

The follow-up period was for a median duration of 8.5 years for the outcome of incident diabetes. Relationship between $PM_{2.5}$ was assessed by the Cox proportional hazards model. Interestingly, a negative control was employed to identify sources of spurious causal inference (in this case, air sodium).

National annual $PM_{2.5}$ exposure estimates were derived from integrating satellite data, surface measurement, geographical data, and a chemical transport model obtained from the 2015 Global Burden of Disease. Estimates of incident rates, years of life with disability, years of life lost, and disability-adjusted life years (DALYs) of diabetes were derived from Global Burden of Disease 2016. The population attributable fraction of diabetes due to $PM_{2.5}$ is the proportion of diabetes that is eliminated, if $PM_{2.5}$ exposure is decreased to levels equal to or less than theoretical minimum risk exposure level.

Global burden of incident diabetes to $PM_{2.5}$ in 2016 was in 1,000s, 3002.9. Global DALYs attributable to $PM_{2.5}$ were 8.2 million. Among the 10 most population nations, India was second to China in attributable burden of disease (ABD) (590.5 in comparison to 600.3 for China). However, among the 10 most populated countries, India had the highest DALYs (1625.8) followed by China (1251.5).[10]

The authors concluded that there was a significant association between the level of $PM_{2.5}$ exposure and diabetes risk. More worrisome is the fact that there was a significant risk even at concentrations below the recommended levels advocated by regulatory agencies.[10]

BURDEN OF AIR POLLUTION IN INDIA

Traditionally, outdoor air pollution has been considered a problem of urban areas, with megacities such as London and Los Angeles in the 20th century and with Beijing, Delhi, and Mexico city in the 21st century.[11] However, rapid industrialization in Asian countries led to expanding geographic areas where $PM_{2.5}$ levels are well in excess of the guideline provided by the WHO. In 2018, Karambelas et al. reported the levels of fine PM and ozone over northern India in the Indo-Gangetic Plain which is reported to be highly polluted.[12] They came to the conclusion that the majority of premature deaths attributable to $PM_{2.5}$ and ozone (O_3) are in rural (383,600) compared to urban (117,200) regions; urban areas were classified as cities and towns having a population of at least 100,000.

Unlike the west, separation of urban and rural areas in India is porous, especially in relation to population densities, which often cluster together in nonurban areas as well. Employing satellite-derived surface $PM_{2.5}$ levels, they reported that outdoor pollution in nonurban areas was just as high as in urban areas.[11]

When annual premature mortality due to $PM_{2.5}$ was estimated for both urban and nonurban areas, it was 1.05 comparable to other studies. The deaths were seen for ischemic heart disease, stroke, lower respiratory infections, chronic obstructive pulmonary disease, lung cancer, and diabetes mellitus. Surprisingly, nonurban regions showed higher mortality perhaps due to the larger population residing in those areas.[11] Higher $PM_{2.5}$ levels were observed both in the urban and nonurban areas. The pollution in nonurban areas could be made worse by the use of household cooking with solid fuels.

Not only does it mandate the estimation of $PM_{2.5}$ levels in both urban and nonurban areas, but measures must be employed to reduce the pollution levels. Even though lowering $PM_{2.5}$ levels is practically difficult, an unintended consequence of the national lockdown in India due to coronavirus disease 2019 (COVID-19) pandemic showed it was possible. Arunkumar and Dhanakumar investigated the impact of COVID-19 pandemic on $PM_{2.5}$ in the national capital city of Delhi. When compared to the years 2018–2019, the spatial pattern of $PM_{2.5}$ between January and April 2020 decreased by 40% during the period of lockdown.[13] Even though the reduction did not reach the standards set up by the WHO, even partial reduction could have beneficial health effects.

MECHANISTIC PROCESSES FOR ASSOCIATION OF AIR POLLUTION, METABOLIC SYNDROME, AND RELATED CONDITIONS

Coronary Artery Disease

Metabolic syndrome is a cluster of conditions, which can eventually lead to coronary artery disease. The biological pathways, which link environmental air pollution to cardiovascular disease, have been charted as inhaled air pollutants leading to their entering the systemic circulation and when chronic leading to oxidative stress and inflammation. This, in turn, interacts with traditional risk factors such as vasoconstriction, elevated blood pressure, insulin resistance, hyperglycemia, and dyslipidemia. There are, in addition, other risk factors such as activation of hypothalamo-pituitary-adrenal axis, endothelial dysfunction, proliferation of smooth muscle cells, and inflammation of central nervous system along with epigenetic modifications.

All these, in turn, lead to the development of subclinical cardiovascular disease, viz., myocardial remodeling and fibrosis, progressive coronary and carotid atherosclerosis, and hypertension.

Acute exposure of air pollutants can lead to acute cardiovascular disease by constriction of the pulmonary and systemic vessels and impaired dilatation of coronary arteries; in addition, endothelial dysfunction, activation of platelets, and thrombotic pathways are associated with reduced fibrinolysis and an increase of myocardial oxygen demand. Alongside, sympathetic tone is increased resulting in tachycardia and decreased variability of heart rate.

Both the acute and chronic pollutants ultimate lead to cardiovascular events such as acute coronary syndrome, decompensated heart failure, stroke, and disturbances in heart rhythm with their associated hospitalization, morbidity, and death.[14]

The adverse effects can be modified by dietary factors, length of exposure to PM, and by their size.[15]

Lipids, Glucose, and Diabetes Mellitus

Shin et al. examined the effect of ambient small PM on fasting glucose and lipid profiles in a nationwide cohort from Korea.[16] Data on 85,869 persons aged 20 years and above was retrieved from the National Health Insurance Service-National Health Cohort. Significant associations were found between increased interquartile range for $PM_{2.5}$ and elevated fasting glucose levels and LDL cholesterol. Such an association was not observed with coarse PM. The authors claimed that this was the first study providing comprehensive direct evidence of size-specific effects of $PM_{2.5}$ from Asia.[16] Additional operating factors include accelerated atherosclerosis following altered coagulation, blood cell responses, and dysfunctional HDL-C with lowered ability to act as antioxidant.[17] Sade et al. assessed the association among $PM_{2.5}$ glucose, glycosylated hemoglobin (HbA1c) levels, and lipids employing a satellite model to assess $PM_{2.5}$ exposure. It was a retrospective cohort study in Southern Israel over 10 years. Average concentrations of $PM_{2.5}$ over 3 months average were associated with increased levels of serum glucose, HbA1c, LDL-C, triglycerides, and decreased HDL-C. The strongest link was seen in subjects having diabetes.[17]

Despite indoor air pollution not factored because of difficulties in measurement, outdoor air pollution has both epidemiological and mechanistic associations with T2DM; subjects with T2DM are more susceptible to the adverse effects of air pollution.[18] Exposure to air pollutants leads to inflammation in the visceral adipose tissue and hepatic insulin resistance.[18] Further studies aim to look at the direct effects of pollutants on β-cell function, counterregulatory hormones such as glucagon, and indirectly on appetite acting through the hypothalamus.[18]

In addition to $PM_{2.5}$, exposure to ozone leads to oxidation of lipid-rich alveolar lining fluid resulting in oxidative stress. Stress kinases can be activated via c-Jun N-terminal kinases along with disturbance of other components of the insulin signaling pathway.[19]

Other putative mechanisms include the association of air pollution and low levels of vitamin D.[20] Interestingly, Eze et al. proposed that genetic risk for T2DM may alter the susceptibility to the adverse effects of air pollution acting via alteration in insulin sensitivity.[21]

Rao et al. summarized the pathways through which air pollutants mediate the development of metabolic syndrome and diabetes.[5] Pollutants along with high-calorie diet lead to systemic inflammation, which, in turn, result in CCR2-dependent and CCR2-independent alterations in distal tissues such as fat, liver, muscle, and endothelium, finally resulting in insulin resistance.[5]

PRACTICAL ISSUES ARISING

In view of the adverse effects of air pollution and the necessarily exposure to outdoor air pollutants with physical activity, what is the cost-benefit of exercise? Do the health benefits of exercise exceed the adverse health outcomes of being exposed to air pollution? Guo et al. provided practical answer to this dilemma. Among a cohort of 156,314 subjects with nondiabetic adults, incidence of T2DM was identified on follow-up examinations.[22] They reported that compared to those who performed high physical activity, those with moderate or low physical activity had higher risk of diabetes, regardless of the levels of exposure to $PM_{2.5}$. It was suggested that habitual physical activity is safer in preventing diabetes even among persons living in relatively polluted areas.[22]

Nevertheless, efforts must be made to lower air pollution, as summarized by Zhang and Day in relation to developing countries: *Clean air is possible from a combination of legislation, technology, and enforcement.*[23]

Developed countries such as USA reported improved air quality following the passage of the Clean Air Act.[24] Ensuring that level of pollutants is lower, it requires simple and cost-effective and implementable methods of measuring the level of pollutants. We propose such a model, which can then be applied to the National Clean Air Programme (NCAP 2019) proposed by Government of India to mitigate air pollution locally and across boundaries.[25]

AMBIENT AIR QUALITY MONITORING: ISSUES, COMPLEXITIES, AND THE SOLUTION

However, the complexities for effectively monitoring ambient air quality led to confusing practices in selection of sensors and systems for air quality monitoring, the siting of systems, and the empirical approaches followed by different stakeholders in arriving at averaging times related to expensive systems for measurements, resulted in different definitions of air quality.

Today, the confusion is worse confounded with the advent of new entrants into the field advocating low cost sensors with lesser accuracies for niche applications.[26]

Against this backdrop of the impetus, complexities, and challenges posed for ambient air quality monitoring, we introduce a novel indigenously developed state of art photonic system for ambient air quality monitoring having higher accuracies and sensitivities with overarching capabilities for diverse applications.

The novel photonic system christened as "Air Unique-quality Monitoring (AUM)" was compared with the conventional imported ambient air quality monitoring stations and found to be far superior in characteristics.

The uniqueness and novelty of AUM (*patent pending*) lie in an innovative application of the principles of laser back scattering, statistical mechanics, optoelectronics, artificial intelligence, machine/deep learning, and internet of things—resulting in a unique system capable of identification, classification, and quantification of various pollutants *simultaneously* (of accuracies of less than 1 ppb, parts per billion) and meteorological parameters with very high precision, sensitivity, and accuracy.

Air Unique-quality Monitoring is a unique photonic system capable of nonintrusive monitoring in real time of all the air quality parameters of interest at one go with very high sampling frequencies. AUM has the additional unique capability of enabling spatial profile sampling information in addition to temporal sampling. The system has embedded intelligent algorithms and software operating on a user selectable remote server with data encryption, which ensures data security as well as free flow of desired information to authorized users as per specific requirements.

Air Unique-quality Monitoring has two options for data communications—a *wired* option or a *wireless* option enabling different sampling frequencies of data from system as per user requirements.

Air Unique-quality Monitoring is integrated with proprietary software that can be deployed on local or cloud server. The software is developed on Apache Cassandra platform, so that it can handle terabytes of data. AUM equipment is robust and can functions day and night in harsh environmental conditions. AUM is Wi-Fi enabled and can seamlessly connect to any Wi-Fi network protocols.

Air Unique-quality Monitoring was successfully evaluated during laboratory trials in a subsonic wind tunnel in the laboratory with gold standards (in collaboration with EffecTech, UK an ISO 17025:2000 International Standards Accredited Laboratory) and also compared in the field with the imported systems from Environment SA, France and Ecotech, Australia operated by Karnataka State Pollution Control Board's Central Environmental Laboratory with ISO 17025:2005 and National Accreditation Board for Testing and Calibration Laboratories (NABL) Accreditation under the aegis of the Central Pollution Control Board of India. In summary, AUM was demonstrated to be very highly sensitive and accurate and capable of simultaneous detection and quantification of all air quality parameters and offers a number of merits over any of the currently available conventional systems having the following features and characteristics:

- *Portable, compact, low powered, and economical*
- *Plug and play* system requires no setting up time and no additional civil infrastructure for housing
- Provides information on all gases and meteorological parameters simultaneously
- *Nonintrusive, remote, in-situ, and real-time monitoring system with very high sensitivities and accuracies*
- *Single system capable of monitoring in both spatial and temporal domains with high sampling rates*
- Data from sensors seamlessly streamed to a cloud server from where encrypted real-time dash board information is pushed to authorized users
- System can work continuously even under extreme weather and climatic conditions
- Embedded intelligent monitoring algorithms to identify and alert impending system failures to enable preventive maintenance
- Spatial sampling as per user requirements dictated by unhindered line of sight conditions in the field

Being an indigenous design and development, AUM is extremely economical compared to the conventional standard reference stations, thus making it ideal for large scale deployment to effectively monitoring the hitherto eluded spatiotemporal variations of ambient air quality (**Table 1, Fig. 1**).

SUMMARY

Environmental pollution, chiefly air pollution, is ubiquitous with adverse health and, thereby, economic impact principally in developing countries. Decades long efforts in developed countries have gradually reduced the levels of air pollution. Air pollutants have varied effects on obesity, insulin resistance, T2DM, and coronary artery disease, which are leading causes of morbidity and mortality in India. Attempts to lower the levels must be preceded by the availability of instruments to measure them. Currently available sensors are difficult to procure and expensive, limiting their use, and, therefore, their effectiveness. We developed an indigenous system,

TABLE 1 Air Unique-quality Monitoring (AUM): Technical data and specifications.

Electrical power supply	230*V*, 50 *Hz* AC, and 15 *A electrical socket*
Current consumption	135 W
System detection range	<10 *m* to >1 *km*; configurable as per user requirements
Accuracy	Less than ppb for gases, <0.1 SI units for temperature, wind, and pressure
Response time	Less than10 *ns*
Sampling frequency	1–10 *kHz* (wired) and 150–200 *Hz* (wireless)
Cable types	22, 24 AWG
Real-time data recording	On designated computer server, encrypted
Data/Information display	Real-time display on PC/smartphone through internet, encrypted
Operational range of temperature	–25°C to +70°C (ruggedized) and 0°C to +55°C (standard)
Operational range of humidity	0–100%
System shape/ Dimensions	Cuboid/563 *mm* × 390 *mm* × 160 *mm* [(L × W × H) – ruggedized version] Cylinder/180 *mm* × 220 *mm* [(Ø × L) – standard version]
Weight	<10.0 *kg*
Protection class/ Deployment	IP65/IP67/IP69/field deployable even in harsh environments

Source: Adapted from Tatavarti R. Ambient Air Quality Monitoring: Impetus, Complexities, Challenges and Solutions. Government of India: Commission for Air Quality Management; 2021. p. 30.

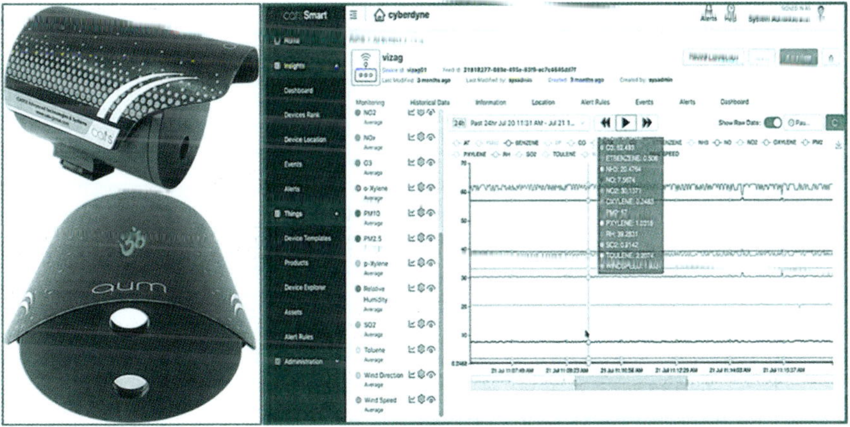

FIG. 1: Side and front views (top and bottom left) of Air Unique-quality Monitoring (AUM) system (180 × 220 mm) and typical real-time dashboard information (right).

Source: Adapted from Tatavarti R. Ambient Air Quality Monitoring: Impetus, Complexities, Challenges and Solutions. Government of India: Commission for Air Quality Management; 2021. p. 30.

which is less expensive and far more superior in accuracy than existing systems. A awareness about the ubiquity of pollutants and a feasible method to measure them would be the first crucial steps in improving the air and environmental quality.

ACKNOWLEDGMENTS

Tatavarti gratefully acknowledges his many mentors, colleagues, and students who helped him graciously in the design and development of the photonic system.

Funding from DST India (Clean Air Research Initiative Program); ADA, Ministry of Defense, India; NIWE, Ministry of New and Renewable Energy, India; and CATS Ecosystem Pvt Ltd, India is gratefully acknowledged.

REFERENCES

1. Logan WP. Mortality in the London fog incident. Lancet. 1952;1:336-8.
2. Liu C, Chen R, Sera F, Vicedo-Cabrera AM, Guo Y, Tong S, et al. Ambient Particulate Air Pollution and Daily Mortality in 652 Cities. N Engl J Med. 2019;381:705-15.
3. Sridhar GR, Kumar PS, Venkata P, Allam AR, Durai VK, Kosuri M, et al. Built Environment Factors, Psychosocial Factors and Diabetes Mellitus: A South Indian Study. Indian J Clin Med. 2010;1:15-22.
4. Dendup T, Feng X, Clingan S, Astell-Burt T. Environmental Risk Factors for Developing Type 2 Diabetes Mellitus: A Systematic Review. Int J Environ Res Public Health. 2018;15:78.
5. Rao X, Liu C, Rajagopalan S. Diabetes and metabolic syndrome. In: Nadadur SS, Hollingsworth JW (Eds). Air Pollution and Health Effects. London: Springer Verlag; 2015. pp. 213-39.
6. Eze IC, Hemkens LG, Bucher HC, Hoffmann B, Schindler C, Künzli N, et al. Association between ambient air pollution and diabetes mellitus in Europe and North America: systematic review and meta-analysis. Environ Health Perspect. 2015;123:381-9.
7. Park SK, Adar SD, O'Neill MS, Auchincloss AH, Szpiro A, Bertoni AG, et al. Long-term exposure to air pollution and type 2 diabetes mellitus in a multiethnic cohort. Am J Epidemiol. 2015;181:327-36.
8. Chen Z, Salam MT, Toledo-Corral C, Watanabe RM, Xiang AH, Buchanan TA, et al. Ambient Air Pollutants Have Adverse Effects on Insulin and Glucose Homeostasis in Mexican Americans. Diabetes Care. 2016;39:547-54.
9. Chuang KJ, Yan YH, Cheng TJ. Effect of air pollution on blood pressure, blood lipids, and blood sugar: a population-based approach. J Occup Environ Med. 2010;52:258-62.
10. Bowe B, Xie Y, Li T, Yan Y, Xian H, Al-Aly Z. The 2016 global and national burden of diabetes mellitus attributable to PM2·5 air pollution. Lancet Planet Health. 2018;2:e301-12.
11. Ravishankara AR, David LM, Pierce JR, Venkataraman C. Outdoor air pollution in India is not only an urban problem. Proc Natl Acad Sci U S A. 2020;117:28640-4.
12. Karambelas A, Holloway T, Kinney PL, Fiore AM, DeFries R, Kiesewetter G, et al. Urban versus rural health impacts attributable to $PM_{2.5}$ and O_3 in northern India. Environ Res Lett. 2018;13:064010.
13. Arunkumar M, Dhanakumar S. Ambient fine particulate matter pollution over the megacity Delhi, India: an impact of COVID-19 lockdown. Curr Sci. 2021;120:304-12.
14. Brauer M, Casadei B, Harrington RA, Kovacs R, Sliwa K, WHF Air Pollution Expert Group. Taking a Stand Against Air Pollution—The Impact on Cardiovascular Disease: A Joint Opinion From the World Heart Federation, American College of Cardiology, American Heart Association, and the European Society of Cardiology. Circulation. 2021;143:e800-4.
15. Araujo JA, Rosenfeld ME. Air pollution, lipids and atherosclerosis. In: Nadadur SS, Hollingsworth JW (Eds). Air Pollution and Health Effects. London: Springer Verlag; 2015. pp. 241-67.

16. Shin WY, Kim JH, Lee G, Choi S, Kim SR, Hong YC, et al. Exposure to ambient fine particulate matter is associated with changes in fasting glucose and lipid profiles: a nationwide cohort study. BMC Public Health. 2020;20:430.
17. Sade YM, Kloog I, Liberty IF, Schwartz J, Novack V. The Association Between Air Pollution Exposure and Glucose and Lipids Levels. J Clin Endocrinol Metab. 2016;101:2460-7.
18. Rajagopalan S, Brook RD. Air pollution and type 2 diabetes: mechanistic insights. Diabetes. 2012;61:3037-45.
19. Kodavanti UP. Air pollution and insulin resistance: do all roads lead to Rome? Diabetes. 2015;64:712-4.
20. Barrea L, Savastano S, Di Somma C, Savanelli MC, Nappi F, Albanese L, et al. Low serum vitamin D-status, air pollution and obesity: a dangerous liaison. Rev Endocrinol Metab Disord. 2017;18:207-14.
21. Eze IC, Imboden M, Kumar A, von Eckardstein A, Stolz D, Gerbase MW, et al. Air pollution and diabetes association: Modification by type 2 diabetes genetic risk score. Environ Int. 2016;94:263-71.
22. Guo C, Yang HT, Chang LY, Bo Y, Lin C, Zeng Y, et al. Habitual exercise is associated with reduced risk of diabetes regardless of air pollution: a longitudinal cohort study. Diabetologia. 2021;64:1298-308.
23. Zhang JJ, Day D. Urban air pollution and health in developing countries. In: Nadadur SS, Hollingsworth JW (Eds). Air Pollution and Health. London: Springer Verlag; 2015. pp. 355-80.
24. Sacks JD, Fann N, Owens EO, Costa DL. Using science to shape policy. In: Nadadur SS, Hollingsworth JW (Eds). Air Pollution and Health. London: Springer Verlag; 2015. pp. 403-36.
25. Anilkumar M, Kashyap S, Mitra SG, Neogi D, Ramaprasad A, Sanjeev A, et al. The pathways to manage air pollution: an ontological assessment of the National Clean Air Programme 2019, India. Curr Sci. 2021;120:1295-302.
26. Tatavarti R. Ambient Air Quality Monitoring: Impetus, Complexities, Challenges and Solutions. Government of India: Commission for Air Quality Management; 2021. p. 30.

CHAPTER 4

Genomics and Diabetes: 20 Years after the Human Genome Project

Ganesh Chauhan, Dwaipayan Bharadwaj

ABSTRACT

One of the greatest achievements in medicine has been unraveling the blueprint of life that is the sequence of the human genome. This has opened doors to multiple research fronts, technologies, and far deeper insight into diseases unparalleled by any other effort by mankind. Here, we visit the advancements in our understanding of the pathophysiology of diabetes that has been possible because of understanding the genetic basis of the disease. We take you through the exciting journey of the first gene discovered for diabetes in 2005 through candidate gene-based studies to hundreds of loci identified using genome-wide association studies and whole-genome sequencing approaches. We visit the international efforts modeled on the basis of the Human Genome Project such as the HapMap and 1,000 Genomes projects and how these have made a difference to the advancement in the field of diabetes genetics. Here, we also highlight the efforts that have gone from simple gene discovery to the functional disease model for diabetes, the population risk based on genetic discoveries, and stepping into the era of precision medicine. A big realization in recent times has been to increase the diversity of the ethnic groups being studied in order to take these advancements to the entire human population. Once genetic discoveries begin to saturate, as we are only able to discover new loci with small effect sizes, the focus has now to change on harvesting the benefits of these discoveries for translational research and simultaneously keep on discovering new genes. We have taken a giant leap into the genetic discoveries for diabetes in the last two decades since the unraveling of the first draft of the human genome and we now need to capitalize on these findings if we have to achieve the goal for precision medicine and find a suitable cure or preventive measures for diabetes.

Keywords: *Human genome project, Genome-wide association studies (GWAS), Whole-genome sequencing, Next generation sequencing (NGS), Precision medicine.*

INTRODUCTION

"Nature" (genes) and "nurture" (environment) together interact to bring about a phenotype. Once deoxyribonucleic acid (DNA) had been identified as the genetic material and the structure was proposed, the interest in the sequence of nucleotide bases that make a gene and code for proteins became an important goal for medicine to tease out the components of "nature" that affected diseases. This led to one of the most ambitious international projects, the "Human Genome Project", that took close to a decade and huge economic and manpower resources across the world to get the first draft of the 3.2 billion base pairs that make us who are as a species (**Fig. 1**).[1,2] Like many other diseases, the field of diabetes has also been reaping the benefits of this huge effort that stands out as one of the brilliant examples of global scientific collaboration. Within 5 years of the release of the human genome sequence, we had our first few genes for diabetes. Once we had access to the human genome, our next challenge was to identify the genetic variations that make each one of us different in physical appearance and physiological response and might predispose us to diseases. On the same lines of the Human Genome Project, another international effort, the "HapMap project", was initiated to identify the haplotype structure of the human genome based on the genetic variations across multiple major ethnic groups of the world.[3] This led to the creation

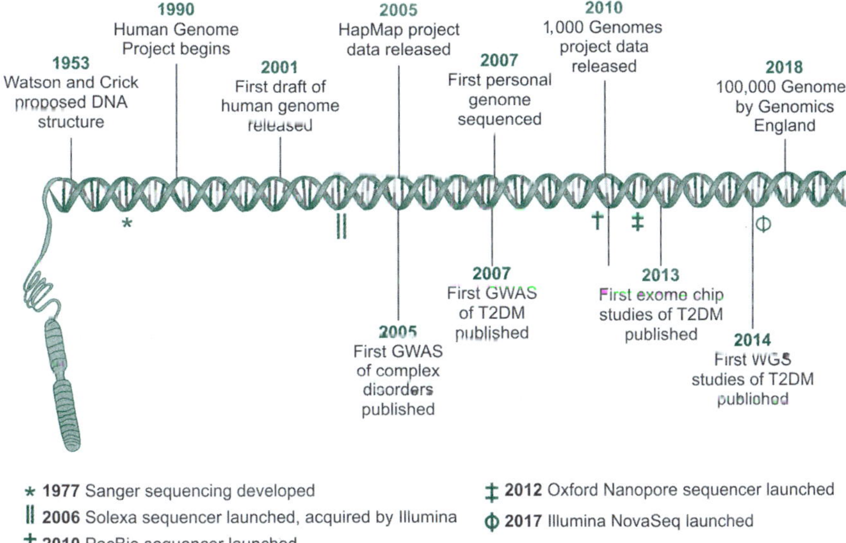

(DNA: deoxyribonucleic acid; GWAS: genome-wide association studies; T2DM: type 2 diabetes mellitus; WGS: whole-genome sequencing)

FIG. 1: Milestones in the era of genomics and diabetes genomics.

of technological platforms where we could interrogate thousands of genetic variations covering the entire genome in one go and this approach today known as genome-wide association study (GWAS) is still the main drivers of gene discovery for complex disorders like diabetes. About 5 years down the lane, further refinement to the HapMap project (genotyping approach) led to the "1,000 Genomes project" (sequencing approach) that led to better coverage and interrogation of genetic variants with lesser frequencies and also included structural variants.[4] More importantly, the 1,000 Genomes project led to the development of tools and techniques that made it possible to sequence large number of genomes. Today with the substantial drop in sequencing cost, the world has seen announcement of national projects where 100,000 to 1 million people are being sequenced (https://www.genengnews.com/insights/the-100000-genomes-club/) and completion of sequencing of 100,000 people by the Genomics England has already been announced in 2018 (https://www.genomicsengland.co.uk/about-genomics-england/the-100000-genomes-project/).

From getting the first draft of the human genome that took 10 years and millions of dollars and international effort to sequencing the human genome in a couple of days by spending <$1,000, we have come a long way in fulfilling the aspirations of the Human Genome Project. The field of diabetes has been one of the direct beneficiaries of these efforts leading to discovery of hundreds of loci for diabetes and its related conditions bringing us closer to the dream of precision medicine. In this review, we will focus on the genes discovered in this span of 20 years since the release of the first draft of the human genome but more importantly, we will also discuss the other outcomes of these gene discoveries and the use of this to further increase our knowledge of the mechanisms leading to the disease and possible treatment options.

CANDIDATE GENES AND LINKAGE STUDIES

Linkage analysis was one of the primary drivers for gene identification. In the initial phases, it had aided in discovery of many monogenic disease-associated genes. The same tool was also applied to complex disorders that yielded multiple candidate genes under the linkage peak with limited success. Follow-up studies of these candidate genes led to the identification of three genes: (1) *KCNJ11*; (2) *PPARG*; and (3) *TCF7L2*.[5-7] Importantly, these three genes have been replicated since then in most of the genetic studies that followed their discovery including GWAS. These loci had high effect sizes and were strong candidates that were involved in monogenic forms of diabetes (*PPARG*) or were targets of drugs (*KCNJ11*) being used to treat diabetes. Although the exception was *TCF7L2* where it opened the doors for the involvement of Wnt signaling pathway that was never a strong candidate prior to the discovery of this gene for type 2 diabetes mellitus (T2DM). *PPARG* and *TCF7L2* have been implicated in many other metabolic conditions with

TCF7L2 often being the lead signal in many diabetes studies conducted across populations.

GENOME-WIDE ASSOCIATION STUDIES ERA

Genome-wide association studies have been the main pivots for gene discovery in complex disorders till date including for diabetes. Finer understanding of the haplotype structure and tagging single nucleotide polymorphisms (SNPs) led to the advent of genome-wide chips where common genetic polymorphisms tagging multiple common variations across the genome were genotyped in one attempt in one individual. The genome-wide approach without bias to focus on a favorite candidate gene or pathway is what popularized this method and earned it the name of an "agnostic approach" or a "hypothesis-free approach". An important outcome of having genome-wide data was the ability to do better quality checks including correction for population stratification that are notorious in giving false positives in association studies. However, we must still keep in mind that the GWAS approach is not an absolute hypothesis-free approach as it was based on the "common disease-common variation" model and in the initial phase the list of genetic variations were biased toward the population groups in the HapMap project and many ethnic groups have only a minor representation including South Asians.

The first GWAS study that identified genes for age-related macular degeneration was published in 2005. About 2 years later, a series of studies on complex metabolic disorders were published including the three studies on T2DM. These studies in total identified close to 10 loci and that was a remarkable achievements considering the fact that prior to this only three genes for T2DM had been identified. However, little did we realize that these would open the flood gates for identifying genetic loci and probably in those times we had never dreamt that there would be hundreds of loci with small effect sizes.

Prior to the GWAS era, genetic studies were notorious for nonreplication of findings in independent studies that were often due to the limited knowledge of disease biology, bias in studying of favorite genes by different groups, smaller sample sizes, and most likely lack of correction for population stratification in the absence of genome-wide data. Another important aspect that led to nonreproducibility of results was the choice of *p*-values of nominal significance ($p < 0.05$ or similar range) for declaring association. The GWAS era changed all of this as it was invariably associated with large sample sizes in order to find anything significant at the genome-wide threshold *p*-value $<5 \times 10^{-8}$. Such a stringent *p*-value is necessary in GWAS to account for correction for multiple testing of approximately 1 million haplotype blocks. The use of standard quality check across studies using genome-wide data was a game changer for GWAS as till date most of the loci identified have been replicated in the next study with a larger sample size.

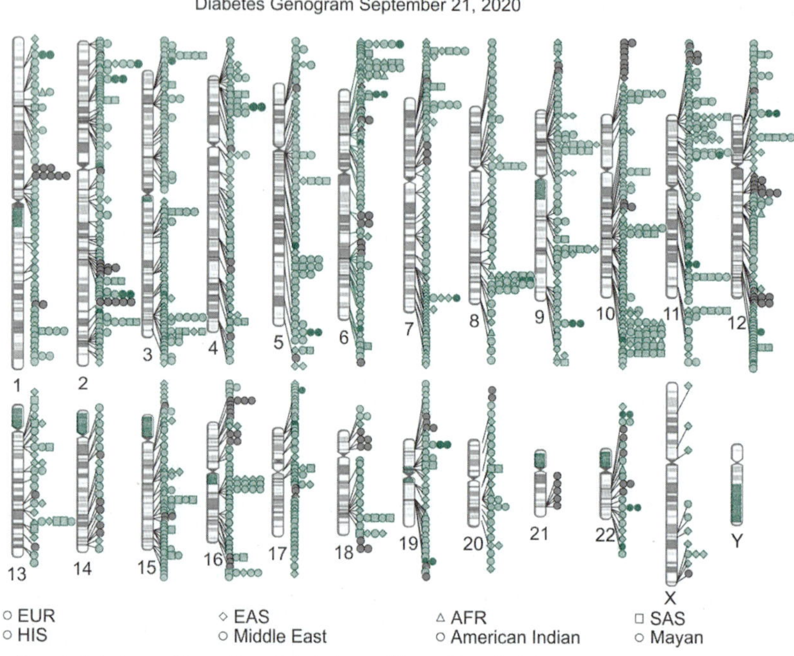

(BMI: body mass index; GWAS: genome-wide association studies)

FIG. 2: Genes identified for diabetes using genome-wide approaches. This figure was generated using the "phenograms" application from Ritchie laboratory (http://visualization.ritchielab.org/home/index). All genetic variations shown to be associated with type 2 diabetes mellitus and type 1 diabetes mellitus were downloaded from the GWAS catalogue (https://www.ebi.ac.uk/gwas/) as on 21st September, 2020. The variations are plotted to show the location of these variations across the autosomes and sex chromosomes. The signals originating from different ethnicities are coded using different shapes and the color denotes the phenotype of interest.

Importantly, all the loci identified by GWAS were replicated in many studies of diverse ancestry.[8-12] This was what built trust in association studies in the post-GWAS era and led to the opening of floodgates for larger GWAS studies including those in non-Europeans. Due to drop in cost in GWAS genotyping chips that can be close to US$ 30, many cohort-based studies have employed genome-wide genotyping on their samples as it is in the similar range to having a detailed blood biochemistry of the samples.

Presently, >400 loci have been identified and majority have very small effect sizes (**Fig. 2**). These loci in-total explain about 20% of the genetic variation for diabetes that is close to half of the genetic variation that has been predicted to be explained by genetic variation on the GWAS chip. This is quite a remarkable achievement considering the fact that many complex disorders are still in the range <5% of the genetic variations explained.

GENOME-WIDE ASSOCIATION STUDIES OF DIABETES IN NON-EUROPEANS

The success of the first series of GWAS for diabetes in the European population encouraged GWAS studies in non-Europeans. The first major non-European study was on Japanese population that led to the identification of *KCNQ1*.[13,14] The discovery of *KCNQ1* was a good example to suggest that difference in allele frequency and linkage disequilibrium pattern between ethnicities would lead to identification of new genes, if we studied multiple ethnicities. Prior to the Japanese study, even larger studies in Europeans could not identify *KCNQ1* due to low allele frequency in their study population.

The other intuitive reason for identifying these novel variants in different populations could also be due to gene-environment interactions like the effect of such variants in carbohydrate metabolism or central obesity that could have a higher impact on Asians rather than Europeans. South Asia including India where there is a high prevalence of diabetes and an earlier year of onset apart from having a higher prevalence of vascular risk factors like central obesity had not been studied for genetics of diabetes. The first GWAS for diabetes from India was published in 2012 that identified a novel locus on 2q21 for T2DM in addition to replicating many loci identified in European.[15] Interestingly, these GWAS findings have now also been validated by functional studies.[16] Similarly, there have been multiple studies on other ethnicities of the world (**Fig. 2**) including the one in the most ancestral populations like the Africans.[17,18] The importance of studying such ancestral populations has been of interest as the size of the linkage disequilibrium block is small in such populations and chances of locating the causal variant are higher on a smaller block.

Another important aspect of studying the same disease in different ethnicities is to use this approach for fine mapping. The linkage disequilibrium block will have varying sizes in different ethnicities, but the causal variant remains the same. By filtering out variants that do not support association in multiple ethnicities, we can reduce the set of variations to a much smaller number that will include the causal variant. This strategy has been effectively used to fine map loci for diabetes.[19] Despite these efforts, the contribution of non European population to disease genetics has been very low.[20] Taking an example of South Asia that accounts for approximately one-fourth of the human populations but the contribution of samples from South Asia for disease identification is only approximately 2%.[20] Similarly, despite realization of the importance of ancestral population in disease genomics, the contribution of African population is again on the same scale as that of South Asians. This has led to increased inclusion of non-Europeans in large national efforts like the National Heart, Lung, and Blood Institute (NHLBI) Trans-Omics for Precision Medicine (TOPMed) program of the United States, where the proportion of non-Europeans subjects is close to 60%

(https://www.nhlbiwgs.org/). The recent use of just the sequencing data from 100,000 participants of this program (https://bravo.sph.umich.edu/freeze8/hg38/) for genotype imputation has given a major boost not only to the number of genetic variations in terms of imputation but a huge jump in the confidence of the imputed variants (https://imputation.biodatacatalyst.nhlbi.nih.gov/#!). This was applicable to all ethnic groups including Europeans.

EXOME AND WHOLE-GENOME SEQUENCING STUDIES

Technological advancements and drop in cost for sequencing led to upliftment of association studies from GWAS to whole exome and genome sequencing. The first large scale whole-genome study did not have much success in identifying new genetic variations as most of the identified loci clustered around known loci.[21] The idea of reaping a large number of rare variants with big effect sizes was also not met. However, this was mainly because of the smaller sample sizes to begin with and not realizing that rare variants would mostly have modest effect sizes. Studies with larger sample sizes are in the pipeline and will definitely lead to novel findings. The largest exome sequencing project for diabetes was successful in identifying new loci including rare variants.[22] This included 12 gene sets that were drug targets of diabetes and candidate genes based on knockout mice studies. The sample sizes for exome and whole-genome sequencing studies for diabetes are yet to catch up with those for GWAS studies but they have clearly implicated new insights both in terms of allelic architecture and actionable genes.

ALLELIC MODEL OF DIABETES

Multiple hypotheses regarding the spectrum of allele frequency of genetic variants implicated in diabetes have been proposed. The most popular hypothesis at the beginning years of diabetes genetics was the "common disease-common variation" hypothesis. This was mainly popular as in the beginning it was believed that rare variants had very high effect size and were more involved in monogenic conditions rather than complex disorders. The natural selection process often excluded these variations due to their high penetrance and they did not find their way into common disorders that affect a large number of people. For the first time, "the mosaic model" was proposed that modified this hypothesis to state that in addition to common variations, rare variations also had a role in complex disorders and till date this is the most accepted model and has been proven by studies on exome chip, exome sequencing, and whole-genome sequencing studies.[23] Interestingly, this hypothesis was proposed even before findings from GWAS studies were known.

Though exome chip, exome sequencing, and whole-genome sequencing-based studies have identified genetic variants in diabetes, the hope for identifying a large number of rare variants with large effect sizes was not met. However, these results have to be interpreted keeping in mind that rare variants may not have large effect sizes as anticipated previously and statistical methods like burden test often used for testing association of rare variants by combining them in groups have limitations. Thus, larger studies and newer statistical approaches are required to better resolve this problem. Thus, the "mosaic model" still prevails albeit with fewer rare variants without large effects and a long chain of common variants with very small effects.

FUNCTIONAL STUDIES OF GENES IDENTIFIED THROUGH GENOME-WIDE ASSOCIATION STUDIES

At the end of the day, GWAS and sequencing approaches only tell us if a genomic region is associated with diabetes or not, they are not designed to infer causality. The outcome of these methods is a region of interest, which often has a large number of genetic variations and we are not sure that one of them is the causal variation. Interestingly, we are also not aware of the functional element this casual variation might affect, i.e., that protein coding gene or regulatory element. Thus, these genetic methods of statistical associations at best give us a "lamp post" to hover around and many times these may be located in "no man's land", i.e., intergenic regions. One of the biggest criticisms of association studies has, thus, been inability to pinpoint causal genes and due to the low effect sizes of the identified variants, straightforward functional studies like those for Mendelian disorders have not been possible.

Again international efforts such as the Encyclopedia of DNA Elements (ENCODE) project[24] and the Genotype-Tissue Expression (GTEx)[25] project have come to the rescue of association studies by giving some guidance by indicating the regulatory nature of the variations present under the "lamp post" and suggesting the genes whose expression might get affected due to the genetic variations under consideration.

Despite the difficulties associated with designing functional studies for signals indicated by association studies, there are multiple success stories. The 2q21 locus that was identified to be associated with diabetes in a study from North India has been successfully resolved to indicate the mechanisms of the causal gene *TMEM163* in pathophysiology of diabetes. Fine mapping of this locus indicated a nonsynonymous variation in *TMEM163* that increased glycemic index. Knocking down of this *TMEM163* in MIN6 cell lines increased the concentration of zinc in the intracellular space and amount of insulin. This silencing of *TMEM163* led to increased glucose uptake by the cells. This is an excellent example from locus identification to fine mapping to understanding mechanisms through which the gene causes the disease.

SLC30A8 is another solute carrier that codes for the islet zinc transporter 8 (ZnT8) and was identified in the first series of GWAS studies to harbor common variants associated with diabetes.[26-28] Studies on diabetes patients and their relatives in Finnish populations followed by functional studies on human-induced pluripotent stem cell (iPSC)-derived β-like cells have suggested rare loss-of-function allele p.Arg138* that results in reduced *SLC30A8* expression.[29] Further, fine mapping of this gene has led to identification of at least 12 protein truncating variants that collectively reduced the risk of diabetes. Studies in animal models have also proved that common variants in this protein destabilize the zinc transport function. Thus, genetic studies in this gene have now suggested that ZnT8 inhibition as a new strategy for diabetes prevention.[29,30]

GENETICS OF DIABETES INFORMING MECHANISMS AND TREATMENT OPTION FOR OTHER DISEASES

Diabetes may be classified as a metabolic disorder, but it has far-reaching consequences on the health of an aging individual. Effects of diabetes on other conditions such as retinopathy, neuropathy, nephropathy, obesity, and cardiac condition are well-known complications that affect the micro- and macrovasculature. There have also been numerous clinical and epidemiological reports that suggest causal relationship between diabetes and mental health like association with psychiatric disease like schizophrenia[31] and neurological diseases like Alzheimer's disease.[31-33] Due to development of new statistical approaches that can interrogate genetic correlation based on summary statistics and many consortia making these statistics freely available, it is now possible to correlate a large number of diseases for genetic basis.[34,35] The linkage disequilibrium score regression (LDSC) tool employed on LD Hub (http://ldsc.broadinstitute.org/) can rapidly do such analysis on hundreds of phenotypes. Such genetic correlation analyses have suggested genetic correlation of diabetes with many of the diseases and especially related risk factors such as intracranial volume, educational attainment, etc. (**Fig. 3**). This knowledge corroborates previous epidemiological and clinical observations, but also pinpoints loci, genes, and pathways that are common to these diseases. There are no medications for treating Alzheimer's diseases, but these types of strong indicators have led to opening of doors for drugs being used for treating diabetes for treating Alzheimer's diseases.[35,36]

GENETIC RISK SCORES

The concept of genetic risk score comes from the idea of predicting a disease based on the genetic variants known for a disease. In Mendelian disorders, it is very simplistic, i.e., if an individual carries the disease-causing allele of

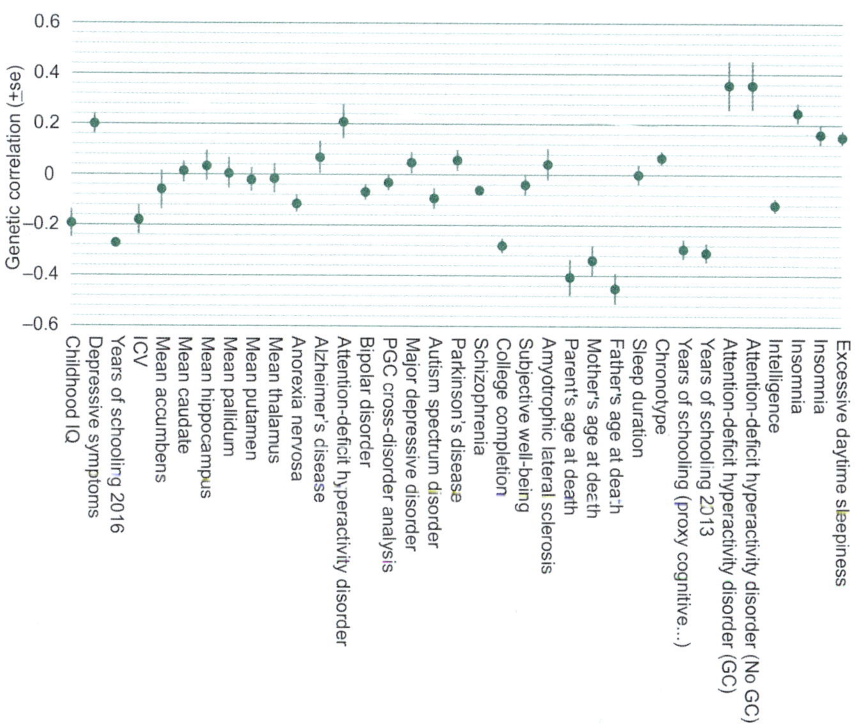

(GWAS: genome-wide association studies; PGC: Psychiatric Genomics Consortium; LDSC: linkage disequilibrium score regression)

FIG. 3: Genetic correlation of diabetes with other disorders. The genetic correlations were calculated using the method implemented in LDSC using the resources on LD Hub (http://ldsc.broadinstitute.org/). Genome-wide association summary statistics for type 2 diabetes mellitus (T2DM) were included from one of the largest GWAS on European ancestry (Mahajan et al. 2018, PMID: 30297969).[41] Genetic correlation was performed on LD Hub for traits grouped as "neurological diseases, sleeping, cognitive, education, brain volume (ENIGMA), psychiatric diseases, and aging" on LD Hub server (Date: 21st September, 2020). These phenotypes were specifically targeted to check association of T2DM genetics on mental health.

the mutation, then the individual will have the disease. However, in complex polygenic disorders like diabetes, there are a large number of polymorphisms involved instead of one mutation. Thus, the probability of an individual to get the disease increases depending upon the number of risk alleles present in the set of polymorphisms being considered for the analysis. Hence, the count of number of risk alleles is used as the exposure variable in the regression analysis to estimate the chance of the individual to get the disease. It is to be noted that the count of the alleles are weighted for the effect size of the polymorphism such that polymorphisms with higher effects get more weightage. The regression coefficient, beta, is used as the weight for effect size and not the popular measure of effect size for case-control studies, i.e., odds ratio. Genetic risk score analyses are also sometimes referred to as polygenic risk scores and these can include a selective set of polymorphisms, all genome-wide polymorphisms, or all polymorphisms with genotypes after filtering based on *p*-value, allele frequency, and degree of linkage disequilibrium. This weighted count of the risk alleles is used as the exposure variable in the regression analysis.

A recent analysis using genome-wide genetic risk score for diabetes has found that it could predict >3-fold increased risk for 3.5% subjects in UK Biobank subjects.[37] The authors suggested that this is more than the number of people being diagnosed for monogenic conditions of diabetes.[38] Providing preventive care for these subjects at increased risk can considerably delay the onset if not prevent diabetes and definitely lowers the public burden of the disease. These genetic risk scores can also be used to perform receiver operating characteristic (ROC) curve analysis for disease predictions and include other covariates such as age, gender, and body mass index (BMI). The area under the curve of ROC (AUROC) is indicative of the chance that such a curve will correctly predict a diabetic subject. Based on results from multiple studies, it seems the predictive power of known diabetes genes (AUROC ~0.7) is still low and definitely not at par with clinical factors (AUROC ~0.9). Improvement has been observed if age, gender, and BMI have been included in the analysis (AUC ~0.8). However, these analyses are more relevant to individuals of European ancestry and power of ROC analysis drops badly for African and other populations, i.e., a clear indicator that these loci identified mainly through genetic studies in Europeans do not predict diabetes in non-European populations. This has led to the speculation that the clinical utility of current genetic findings will have large disparities as it is mainly derived from studying individuals of European ancestry.[20]

PRECISION MEDICINE

The use of multidimensional data to gain precision in prediction, treatment, and diagnosis is often referred to as precision medicine. Though genomics data has mainly been highlighted to play an important role in precision medicine, other sources of omics data and data from wearable devices and medical data from large records have also played an important role in designing strategies for precision medicine. A relatively new entry to this multiomics data is genetic variants affecting protein expression data or protein quantitative trait loci (pQTL) and has been recently used to better inform the disease biology of diabetes.[39] Precision medicine is already a reality in the field of diabetes as genomics data is being used for precise diagnosis and treatment of many monogenic forms of diabetes.[40] Classification of monogenic forms of neonatal diabetes based on genetics can identify sets of individuals who will respond to oral sulfonylureas that often leads to good glucose management. While there are some forms of neonatal diabetes [maturity-onset diabetes of the young type 2 (MODY2)] that will not respond to this therapy and focus should shift other forms of glucose management. However, the same has not been possible for T1DM and T2DM and needs further discoveries in the field of diabetes and related conditions.

ROAD AHEAD

We have had tremendous success in the discovery of loci associated with diabetes and currently this has become a function of number, ethnicity, and genotyping technologies. Saturation has reached in terms of identifying genetic loci with high effect sizes. We still are not sure about the genes through which these genetic variants act and much further from identifying how the identified gene causes or protects us from diabetes. This is a big opportunity for functional studies in various model systems both in vitro and in vivo. Transferability of this genetic knowledge to different ethnicities of the world should be one of the major goals as it has been in other fields of medicine. So far, approximately 2% of the subjects studied are non-European and this must shift somewhere near to the middle line to prevent disparity. The use of these large genetic discoveries will remain limited if more ways to use this in informing the drug discovery process and design of intervention strategies is not found.

CONCLUSION

Twenty years may appear a long time, but it is a much shorter period in the history of disease treatments, and we have seen a tremendous leap in our understanding of the genetic basis of diabetes, thanks to the Human Genome Project. Within this time period we have witnessed the discovery of the first gene for common form of diabetes to large-scale multi-nation studies that have identified hundreds of genetic loci including both common and rare variants. We have witnessed studies involving single gene to whole genomes of thousands of individuals. Today we are convinced that diabetes is a multifactorial disease not just based on environmental exposure but also based on genetic basis as genetic determinants of diabetes are shared across many other metabolic conditions and neurological conditions. This has re-emphasized our previous believes that treating root cause of diabetes could prevent many other diseases. This change in scenario for diabetes; "no gene to hundreds of genes", "common to common and rare", "single gene to whole genome studies", "hundreds of individuals to hundred thousands of individuals" has been made possible in these twenty years greatly due to the Human Genome Project. As we enter the era of precision medicine if we can fill the gap of ethnic inclusion and genetic discovery to functional studies, we will move much closer towards treatment of diabetes and realizing the ultimate goal set by the Human Genome Project.

REFERENCES

1. Lander ES, Linton LM, Birren B, Nusbaum C, Zody MC, Baldwin J, et al. Initial sequencing and analysis of the human genome. Nature. 2001;409(6822):860-921.
2. Venter JC, Adams MD, Myers EW, Li PW, Mural RJ, Sutton GG, et al. The sequence of the human genome. Science. 2001;291(5507):1304-51.
3. The International HapMap Consortium. A haplotype map of the human genome. Nature. 2005;437(7063):1299-320.
4. Human genome: Genomes by the thousand. Nature. 2010;467(7319):1026-7.
5. Gloyn AL, Weedon MN, Owen KR, Turner MJ, Knight BA, Hitman G, et al. Large-scale association studies of variants in genes encoding the pancreatic beta-cell KATP channel subunits Kir6.2 (KCNJ11) and SUR1 (ABCC8) confirm that the KCNJ11 E23K variant is associated with type 2 diabetes. Diabetes. 2003;52(2):568-72.
6. Altshuler D, Hirschhorn JN, Klannemark M, Lindgren CM, Vohl MC, Nemesh J, et al. The common PPARgamma Pro12Ala polymorphism is associated with decreased risk of type 2 diabetes. Nat Genet. 2000;26(1):76-80.
7. Grant SF, Thorleifsson G, Reynisdottir I, Benediktsson R, Manolescu A, Sainz J, et al. Variant of transcription factor 7-like 2 (TCF7L2) gene confers risk of type 2 diabetes. Nat Genet. 2006;38(3): 320-3.
8. Chauhan G, Spurgeon CJ, Tabassum R, Bhaskar S, Kulkarni SR, Mahajan A, et al. Impact of common variants of PPARG, KCNJ11, TCF7L2, SLC30A8, HHEX, CDKN2A, IGF2BP2, and CDKAL1 on the risk of type 2 diabetes in 5,164 Indians. Diabetes. 2010;59(8):2068-74.
9. Omori S, Tanaka Y, Takahashi A, Hirose H, Kashiwagi A, Kaku K, et al. Association of CDKAL1, IGF2BP2, CDKN2A/B, HHEX, SLC30A8, and KCNJ11 with susceptibility to type 2 diabetes in a Japanese population. Diabetes. 2008;57(3):791-5.
10. Chauhan G, Tabassum R, Mahajan A, Dwivedi OP, Mahendran Y, Kaur I, et al. Common variants of FTO and the risk of obesity and type 2 diabetes in Indians. J Hum Genet. 2011;56(10):720-6.
11. Dwivedi OP, Tabassum R, Chauhan G, Ghosh S, Marwaha RK, Tandon N, et al. Common variants of FTO are associated with childhood obesity in a cross-sectional study of 3,126 urban Indian children. PLoS One. 2012;7(10):e47772.
12. Chavali S, Mahajan A, Tabassum R, Dwivedi OP, Chauhan G, Ghosh S, et al. Association of variants in genes involved in pancreatic β-cell development and function with type 2 diabetes in North Indians. J Hum Genet. 2011;56(10):695-700.
13. Unoki H, Takahashi A, Kawaguchi T, Hara K, Horikoshi M, Andersen G, et al. SNPs in KCNQ1 are associated with susceptibility to type 2 diabetes in East Asian and European populations. Nat Genet. 2008;40(9):1098-102.
14. Yasuda K, Miyake K, Horikawa Y, Hara K, Osawa H, Furuta H, et al. Variants in KCNQ1 are associated with susceptibility to type 2 diabetes mellitus. Nat Genet. 2008;40(9):1092-7.
15. Tabassum R, Chauhan G, Dwivedi OP, Mahajan A, Jaiswal A, Kaur I, et al. Genome-wide association study for type 2 diabetes in Indians identifies a new susceptibility locus at 2q21. Diabetes. 2013;62(3): 977-86.
16. Chakraborty S, Vellarikkal SK, Sivasubbu S, Roy SS, Tandon N, Bharadwaj D. Role of Tmem163 in zinc-regulated insulin storage of MIN6 cells: Functional exploration of an Indian type 2 diabetes GWAS associated gene. Biochem Biophys Res Commun. 2020;522(4):1022-9.
17. Chen J, Sun M, Adeyemo A, Pirie F, Carstensen T, Pomilla C, et al. Genome-wide association study of type 2 diabetes in Africa. Diabetologia. 2019;62(7):1204-11.
18. Doumatey AP, Ekoru K, Adeyemo A, Rotimi CN. Genetic Basis of Obesity and Type 2 Diabetes in Africans: Impact on Precision Medicine. Curr Diab Rep. 2019;19(10):105.
19. Horikoshi M, Pasquali L, Wiltshire S, Huyghe JR, Mahajan A, Asimit JL, et al. Transancestral fine-mapping of four type 2 diabetes susceptibility loci highlights potential causal regulatory mechanisms. Hum Mol Genet. 2016;25(10):2070-81.
20. Martin AR, Kanai M, Kamatani Y, Okada Y, Neale BM, Daly MJ. Clinical use of current polygenic risk scores may exacerbate health disparities. Nat Genet. 2019;51(4):584-91.

21. Fuchsberger C, Flannick J, Teslovich TM, Mahajan A, Agarwala V, Gaulton KJ, et al. The genetic architecture of type 2 diabetes. Nature. 2016;536(7614):41-7.
22. Flannick J, Mercader JM, Fuchsberger C, Udler MS, Mahajan A, Wessel J, et al. Exome sequencing of 20,791 cases of type 2 diabetes and 24,440 controls. Nature. 2019;570(7759):71-6.
23. Sharma A, Chavali S, Mahajan A, Tabassum R, Banerjee V, Tandon N, et al. Genetic association, post-translational modification, and protein-protein interactions in Type 2 diabetes mellitus. Mol Cell Proteomics. 2005;4(8):1029-37.
24. Dunham I, Kundaje A, Aldred SF, Collins PJ, Davis CA, Doyle F, et al. An integrated encyclopedia of DNA elements in the human genome. Nature. 2012;489(7414):57-74.
25. Lonsdale J, Thomas J, Salvatore M, Phillips R, Lo E, Shad S, et al. The Genotype-Tissue Expression (GTEx) project. Nat Genet. 2013;45(6):580-5.
26. Sladek R, Rocheleau G, Rung J, Dina C, Shen L, Serre D, et al. A genome-wide association study identifies novel risk loci for type 2 diabetes. Nature. 2007;445(7130):881-5.
27. Scott LJ, Mohlke KL, Bonnycastle LL, Willer CJ, Li Y, Duren WL, et al. A genome-wide association study of type 2 diabetes in Finns detects multiple susceptibility variants. Science. 2007;316(5829):1341-5.
28. Zeggini F, Weedon MN, Lindgren CM, Frayling TM, Elliott KS, Lango H, et al. Replication of genome-wide association signals in UK samples reveals risk loci for type 2 diabetes. Science. 2007;316(5829):1336-41.
29. Dwivedi OP, Lehtovirta M, Hastoy B, Chandra V, Krentz NAJ, Kleiner S, et al. Loss of ZnT8 function protects against diabetes by enhanced insulin secretion. Nat Genet. 2019;51(11):1596-606.
30. Flannick J, Thorleifsson G, Beer NL, Jacobs SBR, Grarup N, Burtt NP, et al. Loss-of-function mutations in SLC30A8 protect against type 2 diabetes. Nat Genet. 2014;46(4):357-63.
31. Mamakou V, Thanopoulou A, Gonidakis F, Tentolouris N, Kontaxakis V. Schizophrenia and type 2 diabetes mellitus. Psychiatriki. 2018;29(1):64-73.
32. Hao K, Di Narzo AF, Ho L, Luo W, Li S, Chen R, et al. Shared genetic etiology underlying Alzheimer's disease and type 2 diabetes. Mol Aspects Med. 2015;43-44:66-76.
33. Paul KC, Jerrett M, Ritz B. Type 2 Diabetes Mellitus and Alzheimer's Disease: Overlapping Biologic Mechanisms and Environmental Risk Factors. Curr Environ Health Rep. 2018;5(1):44-58.
34. Bulik-Sullivan BK, Loh PR, Finucane HK, Ripke S, Yang J, Schizophrenia Working Group of the Psychiatric Genomics C, et al. LD Score regression distinguishes confounding from polygenicity in genome-wide association studies. Nat Genet. 2015;47(3):291-5.
35. Bulik-Sullivan B, Finucane HK, Anttila V, Gusev A, Day FR, Loh PR, et al. An atlas of genetic correlations across human diseases and traits. Nat Genet. 2015;47(11):1236-41.
36. Bendlin BB. Antidiabetic therapies and Alzheimer disease. Dialogues Clin Neurosci. 2019;21(1):83-91.
37. Boccardi V, Murasecco L, Mecocci P. Diabetes drugs in the fight against Alzheimer's disease. Ageing Res Rev. 2019;54:100936.
38. Khera AV, Chaffin M, Aragam KG, Haas ME, Roselli C, Choi SH, et al. Genome-wide polygenic scores for common diseases identify individuals with risk equivalent to monogenic mutations. Nat Genet. 2018;50(9):1219-24
39. Bandesh K, Bharadwaj D. Genetic variants entail type 2 diabetes as an innate immune disorder. Biochim Biophys Acta Proteins Proteomics. 2020;1868(9):140458.
40. Chung WK, Erion K, Florez JC, Hattersley AT, Hivert MF, Lee CG, et al. Precision Medicine in Diabetes: A Consensus Report from the American Diabetes Association (ADA) and the European Association for the Study of Diabetes (EASD). Diabetes Care. 2020;43(7):1617-35.
41. Mahajan A, Taliun D, Thurner M, Robertson NR, Torres JM, Rayner NW, et al. Fine-mapping type 2 diabetes loci to single-variant resolution using high-density imputation and islet-specific epigenome maps. Nat Genet. 2018;50(11):1505-13.

CHAPTER 5

Cerebrovascular Disease in Diabetes

Venkateswarlu Kolichana, Mythili Ayyagari

ABSTRACT

Diabetes is an established risk factor for ischemic stroke, in particular, lacunar stroke. Patients with diabetes who develop a stroke tend to fare worse than those without diabetes despite established therapy with thrombolysis, although rapid control of hyperglycemia seems to improve outcomes. Achieving optimum glycated hemoglobin (HbA1c) is an important and achievable goal of primary and secondary prevention of stroke. Control of coexisting hypertension and dyslipidemia are critical in preventing cerebrovascular disease.

Keywords: *Ischemic stroke, Hypertension, Dyslipidemia, Antiplatelets, Statins, Prevention.*

INTRODUCTION

Stroke affects nearly 15 million people globally, of whom 30% die; another 30% have residual disability with its attendant costs to the family and society.[1] India is home to both communicable and noncommunicable diseases among which stroke is a leading cause of disability and death.

EPIDEMIOLOGY OF STROKE

The estimated adjusted prevalence rate of stroke in India, according to the India stroke factsheet updated in 2012, ranges from 84 to 262/100,000 in rural and 334 to 424/100,000 in urban areas.[2] The incidence rate is 119–145/100,000 based on recent population studies. Variability of case fatality rates is due to differences in the center where study was conducted and whether data was hospital or community based.

In middle- and low-income countries, hypertension contributes to 54% of stroke, hypercholesterolemia to 15%, and tobacco smoking to 12%. In the Trivandrum Stroke Registry which is a part of four population-based stroke epidemiology studies conducted according to the "WHO-STEPS stroke protocol" during the first decade of 21st century (Mumbai, Kolkata, and Bangalore being other centers), nearly 85% had hypertension, 50% had diabetes mellitus (DM), 26% had dyslipidemia, and 26.8% of men smoked tobacco.[3]

PATHOPHYSIOLOGY OF ISCHEMIC STROKE

Diabetes contributes to increased risk of stroke in many ways by accelerating atherosclerosis in large- and medium-sized arteries. Carotid intima-media thickness (CIMT), a marker of early atherosclerosis, can be reliably measured by Doppler study. Increased CIMT is a risk factor for both first as well as recurrent stroke. CIMT is increased in diabetes and with each increase of CIMT by 0.1 mm risk of stroke is increased by 18%.

Nitric oxide (NO) in endothelium of cerebral blood vessels is a potent vasodilator; when released in ischemic conditions, it prevents platelet aggregation and protects tissue injury. In diabetics with accelerated atherosclerosis, the response of the endothelium to NO is blunted where less NO is produced along with alteration in its metabolism. All these lead to vasoconstriction, impairing the ability of brain tissue to tolerate hypoxia. The beneficial effects of statins in reducing the incidence of stroke go beyond cholesterol lowering. They increase the expression of endothelial NO synthase and also decrease the activity of Rho kinase, a proconstrictor enzyme.

In addition, diabetes is associated with increased levels of thrombin (promoted by associated platelet hyperreactivity), prothrombin fragments, and thrombin-antithrombin III complexes which make the blood hypercoagulable. All these increase the risk of thrombo-occlusive complications. Lacunar stroke, more common in diabetes, results from microatheroma in small penetrating arteries.

DIABETES AND HEMORRHAGIC STROKE

While evidence for diabetes being a strong risk factor for ischemic stroke is compelling, epidemiological studies, though sparse, suggest a negative association between diabetes and intracerebral hemorrhage (ICH). In the Honolulu Heart Program data, risk of ICH is not significantly increased in diabetes. There seems to be no association with blood glucose levels at admission and mortality in ICH. In the University of Iowa-Cooperative Aneurysm study, there was a negative correlation between diabetes and subarachnoid hemorrhage.

HYPOGLYCEMIA AND STROKE

Blood glucose level <50 mg/dL is a contraindication for thrombolytic therapy. Hypoglycemia is an uncommon observation in acute stroke; when seen, it is often due to the use of antidiabetic medications. Therefore, it is important to estimate blood glucose at admission in all patients with acute stroke that cannot be overemphasized. Hypoglycemia itself can present as stroke mimic and is an exception to the rule that metabolic encephalopathies do not have lateralizing signs. Blood glucose levels <60 mg/dL in the setting of acute ischemic stroke should be immediately corrected.[4] Prolonged hypoglycemia must be corrected with intravenous (IV) 25% glucose to prevent irreversible brain damage. Though most often autonomic symptoms such as sweating, trembling, and anxiety precede central nervous system (CNS) symptoms, in patients with long-standing poorly controlled diabetes, CNS symptoms may be inaugural. Unless recognized and corrected, critical time is lost while the patient is being shifted for imaging studies.

HYPERGLYCEMIA AND STROKE

Hyperglycemia with blood glucose levels >400 mg/dL is a relative contraindication for thrombolytic therapy for reasons discussed below. High blood glucose can itself cause focal neurological deficits mimicking stroke which is another reason why plasma glucose >400 mg/dL was an exclusion criterion in the NINDS (National Institute of Neurological Disorders and Stroke) trial.[5] It may be reasonable to bring down the blood glucose levels with insulin and give thrombolytic therapy if deficits do not resolve.

Hyperglycemia has an adverse effect on the outcome of acute ischemic stroke, often seen in >40% of patients with acute ischemic stroke in emergency rooms.[3] The adverse outcomes of hyperglycemia at admission extend to nondiabetic individuals also.

Compared to those who are euglycemic at admission, those with hyperglycemia are likely to have larger infarcts, higher rates of symptomatic ICH, lesser chances of recanalization of occluded vessel, and poorer functional grades on recovery.[6] The likelihood of intracranial hemorrhage seems to be related to blood glucose: Higher the level, greater the risk of hemorrhage. Unlike persistent hyperglycemia due to diabetes, transient hyperglycemia as a stress response to acute stroke is not associated with comparable poorer outcomes.

The GIST-UK (United Kingdom Glucose Insulin in Stroke Trial) conducted to show the beneficial effects of insulin to treat hyperglycemia failed to demonstrate positive outcomes probably because of methodological flaws.[7] Pending further clinical trials, it seems prudent to maintain the blood glucose levels between 140 and 180 mg/dL with insulin avoiding hypoglycemia.[8]

TREATMENT OF ACUTE ISCHEMIC STROKE

Brain is vulnerable to ischemia. While the normal brain tissue receives a blood flow of 50 mL/min/100 g of the brain tissue, it can tolerate a reduction of up to 20 mL/100 g without adverse effects. When the blood flow falls under 20 mL/100 g, signs of ischemia begin to appear followed by irreversible damage when the flow drops to <10 mL/100 g/min. Restoration of blood supply to ischemic tissue within a specified window period will salvage the tissue in the penumbra, but not in the fully damaged area.

Intravenous thrombolysis using recombinant tissue plasminogen activator (rtPA), given in the window period of 3 hours, is highly effective and safe therapy for acute ischemic stroke as shown in the NINDS trial.[5] Subsequent, the ECASS III (European Cooperative Acute Stroke Study III) trial confirmed that benefits can be extended up to 4.5 hours with IV therapy.[9] Intra-arterial thrombolysis with urokinase injected into angiographically proven occluded vessel can be done with good outcomes till 6 hours. For every 100 patients treated with IV thrombolysis, 11 more patients are likely to achieve modified Rankin Scale of 0–1 compared to the group treated with placebo. Though the treated group had increased risk of symptomatic ICH (6.4% vs. 0.6% with placebo), mortality rates were not significantly different at 3 months between two groups.[10] The PROACT II (Prolyse in Acute Cerebral Thromboembolism II) trial, which studied the efficacy of intra-arterial therapy within 6-hour window period, showed that with comparable mortality, high recanalization of the occluded vessel was achieved with minimal or no functional disability at 3 months.[11]

But outcomes in patients with diabetes do not match with nondiabetes controls. When recanalization was monitored by transcranial Doppler, none of the 27 patients with diabetes who received thrombolytic therapy achieved recanalization.[12] In another study, presence of diabetes had a negative outcome with IV thrombolysis.[13]

Degree of lowering blood pressure (BP) in acute ischemic stroke remains controversial. Most stroke neurologists believe that systolic blood pressure (SBP) up to 220 mm Hg and diastolic BP up to 120 mm Hg need not be treated in the absence of hypertensive emergency such as dissection or acute left ventricular failure.[4] BP readings higher than mentioned should be treated with either parenteral labetalol, enalapril, and nicardipine with reductions not >15% over 24 hours. The incidence of intracranial hemorrhage after thrombolytic therapy steeply increases with BP >185/100 mm Hg. BP should be lowered with IV labetalol before administering IV rtPA. Fever should be treated aggressively as for every degree rise of temperature mortality doubles.[14] Source of infection should be sought and treated. Attention should be paid to swallowing to prevent aspiration. Feeding via Ryle's tube or percutaneous endoscopic gastrostomy should be planned in case of dysphagia. Dehydration should be corrected while avoiding parenteral fluid overload. Precautions to prevent deep venous thrombosis such as subcutaneous unfractionated heparin or low-molecular-weight heparin should be initiated.

Diabetes predisposes to complications in the immediate poststroke period such as pneumonia and urinary tract infection which may adversely affect good recovery. Persistent hyperglycemia impairs neuronal plasticity leading to poor outcomes.

The prognosis of stroke improves when managed in a stroke unit where comprehensive care can be provided under a dedicated and trained team comprising of neurologist, nurses, physical therapist, occupational therapist, and speech and swallowing specialists.[15]

PREVENTION

Primary Prevention

Glycemic Control

Persons with DM are not only predisposed to atherosclerosis, but also have other proatherogenic factors such as hypertension and dyslipidemia. That diabetes is an independent risk factor for ischemic stroke is proven in both case controlled and epidemiological studies. The relative risk is increased by 1.8—nearly 6-fold. In the Northern Manhattan Study (NOMAS), of the 3,298 community residents without previous history of stroke, 572 had a diagnosis of diabetes and 338 had elevated fasting blood glucose. Those with elevated fasting glucose levels had an increased stroke risk [hazard ratio (HR) 2.7; 95% confidence interval (CI) 2.0–3.8], but not those with a fasting blood glucose level <126 mg/dL.[16]

In Greater Cincinnati/Northern Kentucky Stroke Study, ischemic stroke patients with diabetes tended to be younger, more often have hypertension, coronary artery disease, and dyslipidemia and more likely to be black compared to those without diabetes.[17] The risk is particularly increased ten times in individuals younger than 55 years, although no age group is exempt.

Among the three commonly occurring subtypes of stroke: (1) Large vessel disease; (2) Cardioembolic; and (3) Lacunar strokes, diabetes significantly increases the risk of lacunar stroke.[18]

There are few studies addressing the causal relationship between type 1 diabetes mellitus (T1DM) and stroke. A 10% incidence of stroke and 7% mortality from stroke are reported in a 40-year follow-up study.[19] Similar to type 2 diabetes mellitus (T2DM), intensive treatment of blood glucose does not seem to reduce the risk of stroke.

The United Kingdom Prospective Diabetes Study (UKPDS) identified atrial fibrillation (AF) as a strong risk for cardioembolic stroke in diabetes. Compared to patients in sinus rhythm, those who have both diabetes and AF were eight times are more likely to develop stroke. Their risk has to be categorized as per CHADS2 score and individuals at high risk (score of 2 or more) should be given anticoagulant to maintain international normalized ratio between 2.0 and 3.0. Lower risk category patients may be treated either with aspirin or warfarin.[4]

While majority of the studies failed to demonstrate benefits of intensive lowering of blood glucose in reducing the risk of stroke, some trials showed that risk can be reduced by optimum glycated hemoglobin (HbA1c) levels. In STENO-2 study, 160 patients with T2DM with persistent albuminuria were assigned to either intensive therapy or conventional therapy. The intensive group received antiplatelet, statin, angiotensin-converting enzyme (ACE) inhibitor, and angiotensin receptor blocker (ARB) apart from behavioral risk modification. The mean treatment period was 7.8 years and mean follow-up for an average was 5.5 years. The primary endpoint was time to death from any cause. Apart from reduction in the risk of cardiovascular events by 60% in the intensive treatment group, number of strokes was 6 compared to 30 in conventionally treated group.[20]

Hypertension

While the benefits of lowering blood glucose in reducing the risk of stroke are not convincing, more definite evidence exists that effective management of associated hypertension and dyslipidemia reduces the risk of stroke. In the UKPDS, tight BP control (BP achieved in the study 144/82 mm Hg) in addition to intensive glycemic control resulted in 44% reduction in risk of stroke compared to a group which received less aggressive treatment (BP achieved 154/87 mm Hg).[21] The HOPE (Heart Outcomes Prevention Evaluation) study which evaluated a subgroup of high-risk patients with diabetes with a previous cardiovascular event or an additional risk factor showed a 33% reduction in stroke in the group which received an ACE inhibitor in addition to current medical regimen.[22]

Various studies using thiazide diuretics, ACE inhibitors, ARBs, beta-blockers, and calcium channel blockers have shown benefits on both microvascular and macrovascular endpoints, suggesting that absolute reduction in BP is more important rather than the antihypertensive agent used. However, several recent trials suggest that ACE inhibitors and ARBs extend benefits that cannot be solely explained on the basis of BP reduction alone in preventing and the progression of advanced diabetic kidney disease. Regardless of the initial therapy, majority of people with diabetes will require more than one drug for effective control of hypertension to reach the desired target levels of SBP <130 mm Hg and diastolic BP <80 mm Hg.

The ACCORD (Action to Control Cardiovascular Risk in Diabetes) trial indicates that lowering SBP <140 mm Hg does not offer extra advantage in preventing major adverse cardiovascular events.[23] The American Diabetes Association (ADA) recommends that lower goals for BP control may be adopted for certain specific categories like young individuals who can tolerate without inconvenience of side effects.[24]

Lipids

Compared to those without diabetes, patients with T2DM have a significantly increased risk of atherosclerotic cardiovascular disease (CVD) including stroke. While controlling blood glucose is beneficial in preventing microvascular complications, intensive management of dyslipidemia is essential for reducing the risk of macrovascular disease.

The Medical Research Council/British Heart Foundation Heart Protection Study (HPS), involving 5,963 diabetic individuals, found that addition of a statin to the existing best medical care led to a 22% reduction in major vascular events and 24% reduction in strokes.[25] The CARDS (Collaborative Atorvastatin Diabetes Study) showed that in patients with T2DM who have an additional risk factor (retinopathy, albuminuria, smoking, or hypertension) and low-density lipoprotein cholesterol (LDL-C) level of <160 mg/dL, addition of a statin resulted in 48% reduction in stroke.[26] The TNT (Treating to New Targets) study compared effects of intensive lowering of LDL-C with high dose (80 mg) versus low dose (10 mg) atorvastatin in group of patients with coronary artery disease and diabetes with a follow-up of 4.9 years.[27] High-dose treatment was associated with 40% reduction in cerebrovascular events. In a meta-analysis involving 1,466 patients with T1DM and 17,220 with T2DM, administration of statin with a target of lowering LDL-C by 40 mg/dL approximately resulted in significant reductions in myocardial infarction (MI) and coronary deaths including strokes.[28] In the VA-HIT (Veterans Affairs High-Density Lipoprotein Intervention Trial), use of gemfibrozil (1,200 mg/day) compared to placebo led to a 40% reduction in stroke in subjects with diabetes.[29] However, the FIELD (Fenofibrate Intervention and Event Lowering in Diabetes) study which assessed the effect of fenofibrate on cardiovascular events in patients with T2DM did not find any benefit in reducing the risk of stroke.[30]

Secondary Prevention

All the three principal disorders of glucose metabolism namely, T1DM, pre-DM, and T2DM, seem to increase the risk of first as well as recurrent stroke.

In population studies, DM seems to account for 8% of all first ischemic strokes. About 60–70% of patients with established stroke may have dysglycemia.[31] In a study which included patients with a past history of ischemic stroke (Cardiovascular Health Study), DM was associated with 60% increased risk of recurrent stroke. Insulin resistance as a part of metabolic syndrome doubles the risk of ischemic stroke even without overt DM.

Two stroke cohort studies showed that diabetes is predictor of presence of multiple lacunar strokes.

Glycemic Control

Three randomized clinical trials of intensive glucose management in persons with DM with history of CVD, stroke, or additional vascular risk factors failed to demonstrate any reduction in cardiovascular events or death in the groups receiving intensive insulin therapy. In the ACCORD trial, 10,251 patients with T2DM and vascular disease or multiple risk factors were randomly assigned to intensive insulin regimen with a target HbA1c <6 or less rigorous control with HbA1c between 7 and 7.9.[31] The trial was stopped midway because of increased death in group with intensive regimen. Both groups did not differ in rate of nonfatal stroke or primary endpoint which was a composite of nonfatal stroke or nonfatal heart attack and death due to CVD. In the ADVANCE (Action in Diabetes and Vascular Disease: Preterax and Diamicron Modified Release Controlled Evaluation) trial, 11,140 patients with T2DM and history of macrovascular disease or another vascular risk factors were randomly assigned to either intensive insulin regimen (target HbA1c <6.5%) or standard therapy (target HbA1c <7%).[32] There was no significant difference in occurrence of macrovascular events or nonfatal stroke in either arm.

In the Veterans Affairs Diabetes trial, 1,791 patients with T2DM were randomly assigned to either intensive insulin regimen or standard therapy.[32] The primary outcome was time to occurrence of major cardiovascular event or in rate of death due to any cause. There was no significant difference in outcome between the two groups.

Results of all these trials suggest that in T2DM, there is no evidence that lowering blood glucose levels is associated with better outcomes in reducing the short-term risk of macrovascular disease including stroke. The ADA recommended target HbA1c level of <7.0% to prevent long-term microvascular complications in diabetes. These trials indicate that in patients with presence of vascular risk factors and prior history of CVD, glycemic targets should not be lowered to <6.5%. The ADA, however, states that intensive therapy with target HbA1c level of <6.5% may be recommended for younger individuals in those with short duration diabetes and long life expectancy to decrease the risk of macrovascular complications.[24]

Lipids

The SPARCL (Stroke Prevention by Aggressive Reduction in Cholesterol Levels) study enrolled 4,731 individuals with history of transient ischemic attack (TIA) or stroke without coronary heart disease (CHD), whose LDL C levels were between 100 and 190 mg/dL. They were assigned to either 80 mg of atorvastatin or placebo and followed for 4.9 years.[33] There was a significant reduction in fatal and nonfatal stroke in atorvastatin group. In spite of the exclusion of patients with CHD, number of CHD events prevented exceeded the number of strokes. Unlike some earlier studies which showed increase in number of hemorrhagic strokes, this study showed that these benefits accrued without such adverse event.

In patients who already experienced a TIA or ischemic stroke with or without a history of coronary artery disease, intense lowering of LDL-C by a combination of lifestyle modification, and dietary guidelines, addition of a high-dose statin (atorvastatin 40–80 mg/day or rosuvastatin 20–40 mg/day) to target a reduction of at least 50% in LDL-C or a target LDL-C level of <70 mg/dL gave maximum benefit. Combination therapy of statins and fibrates has not been shown to be superior and is not recommended. However, therapy with statin and fenofibrate may be considered for men with both triglycerides level >204 mg/dL and HDL-C <34 mg/dL.[24] Combination therapy with niacin and statin does not provide additional benefit over statin therapy alone and is not recommended as it may increase the risk of stroke.

It is interesting to consider whether any particular class of oral antidiabetic agents has advantage over others in reducing the incidence of stroke in DM. Preliminary evidence suggests that metformin, pioglitazone, and linagliptin offer some advantage.

In the IRIS (Insulin Resistance Intervention After Stroke) trial, 3,876 patients without diabetes who had insulin resistance along with a recent history of ischemic stroke or TIA were randomly assigned to either pioglitazone or placebo.[34] The primary outcome was fatal or nonfatal stroke or MI. The risk of stroke or MI was lower among patients who received pioglitazone compared to controls. Pioglitazone was also associated with a lower risk of diabetes, but with higher risks of weight gain, edema, and fracture.

Though it is premature to recommend any particular antidiabetic agent for primary or secondary prevention of vascular events, therapy must be tailored to suit individual characteristics of the patient. These may include target HbA1c levels, risk of side effects, cost, and other nonglycemic benefits.

ANTIPLATELETS IN STROKE

The beneficial role of antiplatelet agents in primary prevention of stroke in diabetes has not been convincing.[21] The benefits do not seem to override the risk of bleeding complications in subjects with low risk for cardiovascular events. However, it may be considered in those with high CVD risk, particularly women whose 10-year risk of cardiovascular events is >10%.[24]

The role of aspirin in the immediate treatment of acute ischemic stroke was extensively investigated.[35] The benefits of administering aspirin within 24–48 hours of stroke are modest, more likely due to prevention of recurrent events rather than halting the progression of the primary event. The role of other antiplatelets like clopidogrel and IV agents like glycoprotein IIb/IIIa receptor inhibitors has not been established. Aspirin should not be used as substitute for patients who fulfill the eligibility criterion for IV thrombolysis.

The beneficial effects of antiplatelets in the prevention of recurrent stroke who already had a prior stroke or TIA is convincing.[36] All interventions including aspirin (50–325 mg/day), clopidogrel (75 mg/day), combination of low-dose aspirin (25 mg/day), and extended-release dipyridamole

(200 mg/day) twice daily seem to be effective. The choice has to be individualized on the basis of risk factors, cost, tolerance, etc. Clopidogrel is an effective alternative for aspirin intolerant patients. Combination of aspirin and clopidogrel does not seem to offer extra benefit while increasing the risk of bleeding. The presence of intracranial stenosis may be special case for dual antiplatelet therapy because of high incidence of stroke. The guidelines are not clear on what should be the alternative when stroke or TIA occurs in a patient who is already on aspirin. More stringent control of risk factors is warranted. A Chinese study reported that in Asian population, dual antiplatelet therapy with aspirin and clopidogrel for 30 days followed by aspirin alone is more effective in preventing recurrent stroke than aspirin monotherapy.[37]

CONCLUSION

Diabetes mellitus is an important risk factor for ischemic stroke. Control of hyperglycemia improves outcomes of acute stroke therapy. While adequate treatment of diabetes reduces long-term, microvascular complications related to diabetes, attending to concomitant hypertension and dyslipidemia seem to benefit macrovascular disease. Antiplatelets, antihypertensives, and statins, optimally used to achieve desired goals of BP and LDL-C, can reduce the incidence of stroke and its related morbidity. In summary, although diabetes is recognized as a risk factor for stroke, preventing cerebrovascular disease depends more on correcting other risk factors associated with diabetes (viz., hypertension, cessation of smoking, physical exercise) rather than mere control of glycemia.[38]

REFERENCES

1. Pandian JD, Srikanth V, Read SJ, Thrift AG. Poverty and stroke in India. A time to act. Stroke. 2007;38:3063-9.
2. Sridharan SE, Unnikrishnan JP, Sukumaran S, Sylaja PN, Nayak SD, Sarma PS, et al. Incidence, types, risk factors, and outcome of stroke in a developing country: The Trivandrum Stroke Registry. Stroke. 2009;40:1212-8.
3. Gentile NT, Seftchick MW, Huynh T, Kruus LK, Gaughan J. Decreased mortality by normalizing blood glucose after acute ischemic stroke. Acad Emerg Med. 2006;13:174-80.
4. Jauch EC, Saver JL, Adams HP, Bruno A, Connors JJ, Demaerschalk BM, et al. Guidelines for the early management of patients with acute ischemic stroke: a guideline for healthcare professionals from the American Heart Association/American Stroke Association. Stroke. 2013;44:870-947.
5. National Institute of Neurological disorders and Stroke rt-PA Stroke Study Group. Tissue plasminogen activator for acute stroke. N Engl J Med. 1995;333:1317-29.
6. Bruno A, Levine SR, Frankel MR, Brott TG, Lin Y, Tilley BC, et al. Admission glucose level and clinical outcomes in the NINDS rt-PA Stroke Trial. Neurology. 2002;59:669-74.
7. Gray CS, Hildreth AJ, Sandercock PA, O'Connell JE, Johnston DE, Cartlidge NE, et al. Glucose-potassium-insulin infusions in the management of post-stroke hyperglycaemia: the UK Glucose Insulin in Stroke Trial (GIST-UK). Lancet Neurol. 2007;6:397-406.
8. American Diabetes Association. Standards of Medical Care in Diabetes—2010. Diabetes Care. 2010;33: S11-61.

9. Hacke W, Donnan G, Fieschi C, Kaste M, von Kummer R, Broderick JP, et al. Association of outcome with early stroke treatment: pooled analysis of ATLANTIS, ECASS, and NINDS rt-PA stroke trials. Lancet. 2004;363:768-74.
10. The National Institute of Neurological Disorders and Stroke rt-PA Stroke Study Group. Tissue plasminogen activator for acute ischemic stroke. N Engl J Med. 1995;333:1581-7.
11. Furlan A, Higashida R, Wechsler L, Gent M, Rowley H, Kase C, et al. Intra-arterial prourokinase for acute ischemic stroke: the PROACT II study: a thromboembolism. JAMA. 1999;282:2003-11.
12. Askevold TE, Naess H, Thomassen L. Predictors for recanalisation after intravenous thrombolysis in acute stroke. J Stroke Cerebrovasc Dis. 2007;16:21-4.
13. Leigh R, Zaidat OO, Suri MF, Lynch G, Sundararajan S, Sunshine JL, et al. Predictors of hyperacute clinical worsening in ischemic stroke patients receiving thrombolytic therapy. Stroke. 2004;35;1903-7.
14. Azzimondi G, Bassein L, Nonino F, Fiorani L, Vignatelli L, Re G, et al. Fever in acute stroke worsens prognosis. A prospective study. Stroke. 1995;26:2040-3.
15. Rudd AG, Hoffman A, Irwin P, Lowe D, Pearson MG. Stroke unit care and outcome: results from the 2001 National Sentinel Audit of Stroke (England, Wales, and Northern Ireland). Stroke. 2005;36: 103-6.
16. Boden-Albala B, Cammack S, Chong J, Wang C, Wright C, Rundek T, et al. Diabetes, fasting glucose levels, and risk of ischemic stroke and vascular events: findings from the Northern Manhattan Study (NOMAS). Diabetes Care. 2008;31:1132-7.
17. Kissela BM, Khoury J, Kleindorfer D, Woo D, Schneider A, Alwell K, et al. Epidemiology of ischemic stroke in patients with diabetes: The Greater Cincinnati/Northern Kentucky Stroke Study. Diabetes Care. 2005;28:355-9.
18. Horowitz DR, Tuhrim S, Weinberger JM, Rudolph SH. Mechanisms in lacunar infarction. Stroke. 1992;23:325-7.
19. Tunbridge WMG. Factors contributing to deaths of diabetics under fifty years of age. Lancet. 1981;318:569-72.
20. Gaede P, Lund-Andersen H, Parving HH, Pedersen O. Effect of a multifactorial intervention on mortality in type 2 diabetes. N Engl J Med. 2008;358:580-91.
21. UK Prospective Diabetes Study Group. Tight blood pressure control and risk of macrovascular and microvascular complications in type 2 diabetes: UKPDS 38. UK Prospective Diabetes Study Group. BMJ. 1998;317:703-13.
22. Effects of ramipril on cardiovascular and microvascular outcomes in people with diabetes mellitus: results of the HOPE study and MICRO-HOPE substudy. Heart Outcomes Prevention Evaluation Study Investigators. Lancet. 2000;355:253-9.
23. Barzilay JI, Howard AG, Evans GW, Fleg JL, Cohen RM, Booth GL, et al. Intensive blood pressure treatment does not improve cardiovascular outcomes in centrally obese hypertensive individuals with diabetes: the Action to Control Cardiovascular Risk in Diabetes (ACCORD) Blood Pressure Trial. Diabetes Care. 2012;35:1401-15.
24. American Diabetes Association. Cardiovascular disease and risk management. Sec. 8. In Standards of Medical Care in Diabetes-2016. Diabetes Care. 2016;39:S60-71.
25. Sever PS, Dahlof B, Poulter NR, Wedel H, Beevers G, Caulfield M, et al. Prevention of coronary and stroke events with atorvastatin in hypertensive patients who have average or lower-than-average cholesterol concentrations, in the Anglo-Scandinavian Cardiac Outcomes Trial–Lipid Lowering Arm (ASCOT-LLA): a multicentre randomised controlled trial. Lancet. 2003;361:1149-58.
26. Colhoun HM, Betteridge DJ, Durrington PN, Hitman GA, Neil HA, Livingstone SJ, et al. Primary prevention of cardiovascular disease with atorvastatin in type 2 diabetes in the Collaborative Atorvastatin Diabetes Study (CARDS): multicentre randomised placebo-controlled trial. Lancet. 2004;364:685-96.
27. Shepherd J, Barter P, Carmena R, Deedwania P, Fruchart JC, Haffner S, et al. Effect of lowering LDL cholesterol substantially below currently recommended levels in patients with coronary heart disease and diabetes: the Treating to New Targets (TNT) study. Diabetes Care. 2006;29:1220-6.
28. Cholesterol Treatment Trialists' (CTT) Collaborators, Kearney PM, Blackwell L, Collins R, Keech A, Simes J, et al. Efficacy of cholesterol-lowering therapy in 18,686 people with diabetes in 14 randomised trials of statins: a meta-analysis. Lancet. 2008;371:117-25.

29. Rubins HB, Robins SJ, Collins D, Nelson DB, Elam MB, Schaefer EJ, et al. Diabetes, plasma insulin, and cardiovascular disease: subgroup analysis from the Department of Veterans Affairs High-Density Lipoprotein Intervention Trial (VA-HIT). Arch Intern Med. 2002;162:2597-604.
30. Keech A, Simes RJ, Barter P, Best J, Scott R, Taskinen MR, et al. Effects of long-term fenofibrate therapy on cardiovascular events in 9795 people with type 2 diabetes mellitus (the FIELD study): randomised controlled trial. Lancet. 2005;366:1849-61.
31. Mast H, Thompson JL, Lee SH, Mohr JP, Sacco RL. Hypertension and diabetes mellitus as determinants of multiple lacunar infarcts. Stroke. 1995;26:30-3.
32. Duckworth W, Abraira C, Moritz T, Reda D, Emanuele N, Reaven PD, et al. Glucose control and vascular complications in veterans with type 2 diabetes. N Engl J Med. 2009;360:129-39.
33. Amarenco P, Bogousslavsky J, Callahan AS, Goldstein L, Hennerici M, Sillsen H, et al. Design and baseline characteristics of the stroke prevention by aggressive reduction in cholesterol levels (SPARCL) study. Cerebrovasc Dis. 2003;16:389-95.
34. Kernan WN, Viscoli CM, Furie KL, Young LH, Inzucchi SE, Gorman M, et al. Pioglitazone after ischemic stroke or transient ischemic attack. N Engl J Med. 2016;374:1321-31.
35. Meschia JF, Bushnell C, Boden-Albala B, Braun LT, Bravata DM, Chaturvedi S, et al. Guidelines for the primary prevention of stroke: a statement for healthcare professionals from the American Heart Association/American Stroke Association. Stroke. 2014;45:3754-832.
36. Kernan WN, Ovbiagele B, Black HR, Bravata DM, Chimowitz MI, Ezekowitz MD, et al. Guidelines for the prevention of stroke in patients with stroke and transient ischemic attack: a guideline for healthcare professionals from the American Heart Association/American Stroke Association. Stroke. 2014;45:2160-236.
37. Wang Y, Wang Y, Zhao X, Liu L, Wang D, Wang C, et al. Clopidogrel with aspirin in acute minor stroke or transient ischemic attack. N Engl J Med. 2013;369:11-9.
38. Furie K. Epidemiology and primary prevention of stroke. Continuum (Minneap Minn). 2020;26:260-7.

CHAPTER 6

Peripheral Artery Disease in Diabetes

Chitra Selvan, Prasanna Kumar KM

ABSTRACT

Peripheral artery disease (PAD) is an underdiagnosed condition in patients with diabetes. Presence of PAD increases the likelihood of occurrence of cardiovascular events and also mortality. The risk factors for development of PAD in patients with diabetes are increasing age, duration of diabetes, smoking, dyslipidemia, hypertension, and presence of neuropathy.

All patients with diabetes over 50 years of age need to be screened for PAD. ABI is a noninvasive method of detecting presence of ABI. An ABI value between 0.9 and 1.4 is considered normal. Management of patients with PAD has two components, one risk reduction for cardiovascular events and two, management of symptomatic PAD. The risk reduction is accomplished by smoking cessation, diabetes control, hypertension control, statins, and antiplatelet therapy. The symptomatic PAD is managed by an exercise pain and cilostazol to reduce claudication. Revascularization procedures are reserved for critical limb ischemia and symptomatic PAD which has not responded to medical therapy.

Keywords: *Critical limb ischemia, Ankle branchial index.*

INTRODUCTION

Peripheral artery disease (PAD) is a condition characterized by atherosclerotic occlusive disease of peripheral arteries and classically refers to noncardiac and nonintracranial arteries.[1] While it is obvious that presence of PAD increases risk of foot ulceration and amputation,[2] frequently, PAD coexists with the atherosclerotic disease in other vascular beds, especially coronary and cerebrovascular and the presence of PAD is associated with an increase in ischemic events.[3] Despite its obvious risks, this condition is largely undiagnosed.

Patients with diabetes are at increased risk for atherosclerotic disease, hence, it is of no surprise that diabetes and PAD have been shown to coexist, with a greater risk of limb amputations.[4,5] In addition, cardiovascular and cerebrovascular complications are higher in subjects having PAD and diabetes.[6]

EPIDEMIOLOGY OF PERIPHERAL ARTERY DISEASE IN PATIENTS WITH DIABETES

Among 12 million persons in US who have PAD, nearly 20–30% have coexistent diabetes.[7] Accurate estimates of PAD is made difficult by varying diagnostic tests used and also by certain factors pertinent to the condition that makes assessment difficult. One, the condition is often asymptomatic. These may relate to altered pain perception due to peripheral neuropathy and poor specificity of clinical features such as claudication and absent peripheral pulses.[6] Where ankle-brachial index (ABI) was used to screen, prevalence of PAD (ABI <0.90) in diabetes ranged from 20 to 33%.[8,9]

INDIAN SCENARIO

Studies that assessed for prevalence of PAD in patients with diabetes in India have reported rates ranging from 7.6 to 33%.[10-13] Two early papers from Dr Mohan's center have noted a prevalence rate of PAD among patients with diabetes in their center much lower than other ethnicities,[14,15] but all the other groups have reported prevalence rates comparable to global rates. Sosale et al. noted that one in six asymptomatic patients with type 2 diabetes mellitus (T2DM) in South India had PAD.[12] Eshcol et al. noted that women had a higher prevalence of PAD as compared to men.[10]

In the Framingham study, the risk of intermittent claudication was increased manifold with diabetes: More than 3-fold in men and nearly 9-fold in women.[16] Smoking, advanced age, hypertension, and dyslipidemia are all independent risk factors for PAD.[17] Duration of diabetes has a strong positive association with the risk of developing PAD. Al-Delaimy reported that over a follow-up of 11–25 years, there was a relation between the duration of diabetes and the risk of PAD.[18] Kallio et al. showed that not only is the duration of diabetes an important factor, the advanced age of the patient also increased risk of PAD.[19]

The glycemic levels are also an important risk factor for PAD. In the United Kingdom Prospective Diabetes Study (UKPDS), increased glycated hemoglobin (HbA1c) raised the risk of PAD independent of other risk factors. An increase by 1% led to 28% increased risk of developing PAD.[20]

The presence of neuropathy is a risk factor for PAD. McDermott et al. have demonstrated that patients with severe PAD had poorer perineal nerve conduction.[21] Functional impairment is related to leg muscle and peripheral nerve changes due to ischemia among subjects with PAD.[22]

BOX 1 Peripheral artery disease (PAD) and evidence-based medicine.

Peripheral artery disease: Ten evidence-based facts:

1. The risk of PAD increases substantially with age
2. >50% of PAD patients are usually asymptomatic
3. The presence of PAD is associated with a 2-fold increased prevalence of heart failure
4. 20–30% of individuals with PAD have diabetes mellitus
5. Persons with diabetes have 2–4 times higher risk of developing PAD, coronary artery disease (CAD), and ischemic stroke
6. Smokers have 2.5 times higher risk of developing PAD
7. Atherosclerosis is the cause in >90% of cases of PAD
8. Compared to Whites, the likelihood of developing PAD is 55% lower among Chinese and 50% greater among African Americans
9. The femoral and popliteal arteries are affected in 80–90% of symptomatic PAD patients
10. The prevalence of amputation in PAD patients is 3–4%

Thus to summarize, risk factors for PAD in patients with diabetes are advanced age, smoking, hypertension, dyslipidemia, duration of diabetes, degree of glycemic levels, and presence of neuropathy.

The age-adjusted rate of lower-extremity amputation (LEA) in patients with diabetes is approximately 15 times that of patients without diabetes.[2] Among individuals with diabetes, PAD along with neuropathy is major predisposing factors for LEA.[23] The importance of detecting PAD is in identifying patients at high risk for cardiovascular events and mortality. Patients detected to have PAD have a 30% mortality rate and 20% of them will have a cardiovascular event [myocardial infarction (MI) and stroke] over the next 5-year period.[24] Patients with critical limb ischemia have much graver prognosis, 20% are likely to die within 6 months and 30% will have amputations (**Box 1**).[25]

PATHOPHYSIOLOGY

Diabetes is an important risk factor for atherosclerotic disease in all vascular beds. The underlying metabolic dysfunction in diabetes mellitus (DM) increase vascular inflammation, endothelial dysfunction, vasoconstriction, platelet activation, and thrombotic risk, processes which are important to the pathogenesis of PAD among patients with DM.[26] The distribution of PAD in patients with diabetes is often more distal with greater involvement of infragenicular vessels, especially tibial vessels.[27] Changes preceding atherosclerosis are observed in diabetes; they include inflammation of vessels and impairment of hemostatic factors.[6]

Diabetes is a state of inflammation, which in turn is associated with PAD. The often coexisting components of metabolic syndrome such as hypertension and dyslipidemia also contribute to the state of inflammation in the vessel walls. C-reactive protein (CRP), the most studied marker of inflammation, has been found to be elevated in patient with PAD.[28] In the last few years, it is suggested that CRP may lead to atherosclerotic plaque by mechanisms including lowering the activity of endothelial nitric oxide (NO) synthase, upregulation of cell adhesion molecules, and low-density lipoprotein (LDL) cholesterol phagocytosis by macrophages. These in turn lead to migration of smooth muscle and intimal plaque formation.[29] Each one of the steps is involved in evolution and progression of the atherosclerotic plaque which leads to occlusive disease. Many others markers of inflammation, for instance interleukin-6 (IL-6), have also been seen to be elevated in PAD.[30] The endothelial cells of vessels modulate the relation between blood cell elements and the vessel wall, maintaining a balance between thrombosis and fibrinolysis. Abnormalities of endothelium lead to atherosclerosis.[6] Normal endothelial cells release NO. NO is known to be a vasodilator, which also inhibits aggregation of platelets and of intimal migration of vascular smooth muscle cells. When the endothelium is dysfunction, called endothelial dysfunction, it loses its normal ability to promote vasodilatation, fibrinolysis, and action against aggregation. DM is commonly associated with generalized endothelial dysfunction. Hyperglycemia, inflammation secondary to insulin resistance, fatty acids, and reactive oxygen species are all believed to play a role in causation of endothelial dysfunction in diabetes.[31]

Along with endothelial dysfunction, there are other changes such as activated receptors for receptor for advanced glycation end products (RAGE) and vessel wall inflammation due to increased production of transcription factors such as nuclear factor kappa B (NF-κB) and activator protein-1. Foam cells are formed by increased proinflammatory factors and loss of normal NO function.[32]

Increased platelet aggregation and augmented coagulability are seen in diabetes. Platelets have thrombogenic as a result of increased expression of glycoproteins such as Ib and IIb/IIIa.[33] A hypercoagulable state results from increased expression of tissue factor and decreased antithrombin III and other anticoagulant factors, leading to an unstable plaque and thrombus formation.[34]

CLINICAL PRESENTATION

Although most patients with PAD are asymptomatic, the common symptoms of PAD include intermittent claudication, rest pain, and/or foot ulcers. Claudication is the cramping pain especially the calves, seldom thighs, and buttocks experienced on walking that disappears after rest. It is a specific symptom, although not a very sensitive one for PAD. Rest pain is the pain seen in the muscles of the lower limb even at rest, mostly when limbs are elevated and are relieved by hanging legs down. This is a symptom of more advanced PAD. Patients with diabetes often have coexisting neuropathy, which may mask the presence of painful symptoms. Development of dry gangrene is the end result of compromised vasculature. Symptomatic PAD is clinically staged by the Fontaine staging system:[17] Stage I refers to asymptomatic PAD; stages IIa and IIb when claudication is mild and moderate-to-severe, respectively. More extensive involvement leading to ischemic rest pain has stage III, while distal ulceration and gangrene are termed stage IV.[25]

DIAGNOSIS

Every patient with diabetes should get a relevant history and physical examination specific for detection of PAD. History of smoking should be enquired and recorded. Blood pressure must be recorded and all peripheral pulses must be palpated and auscultated for the presence of bruit. Pulse is graded as normal, diminished, or absent. Absent dorsalis pedis pulse is not sensitive in identifying PAD because 1–15% normal persons have a congenital absence.[5] However, the simultaneous absence of the dorsalis pedis pulse and the posterior tibial pulse suggests PAD, which must be confirmed by further evaluation.

Ankle-brachial Index

Peripheral artery disease can be identified by ABI, a noninvasive and reproducible measure. ABI is defined as ratio of the ankle systolic blood pressure divided by the brachial systolic blood pressure. The normal range is between 1.0 and 1.40.[35] The blood pressure in the lower limbs is normally greater than that in the upper limbs, primarily due to two reasons. One, is the amplification of blood pressure waveforms attributable to the retrograde reflection of waveforms from distal resistant arterioles which are additive to the integrate waveform.[36] Two, the changes in the vessel wall thickness due to the increased hydrostatic pressure in the lower limbs secondary to walking.[37]

Low ABI (<0.9) in PAD is a result of ankle systolic blood pressure being lower than brachial systolic blood pressure. Lower the ratio, more severe the PAD and associated cardiovascular events. The American Diabetes Association consensus recommends all subjects with diabetes above the age of 50 years must undergo ABI study. In those with normal ABI (0.91–1.4), it may be repeated after 5 years.[38] However, the reliability of blood pressure in diagnosis PAD is suspect because ABI may be low in subjects with hypertension and high in those with normotension or hypotension.[39]

An ABI of >1.4 may be indicative of noncompressible tibial arteries due to calcification showing a high ABI. Yet such high index predicts cerebral and cardiac vascular events. One must perform other tests such as toe-brachial pressure to diagnose PAD in this subset of patients.[40,41]

An ABI of <0.9 is generally agreed upon as the diagnostic cutoff for presence of PAD. When this cutoff is compared with imaging methods such as color duplex ultrasound, magnetic resonance angiography, or angiography while the specificity (83–99%) of this cutoff was high, the sensitivity was low (69–79%). An ABI of ≤1.0, as a threshold for diagnosis of PAD, has a sensitivity of nearly 100%. Thus, ABI should, therefore, be interpreted based on the pretest probability of PAD and borderline values between 0.91 and 1.00 should be interpreted taking other clinical criteria into consideration.[42] Patients with intermittent claudication, but normal ABI, repeat measurement after exercise may improve in detection.

MANAGEMENT

Medical Management

The primary objective of management of patients with PAD is to prevent cardiovascular events secondary to the multifocal distribution of the disease. Second, is to address functional status of the limb.

Risk Factor Reduction

The risk factors for atherosclerosis include smoking, diabetes, hypertension, and dyslipidemia. Thus, reducing cardiovascular events begin by addressing these risk factors.

Smoking tobacco is one of the most important risk factors for development and progression of atherosclerosis, both peripheral and coronary. Thus, smoking cessation is essential. A 10-year survival rate was reported to be 82% in those who had quit smoking in contrast to 46% in current smokers.[43] Advice against it from physicians at every clinic visit is necessary and has been shown to be helpful in effecting smoking cessation. Counseling and nicotine patches have been found to be useful.[44] Bupropion[45] and varenicline,[46] a newer nicotinic ligand, have been found to be better than placebo in smoking cessation.

Diabetes

Although diabetes is known to be an atherosclerotic risk factor, there is little evidence that aggressive control of hyperglycemia reduces cardiovascular risk associated with PAD. In the UKPDS, intensive glycemic control led to a nonsignificant 16% risk reduction for MI and sudden death.[47] In the follow-up study after 10 years, subjects who originally received intensified glucose treatment had lower incidence of MI (risk ratio reduction 15%; p = 0.0014) and all-cause death (13%; p = 0.007)[48] indicating that early aggressive glycemic control may lower the risk of macrovascular disease.

Studies aiming to intensity further on while no significant improvement in cardiovascular risk was observed with diabetes therapy in the ADVANCE (Action in Diabetes and Vascular Disease: Preterax and Diamicron MR Controlled Evaluation) trial[49] and the VADT (Veterans Affairs Diabetes Trial)[50] did not reduce the cardiovascular risk; on the contrary, the ACCORD (Action to Control Cardiovascular Risk in Diabetes) trial[51] was stopped prematurely because of increased mortality in the group put on intensive control. Thus, tight glycemic control may be lower cardiovascular risk in the early stages of T2DM, but not in those with established cardiovascular disease (CVD); rather, it may even be detrimental.

One should recognize that there have been no studies specifically for association of PAD and glycemic control. Therefore, glycemic targets should be individualized.

Hypertension

Hypertension associated with diabetes further increases the high risk of CVD. In the UKPDS, diabetes endpoints were reduced by tight blood pressure control, but there was no effect on PAD as assessed by the risk of amputation.[52] Lowering of blood pressure even in those who were normotensive, having both diabetes and PAD reduced cardiovascular events,[53] which underscores the importance of blood pressure control to lower cardiovascular events.

Dyslipidemia

Statins reduce the risk of cardiovascular events in subjects with PAD and coexisting coronary artery disease (CAD).[54] The Scandinavian Simvastatin Survival Study (4S) reported a 43% reduction in mortality in subjects with diabetes compared to 29% in nondiabetics.[55]

Recently, the American College of Cardiology/American Heart Association (ACC/AHA) guidelines recommend that moderate-intensity statins can be given to all subjects with diabetes aged between 40 and 75 years. High-intensity statins are advised in those with cardiovascular risk factors, for which PAD qualifies.[56]

Antiplatelet Therapy

Since the role of abnormalities in platelets in atherosclerosis is established, antiplatelet drugs have an important role in the management of PAD.

In the Antiplatelet Trialists' Collaboration, antiplatelet agents reduced cardiovascular deaths by 25% among those with symptomatic atherosclerotic disease. Subjects with intermittent claudication had a lower reduction of mortality (18%).[57] Data on subjects with diabetes were not analyzed separately. Aspirin is given in a daily dose of 75–325 mg.

Clopidogrel is a second-generation thienopyridine drug which has fewer side effects. The CAPRIE (Clopidogrel versus Aspirin in Patients at Risk of Ischemic Events) study[53] compared clopidogrel 75 mg with aspirin 325 mg. In a large cohort of over 19,000 patients, approximately a fifth had diabetes, there was an overall decrease in the primary endpoints (viz., MI, stroke, or vascular deaths) was 8.7%; clopidogrel reduced the risk of MI by 19.2% over that of aspirin irrespective of the primary CVD. The study also showed that in the subgroup (about 30% of the 19,000 patients) with PAD at baseline, clopidogrel lowered the risk of MI, stroke, or vascular death by 24% compared to aspirin.[58] Thus, clopidogrel may be the preferred to aspirin in subjects with PAD.

Protease-activated receptor-1 (PAR-1) is present on platelets, vascular endothelium, and smooth muscle. It is the primary receptor for thrombin. Vorapaxar is a newer antagonist of PAR-1.[59] In the TRA2°P-TIMI 50 (Trial to Assess the Effects of Vorapaxar in Preventing Heart Attack and Stroke in Patients with Atherosclerosis-Thrombolysis in Myocardial Infarction 50), vorapaxar reduced the rate of first acute limb ischemia events in symptomatic PAD patients who had revascularization earlier.[60-62] Therefore, PAR-1 antagonism may be a useful option for subjects having both diabetes and PAD.

Management of Symptomatic Peripheral Artery Disease

Exercise

Employment of exercise for treating intermittent claudication in PAD is grouped as level A evidence (class I).[63] A systematic review by the Cochrane group from 22 randomized controlled trials that recruited subjects with stable claudication showed that supervised exercise program improved treadmill walking time and distance, even though there was no reduction in major cardiovascular events. The improvement persisted for up to 2 years.[64] Patients with PAD without claudication also showed improvement in functional performance, especially while participating in treadmill exercise as compared to lower extremity resistance training.[64] Thus, subjects with PAD (symptomatic or not) are likely to benefit from an exercise regimen.

Pentoxifylline

It is a hemorheological agent, decreases blood viscosity and improves erythrocyte flexibility, and was a popular choice for relieving symptoms of claudication. However, the evidence from clinical trials in its efficacy in improving treadmill walking distance has been equivocal and hence not recommended.[65]

Cilostazol

Cilostazol is a phosphodiesterase type 3 inhibitor. It is believed to act by increasing intracellular concentrations of cyclic adenosine monophosphate (cAMP) leading to vasodilation and inhibition of platelet aggregation. In a meta-analysis of 2,702 subjects with claudication due to PAD, cilostazol was shown to improve maximum and pain-free treadmill walking distance as well as quality of life.[66] It also lowered triglyceride concentration by 16% and increased high-density lipoprotein levels by 13%. Adverse effects consisted of headache, bowel concerns, and palpitations. It is contraindicated in subjects with congestive heart failure.[67]

Naftidrofuryl

Naftidrofuryl (600 mg daily orally), which is currently available in Europe, can be used for the treatment of claudication. Naftidrofuryl has less side effects than cilostazol.

Naftidrofuryl is a 5-hydroxytryptamine-2-receptor antagonist.[68,69] The putative actions occur through promotion of glucose uptake and raising adenosine triphosphate levels. It leads to clinically meaningful improvements in walking distance.[70]

Revascularization Procedures

Revascularization is indicated in PAD in the presence of disabling PAD which does not respond to medical therapy and for critical limb ischemia. A number of procedures are described: Percutaneous transluminal coronary angioplasty (PTCA) alone or with stenting and endarterectomy or bypass grafting. The choice depends on the site and extent of the lesion, distal run-off, and surgical risk due to other comorbidity such as CVD. Results of proximal, short segment disease in the iliac and femoral segments, amenable to PTCA, are comparable to those without diabetes. For more distal disease in the popliteal and tibial arteries, bypass grafting is preferred, which carries a higher risk of periprocedural morbidity and mortality.[5]

Restenosis rates and graft occlusion rates are higher in subjects with diabetes, along with lower survival.[6]

REFERENCES

1. Kullo IJ, Rooke TW. CLINICAL PRACTICE. Peripheral Artery Disease. N Engl J Med. 2016;374:861-71.
2. Bartus CL, Margolis DJ. Reducing the incidence of foot ulceration and amputation in diabetes. Curr Diab Rep. 2004;4:413-8.
3. Grenon SM, Vittinghoff E, Owens CD, Conte MS, Whooley M, Cohen BE. Peripheral artery disease and risk of cardiovascular events in patients with coronary artery disease: insights from the Heart and Soul Study. Vasc Med. 2013;18:176-84.
4. Donahue RP, Orchard TJ. Diabetes mellitus and macrovascular complications. An epidemiological perspective. Diabetes Care. 1992;15:1141-55.
5. Jude EB, Eleftheriadou I, Tentolouris N. Peripheral arterial disease in diabetes—a review. Diabet Med. 2010;27:4-14.
6. American Diabetes Association. Peripheral arterial disease in people with diabetes. Diabetes Care. 2003;26:3333-41.
7. Marso SP, Hiatt WR. Peripheral arterial disease in patients with diabetes. J Am Coll Cardiol. 2006;47:921-9.
8. Beks PJ, Mackaay AJ, de Neeling JN, de Vries H, Bouter LM, Heine RJ. Peripheral arterial disease in relation to glycaemic level in an elderly Caucasian population: the Hoorn study. Diabetologia. 1995;38:86-96.
9. Elhadd TA, Robb R, Jung RT, Stonebridge PA, Belch JJF. Pilot study of prevalence of asymptomatic peripheral arterial occlusive disease in patients with diabetes attending a hospital clinic. Pract Diabetes Int. 1999;16:163-6.

10. Eshcol J, Jebarani S, Anjana RM, Mohan V, Pradeepa R. Prevalence, incidence and progression of peripheral arterial disease in Asian Indian type 2 diabetic patients. J Diabetes Complications. 2014;28:627-31.
11. Agarwal AK, Singh M, Arya V, Garg U, Singh VP, Jain V. Prevalence of peripheral arterial disease in type 2 diabetes mellitus and its correlation with coronary artery disease and its risk factors. J Assoc Physicians India. 2012;60:28-32.
12. Sosale B, Reddy YJ, Nagbhushana MV, Sosale A, Jude EB. Peripheral arterial disease in patients with type 2 diabetes mellitus in South India: The urban vs rural divide. J Acad Med Sci. 2012;2:105-9.
13. Khurana A, Dhoat P, Marwaha TS. Peripheral vascular disease—a silent assassin: Its rising trend in Punjab. J Indian Acad Clin Med. 2013;14:111-4.
14. Mohan V, Premalatha G, Sastry NG. Peripheral vascular disease in non-insulin-dependent diabetes mellitus in South India. Diab Res Clin Pract. 1995;27:235-40.
15. Premalatha G, Mohan V. Is peripheral vascular disease less common in Indians? Int J Diab Dev Countries. 1995;15:68-9.
16. Kannel WB, McGee DL. Update on some epidemiologic features of intermittent claudication: the Framingham study. J Am Geriatr Soc. 1985;33:13-8.
17. Criqui MH. Peripheral arterial disease—epidemiological aspects. Vasc Med. 2001;6:3-7.
18. Al-Delaimy WK, Merchant AT, Rimm EB, Willett WC, Stampfer MJ, Hu FB. Effect of type 2 diabetes and its duration on the risk of peripheral arterial disease among men. Am J Med. 2004;116:236-40.
19. Kallio M, Forsblom C, Groop PH, Groop L, Lepäntalo M. Development of new peripheral arterial occlusive disease in patients with type 2 diabetes during a mean follow-up of 11 years. Diabetes Care. 2003;26:1241-5.
20. Adler AI, Stevens RJ, Neil A, Stratton IM, Boulton AJ, Holman RR. UKPDS 59: hyperglycemia and other potentially modifiable risk factors for peripheral vascular disease in type 2 diabetes. Diabetes Care. 2002;25:894-9.
21. McDermott MM, Sufit R, Nishida T, Guralnik JM, Ferrucci L, Tian L. Lower extremity nerve function in patients with lower extremity ischemia. Arch Intern Med. 2006;166:1986-92.
22. McDermott MM. Lower extremity manifestations of peripheral artery disease: the pathophysiologic and functional implications of leg ischemia. Circ Res. 2015;116:1540-50.
23. Bild DE, Selby JV, Sinnock P, Browner WS, Braveman P, Showstack JA. Lower-extremity amputation in people with diabetes. Epidemiology and prevention. Diabetes Care. 1989;12:24-31.
24. Weitz JI, Byrne J, Clagett GP, Farkouh ME, Porter JM, Sackett DL, et al. Diagnosis and treatment of chronic arterial insufficiency of the lower extremities: a critical review. Circulation. 1996;94:3026-49.
25. Dormandy JA, Rutherford RB. Management of peripheral arterial disease (PAD). TASC Working Group. TransAtlantic Inter-Society Consensus (TASC). J Vasc Surg. 2000;31;S1-S296.
26. Newman JD, Schwartzbard AZ, Weintraub HS, Goldberg IJ, Berger JS. Primary Prevention of Cardiovascular Disease in Diabetes Mellitus. J Am Coll Cardiol. 2017;70:883-93.
27. Haltmayer M, Mueller T, Horvath W, Luft C, Poelz W, Haidinger D. Impact of atherosclerotic risk factors on the anatomical distribution of peripheral arterial disease. Int Angiol. 2001;20:200-7.
28. Vainas T, Stassen FR, de Graaf R, Twiss EL, Herngreen SB, Welten RJ, et al. C-reactive protein in peripheral arterial disease: relation to severity of the disease and to future cardiovascular events. J Vasc Surg. 2005;42:243-51.
29. Tzoulaki I, Murray GD, Lee AJ, Rumley A, Lowe GD, Fowkes FG. C-reactive protein, interleukin-6, and soluble adhesion molecules as predictors of progressive peripheral atherosclerosis in the general population: Edinburgh Artery Study. Circulation. 2005;112:976-83.
30. Khawaja FJ, Kullo IJ. Novel markers of peripheral arterial disease. Vasc Med. 2009;14:381-92.
31. Roberts AC, Porter KE. Cellular and molecular mechanisms of endothelial dysfunction in diabetes. Diab Vasc Dis Res. 2013;10:472-82.
32. Tsao PS, Wang B, Buitrago R, Shyy JY, Cooke JP. Nitric oxide regulates monocyte chemotactic protein-1. Circulation. 1997;96:934-40.
33. Vinik AI, Erbas T, Park TS, Nolan R, Pittenger GL. Platelet dysfunction in type 2 diabetes. Diabetes Care. 2001;24:1476-85.
34. Carr ME. Diabetes mellitus: a hypercoagulable state. J Diabetes Complications. 2001;15:44-54.

35. Hiatt WR. Medical treatment of peripheral arterial disease and claudication. N Engl J Med. 2001;344:1608-21.
36. Safar ME, Protogerou AD, Blacher J. Statins, central blood pressure, and blood pressure amplification. Circulation. 2009;119:9-12.
37. Katz S, Globerman A, Avitzour M, Dolfin T. The ankle-brachial index in normal neonates and infants is significantly lower than in older children and adults. J Pediatr Surg. 1997;32:269-71.
38. Rooke TW, Hirsch AT, Misra S, Sidawy AN, Beckman JA, Findeiss L, et al. Management of patients with peripheral artery disease (compilation of 2005 and 2011 ACCF/AHA Guideline Recommendations): a report of the American College of Cardiology Foundation/American Heart Association Task Force on Practice Guidelines. J Am Coll Cardiol. 2013;61(14):1555-70.
39. Carser DG. Do we need to reappraise our method of interpreting the ankle brachial pressure index? J Wound Care. 2001;10:59-62.
40. Hiatt WR, Hoag S, Hamman RF. Effect of diagnostic criteria on the prevalence of peripheral arterial disease. Circulation. 1995;91:1472-9.
41. Resnick HE, Lindsay RS, McDermott MM, Devereux RB, Jones KL, Fabsitz RR, et al. Relationship of high and low ankle brachial index to all-cause and cardiovascular disease mortality: the Strong Heart Study. Circulation. 2004;109:733-9.
42. Aboyans V, Criqui MH, Abraham P, Allison MA, Creager MA, Diehm C, et al. Measurement and interpretation of the ankle-brachial index: a scientific statement from the American Heart Association. Circulation. 2012;126:2890-909.
43. Jonason T, Bergström R. Cessation of smoking in patients with intermittent claudication. Effects on the risk of peripheral vascular complications, myocardial infarction and mortality. Acta Med Scand. 1987;221:253-60.
44. Anthonisen NR, Skeans MA, Wise RA, Manfreda J, Kanner RE, Connett JE, et al. The effects of a smoking cessation intervention on 14.5-year mortality: a randomized clinical trial. Ann Intern Med. 2005;142:233-9.
45. Jorenby DE, Leischow SJ, Nides MA, Rennard SI, Johnston JA, Hughes AR, et al. A controlled trial of sustained-release bupropion, a nicotine patch, or both for smoking cessation. N Engl J Med. 1999;340:685-91.
46. Wang C, Xiao D, Chan KPW, Pothirat C, Garza D, Davies S. Varenicline for smoking cessation: A placebo-controlled, randomized study. Respirology. 2009;14:384-92.
47. UK Prospective Diabetes Study (UKPDS) Group. Intensive blood-glucose control with sulphonylureas or insulin compared with conventional treatment and risk of complications in patients with type 2 diabetes (UKPDS 33). Lancet. 1998;352:837-53.
48. Holman RR, Paul SK, Bethel MA, Matthews DR, Neil HA. 10-year follow-up of intensive glucose control in type 2 diabetes. N Engl J Med. 2008;359:1577-89.
49. ADVANCE Collaborative Group, Patel A, MacMahon S, Chalmers J, Neal B, Billot L, et al. Intensive blood glucose control and vascular outcomes in patients with type 2 diabetes. N Engl J Med. 2008;358: 2560-72.
50. Duckworth W, Abraira C, Moritz T, Reda D, Emanuele N, Reaven PD, et al. Glucose control and vascular complications in veterans with type 2 diabetes. N Engl J Med. 2009;360:129-39.
51. Action to Control Cardiovascular Risk in Diabetes Study Group, Gerstein HC, Miller ME, Byington RP, Goff DC, Bigger JT, et al. Effects of intensive glucose lowering in type 2 diabetes. N Engl J Med. 2008;358:2545-59.
52. UK Prospective Diabetes Study Group. Tight blood pressure control and risk of macrovascular and microvascular complications in type 2 diabetes: UKPDS 38. UK Prospective Diabetes Study Group. BMJ. 1998;317:703-13.
53. Mehler PS, Coll JR, Estacio R, Esler A, Schrier RW, Hiatt WR. Intensive blood pressure control reduces the risk of cardiovascular events in patients with peripheral arterial disease and type 2 diabetes. Circulation. 2003;107:753-6.
54. Cannon CP, Braunwald E, McCabe CH, Rader DJ, Rouleau JL, Belder R, et al. Intensive versus moderate lipid lowering with statins after acute coronary syndromes. N Engl J Med. 2004;350: 1495-504.

55. Pedersen TR, Kjekshus J, Pyörälä K, Olsson AG, Cook TJ, Musliner TA, et al. Effect of simvastatin on ischemic signs and symptoms in the Scandinavian simvastatin survival study (4S). Am J Cardiol. 1998;81:333-5.
56. Stone NJ, Robinson JG, Lichtenstein AH, Merz CNB, Blum CB, Eckel RH, et al. 2013 ACC/AHA guideline on the treatment of blood cholesterol to reduce atherosclerotic cardiovascular risk in adults: a report of the American College of Cardiology/American Heart Association Task Force on Practice Guidelines. J Am Coll Cardiol. 2014;63:2889-934.
57. Collaborative overview of randomised trials of antiplatelet therapy—I: Prevention of death, myocardial infarction, and stroke by prolonged antiplatelet therapy in various categories of patients. Antiplatelet Trialists' Collaboration. BMJ. 1994;308:81-106.
58. CAPRIE Steering Committee. A randomised, blinded, trial of clopidogrel versus aspirin in patients at risk of ischaemic events (CAPRIE). CAPRIE Steering Committee. Lancet. 1996;348:1329-39.
59. Kluwer W, Adis O. Vorapaxar. Am J Cardiovasc Drugs. 2010;10:413-8.
60. Bonaca MP, Gutierrez JA, Creager MA, Scirica BM, Olin J, Murphy SA, et al. Acute Limb Ischemia and Outcomes With Vorapaxar in Patients With Peripheral Artery Disease: Results From the Trial to Assess the Effects of Vorapaxar in Preventing Heart Attack and Stroke in Patients With Atherosclerosis-Thrombolysis in Myocardial Infarction 50 (TRA2°P-TIMI 50). Circulation. 2016;133:997-1005.
61. Morrow DA, Braunwald E, Bonaca MP, Ameriso SF, Dalby AJ, Fish MP, et al. Vorapaxar in the secondary prevention of atherothrombotic events. N Engl J Med. 2012;366:1404-13.
62. Bonaca MP, Scirica BM, Creager MA, Olin J, Bounameaux H, Dellborg M, et al. Vorapaxar in patients with peripheral artery disease: results from TRA2{degrees}P-TIMI 50. Circulation. 2013;127:1522-9.
63. Olin JW, Allie DE, Belkin M, Bonow RO, Casey DE, Creager MA, et al. ACCF/AHA/ACR/SCAI/SIR/SVM/SVN/SVS 2010 performance measures for adults with peripheral artery disease: a report of the American College of Cardiology Foundation/American Heart Association Task Force on performance measures, the American College of Radiology, the Society for Cardiac Angiography and Interventions, the Society for Interventional Radiology, the Society for Vascular Medicine, the Society for Vascular Nursing, and the Society for Vascular Surgery (Writing Committee to Develop Clinical Performance Measures for Peripheral Artery Disease). Circulation. 2010;122:2583-618.
64. Watson L, Ellis B, Leng GC. Exercise for intermittent claudication. Cochrane Database Syst Rev. 2008;1:CD000990.
65. McDermott MM, Ades P, Guralnik JM, Dyer A, Ferrucci L, Liu K, et al. Treadmill exercise and resistance training in patients with peripheral arterial disease with and without intermittent claudication: a randomized controlled trial. JAMA. 2009;301:165-74.
66. Jackson MR, Clagett GP. Antithrombotic therapy in peripheral arterial occlusive disease. Chest. 2001;119:283S-99.
67. Thompson PD, Zimet R, Forbes WP, Zhang P. Meta-analysis of results from eight randomized, placebo-controlled trials on the effect of cilostazol on patients with intermittent claudication. Am J Cardiol. 2002;90:1314-9.
68. Lehert P, Comte S, Gamand S, Brown TM. Naftidrofuryl in intermittent claudication: a retrospective analysis. J Cardiovasc Pharmacol. 1994;23:S48.
69. Stevens JW, Simpson E, Harnan S, Squires H, Meng Y, Thomas S, et al. Systematic review of the efficacy of cilostazol, naftidrofuryl oxalate and pentoxifylline for the treatment of intermittent claudication. Br J Surg. 2012;99:1630-8.
70. Shu J, Santulli G. Update on peripheral artery disease: Epidemiology and evidence-based facts. Atherosclerosis. 2018;275:379-81.

CHAPTER 7

Diabetic Nephropathy

Kudugunti Neelaveni, Ajay Raj Mallela

ABSTRACT

Diabetic nephropathy (DN) is a common and serious complication of both type 1 diabetes mellitus (T1DM) and type 2 diabetes mellitus (T2DM). It results from a combination of hyperglycemia and hypertension upon an underlying genetic predisposition. Because T2DM is more common, it leads to greater burden of DN compared to T1DM. Nephropathy may march from a stage of microalbuminuria to reduced glomerular filtration rate (GFR) and frank renal failure; reduced GFR without passing through microalbuminuria is being recognized. Coexistence of retinopathy is indicative of nephropathy being due to diabetes and not due to other causes; one must consider nondiabetic patients causes of renal involvement, particularly in T2DM. Prevention and management comprise of controlling glucose levels, blood pressure, use of angiotensin-converting enzyme inhibitors, angiotensin receptor blockers, and sodium-glucose cotransporter-2 (SGLT-2) inhibitors; the last have favorable on both renal and cardiovascular outcomes. Newer group of drugs are in the pipeline.

Keywords: *Podocytes, Microalbuminuria, eGFR, Retinopathy, ACE inhibitors, ARBs, SGLT-2 inhibitors.*

INTRODUCTION

Diabetic nephropathy (DN) is a long-term microvascular complication and an important cause of chronic kidney disease (CKD). It frequently leads to end-stage renal disease (ESRD), which is devastating to the individual with enormous social and financial burden. Classic DN develops and progresses over many years with gradual increase in urinary albumin excretion (UAE), blood pressure, and decline in glomerular filtration rate (GFR).

As nephropathy progresses, the risk of other complications increases, in particular the risk of cardiovascular disease with significant mortality and morbidity. DN occurs in approximately 20–40% of type 2 diabetes mellitus (T2DM) and 30% of type 1 diabetes mellitus (T1DM).[1-3] Occurrence of DN has been reported even in patients with prediabetes.[4] With the improvement in management of diabetes, the prevalence of classic DN has come down in T1DM but not so in T2DM which is attributed to its increased prevalence, obesity, and aging population.[5] Optimized glycemic, blood pressure, lipid control, and the use of renin–angiotensin–aldosterone system (RAAS) inhibitors are proven to be beneficial, still they remain suboptimal with an unmet need for effective therapies. Hence, early diagnosis is very essential to deliver appropriate therapy to prevent the occurrence and progression of the disease, thereby reducing morbidity and mortality.

RISK FACTORS

Diabetic nephropathy is the result of interplay between genetic and environmental factors. Hyperglycemia, hypertension, dyslipidemia, anemia, and lifestyle factors such as obesity and smoking are considered as major risk factors. The extent of albuminuria is also an independent predictor at each stage of nephropathy.[6] T2DM patients with nonalcoholic fatty liver disease (NAFLD) are more likely to have CKD.[7] Although several studies noted strong genetic predisposition to DN in T1DM and T2DM siblings concordant for diabetes,[8,9] genetic factors related to DN are not clearly understood. Studies for identification of genetic loci are ongoing with genome scanning and candidate gene approaches.

PATHOGENESIS

Though many factors play a role in the pathogenesis of DN, it is well known that hyperglycemia is a prime factor and it can trigger metabolic injury mediated by increased advanced glycation end products (AGEs), polyol pathway, and protein kinase C activation in both the glomerular and interstitial cells, with resultant increase in intraglomerular pressure, which upregulates the diverse intracellular signaling pathways including RAAS. This results in enhanced production of reactive oxygen species, inflammatory mediators [nuclear factor-κβ (NF-κβ) and Toll-like receptor (TLR)], growth factors [vascular endothelial growth factor (VEGF) and connective tissue growth factor],[5,10] transforming growth factor-β (TGF-β), proinflammatory, and profibrotic cytokines causing structural and functional renal injury. The growing data suggest the role of elevated fibroblast growth factor 23 (FGF23) and deficient alpha-Klotho in the pathogenesis.[11-13]

ROLE OF PODOCYTES IN DIABETIC NEPHROPATHY

Glomerular hypertension increases the burden on podocytes to cover a larger area of glomerular basement membrane (GBM), resulting in foot process widening, decreased ability to bind to GBM leading to bare areas and consequent protein excretion, as evidenced in several studies.[14-16] Further studies on molecular structure of podocyte and slit diaphragm proteins expression are needed to recognize their role in the pathogenesis of DN.

PATHOLOGY

- *Glomeruli*: Thickening of GBM and mesangial expansion due to accumulation of matrix causing diffuse mesangial sclerosis are the hallmark lesion of DN. The distinctive nodular accumulations of mesangial matrix are known as Kimmelstiel–Wilson nodules
- *Capsular drop*: Hyaline is located between the basement membranes of Bowman's capsule and the adjacent parietal epithelium
- *Fibrin cap*: Hyaline is found within capillary lumina and particularly when it is adherent to the capillary wall
- *Tubules*: Tubular basement thickening, Armani–Ebstein changes (accumulation of glycogen in cells of pars recta), and tubular atrophy
- *Interstitium*: Infiltration with inflammatory cells and fibrosis
- *Blood vessels*: Afferent and efferent arteriolar hyalinosis

In T1DM, most important structural changes are seen in glomerulus, although tubular, interstitial, and arteriolar lesions are present. In contrast, Fioretto P et al. reported heterogeneity in renal structure in a large cohort of T2DM patients with albuminuria. Majority of the patients in that cohort had normal or near-normal glomerular structure with or without tubulointerstitial and arteriolar abnormalities.[17-20]

NATURAL HISTORY

Type 1 Diabetes Mellitus

The stages of diabetic kidney disease (DKD) in T1DM can be divided into five stages:

- *Stage 1*: Renal hypertrophy and hyperfunction, which occur with the onset of diabetes. Some studies showed that glomerular hyperfiltration is a risk factor for DN.[21-25]
- *Stage 2*: A stage of clinical quiescence associated with thickening of basement membrane and mesangial expansion. GFR is normal or may be higher. Patients with upper limit of normoalbuminuria and structural changes of diabetic glomerulosclerosis have a higher chance of developing microalbuminuria.[6,26] Nocturnal nondipping on 24-hour

ambulatory blood pressure monitoring may be an early indicator, which precedes the development of stage 3.[27]

- *Stage 3*: Incipient nephropathy stage, characterized by persistent microalbuminuria. It starts 5-10 years after the onset of T1DM.[28] Approximately, in one-third of type 1 diabetic patients, microalbuminuria can regress toward normoalbuminuria, it can persist as such, or it can progress toward macroalbuminuria.[29,30] GFR may be normal or may show decline. Persistent microalbuminuria is an independent predictor of future cardiovascular risk[31] and progression to macroalbuminuria is associated with arterial hypertension and decrease in GFR.[32]
- *Stage 4*: It is characterized by overt proteinuria. This stage manifests 10–20 years after the onset of T1DM and if untreated, GFR decline progresses at mean annual rate of 10-12 mL/min/1.73 m^2.[33,34] At this stage, diabetes-associated chronic vascular complications are noted in most patients.
- *Stage 5*: Progression to ESRD occurs 5–15 years after the onset of proteinuria.

In T2DM, the natural history of nephropathy is similar to T1DM with the exception that microalbuminuria or proteinuria may be present at diagnosis because onset of diabetes may go undetected for many years. Hence, the relationship of microalbuminuria to T2DM duration is not precisely known.

DIAGNOSIS

Diabetic nephropathy diagnosis is based on clinical features and assessment of estimated glomerular filtration rate (eGFR) and UAE.[2,35]

Nondiabetic kidney is suspected in the following situations and needs appropriate evaluation, if required with renal biopsy except in contracted kidneys.

- Proteinuria in patients with short duration of T1DM
- Absence of retinopathy in T1DM; however, absence in T2DM does not rule out nephropathy
- Presence of active urinary sediment
- Significant drop in GFR than expected with angiotensin-converting enzyme inhibitor/angiotensin receptor blockers (ACEI/ARBs)
- Contracted kidneys
- Presence of other systemic features

Albuminuria

First clinical indicator of DN is albuminuria. It is measured in the following ways:

- 24-hour urine collection—excretion < 30 mg/day is normal, 30–300 mg/day is microalbuminuria, and >300 mg/day is macroalbuminuria

- Timed overnight UAE—excretion < 20 μg/min is normal, 20–200 μg/min is microalbuminuria and >200 μg/min is macroalbuminuria
- Albumin-creatinine ratio (ACR)—<30 mg/g is normal, 30–300 mg/g is microalbuminuria, and >300 mg/g is macroalbuminuria

Recent guidelines recommend use of ACR, as it is performed easily on spot urine sample.[36,37] A patient is considered to have persistent albuminuria when at least two of three measurements of urine ACR examined within 3–6 months are abnormal.

Kidney Disease: Improving Global Outcomes (KDIGO) uses different terminologies to indicate severity of albuminuria and classifies patients into three categories based on ACR.

1. A1: Normal to mildly increased albuminuria—defined as <30 mg/g creatinine, i.e., normoalbuminuria
2. A2: Moderately increased albuminuria—defined as 30–300 mg/g creatinine, i.e., microalbuminuria
3. A3: Severely increased albuminuria—defined as >300 mg/g creatinine, i.e., macroalbuminuria

Estimated Glomerular Filtration Rate

Glomerular filtration rate is considered as the better index of renal function.[38] Regularly used equations for estimation of GFR include the Modification of Diet in Renal Disease (MDRD) study equation or the Chronic Kidney Disease Epidemiology Collaboration equation.[39-41] Serum creatinine is used to estimate these GFRs.

The CKD has been categorized into five stages according to eGFR:[38]

- G1: GFR ≥ 90 mL/min/1.73 m^2
- G2: GFR 60–89 mL/min/1.73 m^2
- G3a: GFR 45–59 mL/min/1.73 m^2
- G3b: GFR 30–44 mL/min/1.73 m^2
- G4: GFR 15–29 mL/min/1.73 m^2
- G5: GFR < 15 mL/min/1.73 m^2

Cystatin C, a cysteine protease inhibitor, is filtered freely by the glomerulus and absorbed in the proximal tubule and considered to be a reliable marker of renal function.[42,43] Cystatin C-based estimation of GFR was demonstrated to be superior.[44] As it is not widely available in routine practice, most guidelines use serum creatinine-based eGFR for diagnosing and monitoring DKD.

Risk Assessment and Monitoring

Annual monitoring of GFR and albuminuria is recommended in stable DKD patients as per the latest KDIGO and American Diabetes Association (ADA) guidelines. As progression of kidney disease is more rapid in patients with low GFR and higher albuminuria, increased frequency of their measurement should be considered.

Early Diagnosis with New Biomarkers

Limitation of Measurement of Urinary Albumin Excretion

- Significant glomerular damage has already occurred by the time albuminuria is evident[45]
- Decline in renal function is not always associated with increased albuminuria[46]

  Several new biomarkers of glomerular and tubular injury, inflammation, and oxidative stress are being investigated.[47-51]

  Albumin accounts for minor fraction of total urinary protein and becomes unreliable in normoalbuminuria.[52] Hence, nonalbumin proteinuria (NAP) may be considered as a marker for early detection of DN.[53-55] The source of urinary NAP includes:[56-62]

  - *Glomerular biomarkers*: Transferrin, immunoglobulin G, ceruloplasmin, type IV collagen, laminin, podocalyxin, and VEGF
  - *Tubular biomarkers*: Neutrophil gelatinase-associated lipocalin (NGAL), alpha-1-microglobulin, kidney injury molecule-1 (KIM-1), N-acetyl-β-D-glucosaminidase (NAG), cystatin C, angiotensinogen, and liver-type fatty acid binding protein
  - *Inflammatory markers*: Tumor necrosis factor-alpha (TNF-α) and orosomucoid

Though small studies showed promise of multiple biomarkers in early diagnosis of DN, larger longitudinal trials are required to validate their clinical use in day-to-day practice.[63]

TREATMENT

The progression of DN takes several years and several factors are known to modulate the course of nephropathy. The "multifactorial" presence of treatable factors has led to the recommendation of "multifactorial approach" of therapeutic interventions for prevention at different stages of nephropathy.

Optimization of Glycemic Control

Studies in T1DM and T2DM have showed favorable impact of blood glucose control on progression of DKD at every stage, i.e., from normoalbuminuria to microalbuminuria (primary prevention), micro- to macroalbuminuria (secondary prevention), and macroalbuminuria to ESRD (tertiary prevention). The Diabetes Control and Complications Trial (DCCT)[64] in T1DM, UKPDS in T2DM,[65] clearly demonstrated that intensive glycemic control delayed the development and progression of microalbuminuria. The follow-up studies of DCCT [EDIC (Epidemiology of Diabetes Interventions and Complications) trial] and UKPDS[65,66] also demonstrated that of initial strict glycemic control persisted far beyond, which is due to metabolic memory or legacy effect.

The more recent ADVANCE (Action in Diabetes and Vascular Disease: Preterax and Diamicron Modified Release Controlled Evaluation), ACCORD (Action to Control Cardiovascular Risk in Diabetes), and Veterans Affairs Diabetes trials also confirmed the same.[67-69] Fioretto P et al. demonstrated regression of established diabetic glomerular lesions in the native kidneys of type 1 diabetic patients with prolonged normalization of glucose levels after successful pancreas transplantation.[70] Though stricter glycemic control is important, it is associated with risk of hypoglycemia in more advanced stages of DN with excess mortality as observed in ADVANCE and ACCORD. Hence, glycemic targets should be individualized aiming to strike a balance between the risk of hypoglycemia and clear benefit of renoprotection.

Pleotropic Renoprotective Benefits of Antidiabetic Drugs beyond Glycemic Control

Glucagon-like peptide-1 (GLP-1) agonist, liraglutide (1.8 mg for 3.8 years) in LEADER (Liraglutide Effect and Action in Diabetes: Evaluation of Cardiovascular Outcome Results) trial, and sodium-glucose cotransporter-2 (SGLT-2) inhibitor, empagliflozin (10 mg or 25 mg for 3.1 years) in EMPA-REG renal study, reduced incident or worsening nephropathy by 22% and 39%, respectively[71-73] and whether these results can be extrapolated to long-term benefits need to be verified. The renal benefits of dipeptidyl peptidase-4 (DPP-4) inhibitors also have been observed in some studies; future trials adequately are powered and designed are needed.[74]

Blood Pressure Control

Hypertension is an independent modifiable risk factor for the onset and progression of diabetic nephropathy. Glomerular hypertension plays a key role in the pathogenesis of DN even in normotensive diabetic animals, indicating that effectively managing systemic blood pressure without reduction in intraglomerular pressure may not be enough to prevent glomerular injury.[75,76] RAAS blockers are known to reduce both systemic and glomerular hypertension and have a dose-dependent action in reducing proteinuria.

Pronounced RAAS blockade using ACEI and ARBs showed increased adverse events and hyperkalemia.[77,78] Similarly, usage of direct renin inhibitor aliskiren along with combination of ACEI/ARB has been contraindicated following the adverse outcomes noted in ATTITUDE trial.[79] RAAS blockers did not prevent the occurrence of the earliest renal histologic lesions of

DKD.[80] Though RAAS blockers are used as first-line therapy for hypertension in patients with diabetes, marked reduction in the development of DN is less likely. Guidelines do not recommend RAAS blockers in normotensive, normoalbuminuric patients with diabetes, although usage of ACEI and ARBs is suggested in normotensive diabetic patients with microalbuminuria who are at risk for development of DKD in the future.[79]

Nondihydropyridine calcium channel blockers (diltiazem or verapamil) are a better choice, if albuminuria persists along with uncontrolled blood pressure on ACEI/ARB monotherapy.[81] Dihydroxypyridine derivatives and diuretics may be used as add-on agents to achieve blood pressure targets.[79] Aldosterone receptor antagonists such as spironolactone, eplerenone, and finerenone are reported to have renoprotective effects[82-84] but combination with RAAS inhibition found greater risk of hyperkalemia. Stricter BP control is very important and must be continued long term, if the benefits are to be maintained.

Lipid-lowering Therapy

The renoprotective effects of statins in T1DM and T2DM patients with micro- and macroalbuminuria are variable and randomized controlled trials (RCTs) with statistically significant results are lacking. The statin therapies in DN showed reduction in the risk of major atherosclerotic events in CKD stages 1–4 or postrenal transplant patients, but not in patients on maintenance hemodialysis as evidenced in AURORA trial.[85] For patients who are intolerant to higher doses of statins, ezetimibe can be added.[86]

For patients with ESRD, both continuous ambulatory peritoneal dialysis (CAPD) and hemodialysis have similar outcomes and kidney transplantation is an option provided cardiovascular status is good.

Other nonpharmacological measures include cessation of smoking, salt restriction (<6 g/day), and appropriate protein consumption (0.6–0.8 g/kg depending on CKD stage).

Newer Therapies

The suboptimal preventive effect of current medication led to studies testing novel medications for DN, including inhibitors of AGE formation and agents to reduce oxidative stress and inflammation. Many newer agents such as ruboxistaurin, bardoxolone methyl, and sulodexide have shown negative outcomes in RCTs and the role of aldose reductase inhibitors is still unsatisfactory.

Vitamin D receptor activators—findings from phase III VITAL study[87] showed that paricalcitol seems effective only at a high dose (2 μg) and its effect in slowing the progression of CKD is still awaited.

Xanthine oxidase inhibitors and pentoxifylline showed renoprotective benefits in smaller trials, which need to be validated in a larger population.[88,89]

Endothelin receptor antagonists—the ASCEND trial using avosentan was terminated due to increased risk of fluid overload and congestive heart failure, despite its favorable effects of reducing albuminuria.[90] A phase III trial (SONAR) with atrasentan is ongoing, which aims to clarify the cardiovascular and renal protective effects of endothelin receptor antagonists.[90]

5′ adenosine monophosphate-activated protein kinase (AMPK) activators and exogenous Klotho[91] showed renoprotective effects in animals models. Human data is not available.

Stem cell therapy in animal DN models has not yet shown efficacy.[92]

CONCLUSION

Although the recent advances in therapeutic strategy have meaningfully improved outcomes for diabetes complications, these improvements have not translated nearly as well to DN. The ongoing robust researches to explore the unanswered questions may provide new insights on the complex pathogenesis, to facilitate early diagnosis, prevention and tailored intervention to reduce the incidence, and minimize progression, so as to relieve the huge burden of CKD.

REFERENCES

1. Reutens AT. Epidemiology of diabetic kidney disease. Med Clin North Am. 2013;97:1-18.
2. Tuttle KR, Bakris GL, Bilous RW, Chiang JL, de Boer IH, Goldstein-Fuchs J, et al. Diabetic Kidney Disease: A Report From an ADA Consensus Conference. Am J Kidney Dis. 2014;64:510-33.
3. Ahn JH, Yu JH, Ko SH, Kwon HS, Kim DJ, Kim JH, et al. Prevalence and Determinants of Diabetic Nephropathy in Korea: Korea National Health and Nutrition Examination Survey. Diabetes Metab J. 2014;38:109-19.
4. Plantinga LC, Crews DC, Coresh J, Miller ER, Saran R, Yee J, et al. Prevalence of Chronic Kidney Disease in US Adults with Undiagnosed Diabetes or Prediabetes. Clin J Am Soc Nephrol. 2010;5:673-82.
5. Tang SCW, Chan GCW, Lai KN. Recent advances in managing and understanding diabetic nephropathy. F1000Res. 2016;5:F1000.
6. Murussi M, Campagnolo N, Beck MO, Gross JL, Silveiro SP. High-normal levels of albuminuria predict the development of micro- and macroalbuminuria and increased mortality in Brazilian type 2 diabetic patients: an 8-year follow-up study. Diabet Med. 2007;24:1136-42.
7. Targher G, Bertolini L, Rodella S, Zoppini G, Lippi G, Day C, et al. Non-alcoholic fatty liver disease is independently associated with an increased prevalence of chronic kidney disease and proliferative/laser-treated retinopathy in type 2 diabetic patients. Diabetologia. 2008;51:444-50.
8. Seaquist ER, Goetz FC, Rich S, Barbosa J. Familial clustering of diabetic kidney disease. Evidence for genetic susceptibility to diabetic nephropathy. N Engl J Med. 1989;320:1161-5.
9. Freedman BI, Tuttle AB, Spray BJ. Familial predisposition to nephropathy in African-Americans with non-insulin-dependent diabetes mellitus. Am J Kidney Dis. 1995;25:710-3.
10. Alicic RZ, Rooney MT, Tuttle KR. Diabetic Kidney Disease: Challenges, Progress, and Possibilities. Clin J Am Soc Nephrol. 2017;12:2032-45.
11. Lee EY, Kim SS, Lee JS, Kim IJ, Song SH, Cha SK, et al. Soluble α-klotho as a novel biomarker in the early stage of nephropathy in patients with type 2 diabetes. PLoS One. 2014;9:e102984.
12. Karalliedde J, Maltese G, Hill B, Viberti G, Gnudi L. Effect of renin-angiotensin system blockade on soluble Klotho in patients with type 2 diabetes, systolic hypertension, and albuminuria. Clin J Am Soc Nephrol. 2013;8:1899-905.

13. Lim SC, Liu JJ, Subramaniam T, Sum CF. Elevated circulating alpha-klotho by angiotensin II receptor blocker losartan is associated with reduction of albuminuria in type 2 diabetic patients. J Renin Angiotensin Aldosterone Syst. 2011;15:487-90.
14. Bjørn SF, Bangstad HJ, Hanssen KF, Nyberg G, Walker JD, Viberti GC, et al. Glomerular epithelial foot processes and filtration slits in IDDM patients. Diabetologia. 1995;38:1197-204.
15. Meyer TW, Bennett PH, Nelson RG. Podocyte number predicts long-term urinary albumin excretion in Pima Indians with type II diabetes and microalbuminuria. Diabetologia. 1999;42:1341-4.
16. Dalla VM, Masiero A, Roiter AM, Saller A, Crepaldi G, Fioretto P. Is podocyte injury relevant in diabetic nephropathy? Studies in patients with type 2 diabetes. Diabetes. 2003;52:1031-5.
17. Parving HH, Mauer M, Fioretto P, Rossing P, Ritz E. Diabetic nephropathy. In: Brenner BM (Ed). Brenner & Rector's The Kidney, 9th edition. Philadelphia: Elsevier Saunders, Inc.; 2012. pp. 1411-145.
18. Fioretto P, Caramori ML, Mauer M. The kidney in diabetes: dynamic pathways of injury and repair. The Camillo Golgi lecture 2007. Diabetologia. 2008;51:1347-55.
19. Fioretto P, Mauer M, Brocco F, Velussi M, Frigato F, Muollo B, et al. Patterns of renal injury in NIDDM patients with microalbuminuria. Diabetologia. 1996;39:1569-76.
20. Fioretto P, Mauer M. Histopathology of diabetic nephropathy. Semin Nephrol. 2007;27:195-207.
21. Mogensen CE. Early glomerular hyperfiltration in insulin-dependent diabetics and late nephropathy. Scand J Clin Lab Invest. 1986;46:201-6.
22. Magee GM, Bilous RW, Cardwell CR, Hunter SJ, Kee F, Fogarty DG. Is hyperfiltration associated with the future risk of developing diabetic nephropathy? A meta-analysis. Diabetologia. 2009;52:691-7.
23. Chiarelli F, Verrotti A, Morgese G. Glomerular hyperfiltration increases the risk of developing microalbuminuria in diabetic children. Pediatr Nephrol. 1995;9:154-8.
24. Steinke JM, Sinaiko AR, Kramer MS, Suissa S, Chavers BM, Mauer M, et al. The early natural history of nephropathy in Type 1 Diabetes: III. Predictors of 5-year urinary albumin excretion rate patterns in initially normoalbuminuric patients. Diabetes. 2005;54:2164-71.
25. Caramori ML, Gross JL, Pecis M, de Azevedo MJ. Glomerular filtration rate, urinary albumin excretion rate, and blood pressure changes in normoalbuminuric normotensive type 1 diabetic patients: an 8-year follow-up study. Diabetes Care. 1999;22:1512-6.
26. Caramori ML, Fioretto P, Mauer M. Long-term follow-up of normoalbuminuric longstanding type 1 diabetic patients: progression is associated with worse baseline glomerular lesions and lower glomerular filtration rate. J Am Soc Nephrol. 1999;10:126A.
27. Lurbe E, Redon J, Kesani A, Pascual JM, Tacons J, Alvarez V. Increase in nocturnal blood pressure and progression to microalbuminuria in type 1 diabetes. N Engl J Med. 2002;347:797-805.
28. Warram JH, Scott LJ, Hanna LS, Wantman M, Cohen SF, Laffel LM, et al. Progression of microalbuminuria to proteinuria in type 1 diabetes: nonlinear relationship with hyperglycemia. Diabetes. 2000;49:94-100.
29. de Boer IH, Rue TC, Cleary PA, Lachin JM, Molitch ME, Steffes MW, et al. Long-term renal outcomes of patients with type 1 diabetes mellitus and microalbuminuria: an analysis of the Diabetes Control and Complications Trial/Epidemiology of Diabetes Interventions and Complications cohort. Arch Intern Med. 2011;171:412-20.
30. Hovind P, Tarnow L, Rossing P, Jensen BR, Graae M, Torp I, et al. Predictors for the development of microalbuminuria and macroalbuminuria in patients with type 1 diabetes: inception cohort study. Br Med J. 2004;328:1105-8.
31. McKenna K, Thompson C. Microalbuminuria: a marker to increased renal and cardiovascular risk in diabetes mellitus. Scott Med J. 1997;42:99-104.
32. Zoppini G, Targher G, Chonchol M, Ortalda V, Negri C, Stoico V, et al. Predictors of estimated GFR decline in patients with type 2 diabetes and preserved kidney function. Clin J Am Soc Nephrol. 2012;7:401-8.
33. Kuboki K, Tada H, Shin K, Oshima Y, Isogai S. Relationship between urinary excretion of fibronectin degradation products and proteinuria in diabetic patients, and their suppression after continuous subcutaneous heparin infusion. Diabetes Res Clin Pract. 1993;21:61-6.
34. Schmidt-Ott KM, Mori K, Li JY, Kalandadze A, Cohen DJ, Devarajan P, et al. Dual action of neutrophil gelatinase-associated lipocalin. J Am Soc Nephrol. 2007;18:407-13.
35. American Diabetes Association. Microvascular Complications and Foot Care: Standards of Medical Care in Diabetes—2021. Diabetes Care. 2021;44:S151-67.

37. Eknoyan G, Hostetter T, Bakris GL, Hebert L, Levey AS, Parving HH, et al. Proteinuria and other markers of chronic kidney disease: a position statement of the National Kidney Foundation (NKF) and the National Institute of Diabetes and Digestive and Kidney Diseases (NIDDK). Am J Kidney Dis. 2003;42:617-22.
38. KDIGO. Chapter 2: definition, identification, and prediction of CKD progression. Kidney Int Suppl. 2013;3:63-72.
39. Levey AS, Bosch JP, Lewis JB, Greene T, Rogers N, Roth D. A more accurate method to estimate glomerular filtration rate from serum creatinine: a new prediction equation. Modification of Diet in Renal Disease Study Group. Ann Intern Med. 1999;130:461-70.
40. Lee CS, Cha RH, Lim YH, Kim H, Song KH, Gu N, et al. Ethnic coefficients for glomerular filtration rate estimation by the Modification of Diet in Renal Disease study equations in the Korean population. J Korean Med Sci. 2010;25:1616-25.
41. Levey AS, Stevens LA, Schmid CH, Zhang YL, Castro AF, Feldman HI, et al. A new equation to estimate glomerular filtration rate. Ann Intern Med. 2009;150:604-12.
42. Chudleigh RA, Dunseath G, Evans W, Harvey JN, Evans P, Ollerton R, et al. How reliable is estimation of glomerular filtration rate at diagnosis of type 2 diabetes? Diabetes Care. 2007;30:300-5.
43. Knight EL, Verhave JC, Spiegelman D, Hillege HL, de Zeeuw D, Curhan GC, et al. Factors influencing serum cystatin C levels other than renal function and the impact on renal function measurement. Kidney Int. 2004;65:1416-21.
44. Mussap M, Vestra DM, Fioretto P, Saller A, Varagnolo M, Nosadini R, et al. Cystatin C is a more sensitive marker than creatinine for the estimation of GFR in type 2 diabetic patients. Kidney Int. 2002;61: 1453-61.
45. Barratt J, Topham P. Urine proteomics: the present and future of measuring urinary protein components in disease. CMAJ. 2007;177:361-8.
46. MacIsaac RJ, Tsalamandris C, Panagiotopoulos S, Smith TJ, McNeil KJ, Jerums G. Nonalbuminuric renal insufficiency in type 2 diabetes. Diabetes Care. 2004;27:195-200.
47. Kamijo-Ikemori A, Sugaya T, Kimura K. Novel urinary biomarkers in early diabetic kidney disease. Curr Diab Rep. 2014;14:513.
48. Nauta FL, Boertien WE, Bakker SJ, van Goor H, van Oeveren W, de Jong PE, et al. Glomerular and tubular damage markers are elevated in patients with diabetes. Diabetes Care. 2011;34:975-81.
49. Jeon YK, Kim MR, Huh JE, Mok JY, Song SH, Kim SS, et al. Cystatin C as an early biomarker of nephropathy in patients with type 2 diabetes. J Korean Med Sci. 2011;26:258-63.
50. Kim SS, Song SH, Kim IJ, Yang JY, Lee JG, Kwak IS, et al. Clinical implication of urinary tubular markers in the early stage of nephropathy with type 2 diabetic patients. Diabetes Res Clin Pract. 2012;97: 251-7.
51. Matheson A, Willcox MD, Flanagan J, Walsh BJ. Urinary biomarkers involved in type 2 diabetes: a review. Diabetes Metab Res Rev. 2010;26:150-71.
52. Ballantyne FC, Gibbons J, O'Reilly DS. Urine albumin should replace total protein for the assessment of glomerular proteinuria. Ann Clin Biochem. 1993;30:101-3.
53. Halimi JM, Matthias B, Al-Najjar A, Laouad I, Chatelet V, Marliere JF, et al. Respective predictive role of urinary albumin excretion and nonalbumin proteinuria on graft loss and death in renal transplant recipients. Am J Transplant. 2007;7:2775-81.
54. Kim SS, Song SH, Kim IJ, Kim WJ, Jeon YK, Kim BH, et al. Nonalbuminuric proteinuria as a biomarker for tubular damage in early development of nephropathy with type 2 diabetic patients. Diabetes Metab Res Rev. 2014;30:736-41.
55. Kim SS, Song SH, Kim IJ, Jeon YK, Kim BH, Kwak IS, et al. Urinary cystatin C and tubular proteinuria predict progression of diabetic nephropathy. Diabetes Care. 2013;36:656-61.
56. Lioudaki E, Stylianou KG, Petrakis I, Kokologiannakis G, Passam A, Mikhailidis DP, et al. Increased urinary excretion of podocyte markers in normoalbuminuric patients with diabetes. Nephron. 2015;131:34-42.
57. Banu N, Hara H, Okamura M, Egusa G, Yamakido M. Urinary excretion of type IV collagen and laminin in the evaluation of nephropathy in NIDDM: comparison with urinary albumin and markers of tubular dysfunction and/or damage. Diabetes Res Clin Pract. 1995;29:57-67.
58. Kubisz P, Stanciaková L, Stâsko J, Galajda P, Mokán M. Endothelial and platelet markers in diabetes mellitus type 2. World J Diabetes. 2015;6:423-31.

59. Tramonti G, Kanwar YS. Tubular biomarkers to assess progression of diabetic nephropathy. Kidney Int. 2011;79:1042-4.
60. Terami T, Wada J, Inoue K, Nakatsuka A, Ogawa D, Teshigawara S, et al. Urinary angiotensinogen is a marker for tubular injuries in patients with type 2 diabetes. Int J Nephrol Renovasc Dis. 2013;6:233-40.
61. Eriguchi M, Yotsueda R, Torisu K, Kawai Y, Hasegawa S, Tanaka S, et al. Assessment of urinary angiotensinogen as a marker of podocyte injury in proteinuric nephropathies. Am J Physiol Renal Physiol. 2016;310:F322-33.
62. Gluhovschi C, Gluhovschi G, Petrica L, Timar R, Velciov S, Ionita I, et al. Urinary Biomarkers in the Assessment of Early Diabetic Nephropathy. J Diabetes Res. 2016;2016:4626125.
63. Kim SS, Kim JH, Kim IJ. Current Challenges in Diabetic Nephropathy: Early Diagnosis and Ways to Improve Outcomes. Endocrinol Metab Seoul Korea. 2016;31:245-53.
64. Effect of intensive therapy on the development and progression of diabetic nephropathy in the Diabetes Control and Complications Trial. The Diabetes Control and Complications (DCCT) Research Group. Kidney Int. 1995;47:1703-20.
65. Intensive blood-glucose control with sulphonylureas or insulin compared with conventional treatment and risk of complications in patients with type 2 diabetes (UKPDS 33). UK Prospective Diabetes Study (UKPDS) Group. Lancet Lond Engl. 1998;352:837-53.
66. Writing Team for the Diabetes Control and Complications Trial/Epidemiology of Diabetes Interventions and Complications Research Group. Sustained effect of intensive treatment of type 1 diabetes mellitus on development and progression of diabetic nephropathy: the Epidemiology of Diabetes Interventions and Complications (EDIC) study. JAMA. 2003;290:2159-67.
67. Ismail-Beigi F, Craven T, Banerji MA, Basile J, Calles J, Cohen RM, et al. Effect of intensive treatment of hyperglycaemia on microvascular outcomes in type 2 diabetes: an analysis of the ACCORD randomised trial. Lancet Lond Engl. 2010;376:419-30.
68. ADVANCE Collaborative Group, Patel A, MacMahon S, Chalmers J, Neal B, Billot L, et al. Intensive blood glucose control and vascular outcomes in patients with type 2 diabetes. N Engl J Med. 2008; 358:2560-72.
69. Duckworth W, Abraira C, Moritz T, Reda D, Emanuele N, Reaven PD, et al. Glucose control and vascular complications in veterans with type 2 diabetes. N Engl J Med. 2009;360:129-39.
70. Fioretto P, Steffes MW, Sutherland DE, Goetz FC, Mauer M. Reversal of lesions of diabetic nephropathy after pancreas transplantation. N Engl J Med. 1998;339:69-75.
71. Marso SP, Daniels GH, Brown-Frandsen K, Kristensen P, Mann JFE, Nauck MA, et al. Liraglutide and Cardiovascular Outcomes in Type 2 Diabetes. N Engl J Med. 2016;375:311-22.
72. Marso SP, Daniels GH, Brown-Frandsen K, Kristensen P, Mann JFE, Nauck MA, et al. Liraglutide and cardiovascular outcomes in type 2 diabetes. N Engl J Med. 2016;375:311-22.
73. Wanner C, Inzucchi SE, Lachin JM, EMPA-REG OUTCOME Investigators. Empagliflozin and progression of kidney disease in type 2 diabetes. N Engl J Med. 2016;375:323-34.
74. Selby NM, Taal MW. An updated overview of diabetic nephropathy: diagnosis, prognosis, treatment goals and latest guidelines. Diabetes Obes Metab. 2020;22:3-15.
75. Anderson S, Rennke HG, Garcia DL, Brenner BM. Short and long term effects of antihypertensive therapy in the diabetic rat. Kidney Int. 1989;36:526-36.
76. Flyihara CK, Padilha RM, Zatz R. Glomerular abnormalities in long-term experimental diabetes. Diabetes. 1992;41:286-93.
77. Kunz R, Friedrich C, Wolbers M, Mann JF. Meta-analysis: effect of monotherapy and combination therapy with inhibitors of the renin angiotensin system on proteinuria in renal disease. Ann Intern Med. 2008;148:30-48.
78. Mann JFE, Schmieder RE, McQueen M, Dyal L, Schumacher H, Pogue J, et al. Renal outcomes with telmisartan, ramipril, or both, in people at high vascular risk (the ONTARGET study): a multicentre, randomised, double-blind, controlled trial. Lancet. 2008;372:547-53.
79. National Kidney Foundation. KDOQI clinical practice guideline for diabetes and CKD: 2012 update. Am J Kidney Dis. 2012;60:850-86.
80. Mauer M, Zinman B, Gardiner R, Suissa S, Sinaiko A, Strand T, et al. Renal and retinal effects of enalapril and losartan in type 1 diabetes. N Engl J Med. 2009;361:40-51.

81. Balakumar P, Arora MK, Ganti SS, Reddy J, Singh M. Recent advances in pharmacotherapy for diabetic nephropathy: current perspectives and future directions. Pharmacol Res. 2009;60:24-32.
82. Epstein M, Williams GH, Weinberger M, Lewin A, Krause S, Mukherjee R, et al. Selective aldosterone blockade with eplerenone reduces albuminuria in patients with type 2 diabetes. Clin J Am Soc Nephrol. 2006;1:940-51.
83. Navaneethan SD, Nigwekar SU, Sehgal AR, Strippoli GFM. Aldosterone Antagonists for Preventing the Progression of Chronic Kidney Disease: A Systematic Review and Meta-analysis. Clin J Am Soc Nephrol. 2009;4:542-51.
84. Bakris GL, Agarwal R, Chan JC, Cooper ME, Gansevoort RT, Haller H, et al. Effect of Finerenone on Albuminuria in Patients With Diabetic Nephropathy: A Randomized Clinical Trial. JAMA. 2015;314: 884-94.
85. Holdaas H, Holme I, Schmieder RE, Jardine AG, Zannad F, Norby GE, et al. Rosuvastatin in diabetic hemodialysis patients. J Am Soc Nephrol. 2011;22:1335-41.
86. Baigent C, Landray MJ, Reith C, Emberson J, Wheeler DC, Tomson C, et al. The effects of lowering LDL cholesterol with simvastatin plus ezetimibe in patients with chronic kidney disease (Study of Heart and Renal Protection): a randomised placebo-controlled trial. Lancet Lond Engl. 2011;377:2181-92.
87. Coyne DW, Andress DL, Amdahl MJ, Ritz E, de Zeeuw D. Effects of paricalcitol on calcium and phosphate metabolism and markers of bone health in patients with diabetic nephropathy: results of the VITAL study. Nephrol Dial Transplant. 2013;28:2260-8.
88. Sircar D, Chatterjee S, Waikhom R, Golay V, Raychaudhury A, Chatterjee S, et al. Efficacy of Febuxostat for Slowing the GFR Decline in Patients With CKD and Asymptomatic Hyperuricemia: A 6-Month, Double-Blind, Randomized, Placebo-Controlled Trial. Am J Kidney Dis. 2015;66:945-50.
89. Mann JFE, Green D, Jamerson K, Ruilope LM, Kuranoff SJ, Littke T, et al. Avosentan for overt diabetic nephropathy. J Am Soc Nephrol. 2010;21:527-35.
90. Schievink B, de Zeeuw D, Smink PA, Andress D, Brennan JJ, Coll B, et al. Prediction of the effect of atrasentan on renal and heart failure outcomes based on short-term changes in multiple risk markers. Eur J Prev Cardiol. 2016;23:758-68.
91. Deng M, Luo Y, Li Y, Yang Q, Deng X, Wu P, et al. Klotho gene delivery ameliorates renal hypertrophy and fibrosis in streptozotocin-induced diabetic rats by suppressing the Rho-associated coiled-coil kinase signaling pathway. Mol Med Rep. 2015;12:45-54.
92. Ezquer F, Giraud-Billoud M, Carpio D, Cabezas F, Conget P, Ezquer M. Proregenerative Microenvironment Triggered by Donor Mesenchymal Stem Cells Preserves Renal Function and Structure in Mice with Severe Diabetes Mellitus. BioMed Res Int. 2015;2015:164703.

CHAPTER 8

Vascular Involvement of the Skin in Diabetes

Vidya D Kharkar, Nitya SN Malladi, Sujatha RL Malladi, GR Sridhar

ABSTRACT

Diabetes is a common metabolic disorder leading to disability and death. Involvement of the skin in diabetes is often related to superficial and deep-seated infections and signs of insulin resistance. Attention is not given to other related and important changes in the vasculature: Vascular endothelial cells are damaged. They cause reduction of skin blood flow, altered thermoregulation, and abnormal response to skin pressure. It is also damaged easily due to easy occlusion of skin circulation. The reaction to locally applied skin pressure as in standing is also altered. The ability to sweat is reduced and leads to increased body temperature when the whole body is heated. The exercise performance is impaired due to organ damage. Impaired vascular endothelial function is a common factor in many of the diabetic complications.

Keywords: *Nitric oxide, Reactive oxidative species, Microcirculation, Videocapillaroscopy.*

INTRODUCTION

Diabetes is increasing globally and particularly so in developing countries from the Asian continent due to a variety of factors.[1-4]

The vascular lumen is covered by a single cell layer, the endothelium. Forming a barrier between blood and the tissues, it has a key role in maintaining vascular homeostasis.[5,6] It helps to control tissue blood flow, maintains fluidity of blood, and also responses to inflammation.[7-9]

Equilibrium between vasoconstriction and vasodilatation is maintained by the endothelium. It also has a role in thrombogenesis and fibrinolysis and regulates platelet aggregation and adhesion.[10] Dysfunction results, if this finely regulated balance is disturbed.

ETIOPATHOGENESIS OF VASCULAR INVOLVEMENT IN DIABETES

The alterations of cutaneous microvessels constitute the earliest manifestations of diabetes. The cells of endothelium and smooth muscle of the walls of blood vessels get metabolically altered by chronic hyperglycemia. Permeability and contractility are impaired, modifying the hemodynamics leading to ectasia and microaneurysms result.[11]

Role of Nitric Oxide

Endothelial cells synthesize nitric oxide (NO), which has a pivotal role in vascular homeostasis. An enzyme, endothelial nitric oxide synthase (eNOS), helps to synthesize NO in the endothelium.[12] Circulating substances such as serotonin and bradykinin elicit shear stress and endothelial cells release NO in response.[13]

Microcirculatory blood flow is tuned by NO.[14] Endothelial dysfunction results if eNOS expression is reduced or NO is not bioavailable.[15-17]

Insulin modulates activity of eNOS. In people having insulin resistance, vasodilatation is impaired. Insulin sensitivity is principally regulated by eNOS.[18-20]

Endothelial Dysfunction

There is a functional alteration in the endothelium in the early stages, which is observed in type 2 diabetes mellitus (T2DM) and insulin resistance.[18] Lack of bioavailable NO is the major feature of endothelial dysfunction. Some other features of this dysfunction are deregulation of hemodynamics, increase of reactive oxygen species (ROS) generation, oxidative stress, and cell layer permeability.[21-25]

Impact of Diabetes on the Vasculature

Etiopathogenesis of endothelial dysfunction could vary between type 1 diabetes mellitus (T1DM) and T2DM;[26] T2DM is clinically diagnosed a few years after endothelial dysfunction begins.[27] The circulating excess glucose and insulin resistance along with the increased release of free fatty acids (FFAs) in diabetes triggers a cascade of changes in the walls of the vessels. Endothelial function is compromised and risk predisposing to inflammation, vasoconstriction, and thrombosis.[28,29]

Hyperglycemia

Prolonged and acute transient hyperglycemia impairs endothelial function in both macro- and microvascular beds.[30-32] The effect of intensive glycemic control on the prevention of microvascular complications has been more directly demonstrated than on macrovascular disease.[33]

Reactive oxygen species is produced by oxidative stress due to hyperglycemia, which triggers damage to DNA and activates enzymes such as poly (ADP-ribose) polymerase (PARP). Intermediates of glycolytic pathway accumulate and damaging mechanisms get activated. Vascular permeability and oxidative stress also get increased.[34,35]

Accelerated formation of multiple biochemical species under hyperglycemic conditions greatly contribute to endothelial dysfunction. The increased oxidative stress is the common alteration triggered by a T2DM. Hyperglycemia is a recognized component of metabolic syndrome.[36]

Insulin Resistance

Insulin resistance is the impaired insulin ability to increase glucose uptake in tissues and to reduce glucose output by the liver.[37] Endothelial dysfunction results from increased inflammatory markers such as tumor necrosis factor-α (TNF-α) and interleukin-6 in the serum.[38]

Free Fatty Acids

Increased circulatory levels of FFAs occur in diabetes due to their release from adipose tissue along with reduced uptake by skeletal muscles.[39,40] Hyperglycemia is associated with increased levels of proinflammatory cytokines and ROS leading to vascular dysfunction.[41-45]

Oxidative Stress

Oxidative stress results from the overproduction of ROS such as superoxide anion, NO, and lipid radicals, while natural antioxidant mechanisms are overwhelmed.[46,47]

Some of the important antioxidants in the endothelium are direct scavengers of ROS such as vitamin C (ascorbic acid), vitamin E (α-tocopherol), glutathione, thioredoxins, superoxide dismutase (SOD), and glutathione peroxidase.[48-50] SODs are primarily important to neutralize ROS. Studies on gene transfer have revealed that endothelial function is improved by overexpression of SOD.[51,52]

There are, thus, many risk factors, which contribute to endothelial dysfunction.[53-56]

SKIN MICROVASCULATURE AS A PARADIGM FOR DIABETIC MICROANGIOPATHY

The components of microcirculation are arteries measuring about 150 μm in diameter, venules, arterioles, and capillaries.[57] Capillaries are responsible for exchange of gases and nutrients, whereas arterioles principally regulate the flow of blood. Vascular smooth muscle cells lie adjacent to vascular endothelium, which release mediators of relaxation and contraction of vessels. As mentioned earlier, NO is a strong vasodilator and is regulated by ROS.

Abnormalities in microvasculature in subjects can occur as a result of both endothelium-dependent and endothelium-independent pathways.[58,59] Studies have shown that microvascular dysfunction leads to higher prevalence of diabetes mellitus as a result of impaired recruitment of capillaries leading to insulin resistance and pancreatic β-cell apoptosis due to microvascular dysfunction in pancreas.[57]

Being accessible, skin microcirculation has been proposed to represent general microvascular function.[60] Endothelial dysfunction consists of impaired endothelium-dependent vasodilation, increased vasoconstriction, and structural remodeling of microvascular structure simultaneously in many vascular beds.[60] Studies have suggested that function of skin microvasculature in diabetes could be a marker of cardiovascular dysfunction and end-stage renal disease.[61,62] Therefore, vasculature of the skin is an accessible correlate for markers of cardiovascular disease.[57]

Noninvasive Assessment of Skin Microvasculature

In view of the cutaneous microvasculature, being a surrogate for status of microvessels in the body, a number of noninvasive technologies have been developed to study them such as optimal microscopy, laser Doppler, capillaroscopy, orthogonal polarization spectral imaging and sidestream dark field imaging.[63]

STUDIES IN SUBJECTS WITH DIABETES

Considering the critical role of microvascular control by local interplay of endothelium, nerves, and myocytes, any imbalance can lead to impaired tissue function and, thereby, diabetic complications.[64] Dysfunction of local motion activity can lead to impaired microvascular blood flow and poor tissue oxygenation, thus providing evidence for abnormalities in the regulatory function of microvasculature. Jonasson et al. evaluated microcirculatory function in T2DM subjects with and without microalbuminuria. Reduced nutritional perfusion and red cell tissue fraction in diabetes were related to long-term glycemic control that was independent of renal microvascular changes.[65]

VISUALIZING THE SKIN VASCULATURE IN DIABETES BY VIDEOCAPILLAROSCOPY

Capillaroscopy is a method to study the morphological and functional abnormalities of the microcirculation. Videocapillaroscopy is indicated in all diseases whose pathogenesis recognizes anatomical and/or functional abnormalities in microcirculation.[3]

Nailfold videocapillaroscopy (NVC) is one of the best diagnostic noninvasive imaging techniques to evaluate microcirculation in vivo.[66,67] It is applied to the study of rheumatic and many extra rheumatic diseases such as arterial hypertension, diabetes mellitus, and psoriasis, among others.

The advantages of capillaroscopy are that it is noninvasive with good sensitivity and specificity. Besides, it is easy to perform and is not time-consuming. Capillary abnormalities are observed in diabetes mellitus.

In NVC, the nail bed is utilized to study microvessels due to its easy approach with the probe. Valuable images can be easily obtained as the capillary vessels of the nail bed are parallel to cutaneous vessels. The fourth and fifth fingers of the nondominant hand enable clear visualization of the nailfold capillaries. NVC helps to evaluate: (a) Architecture of capillary vessels, (b) Number and distribution of the vessels, and (c) Capillary inflow and outflow.

The normal pattern of capillary vessels is as follows (**Fig. 1**):

- Hairpin appearance
- Small vessels distributed regularly and are homogeneous
- One dermal papilla contains one to three capillary vessels
- Arterial border blood column diameter is from 5 to 16 microns
- Venule border blood column diameter is from 7 to 18 microns

A typical "diabetic pattern" of NVC is not yet fully described. It detects some features of diabetic microangiopathy such as a homogeneous increase in capillary diameter (especially at the venous limb level) and convoluted loops

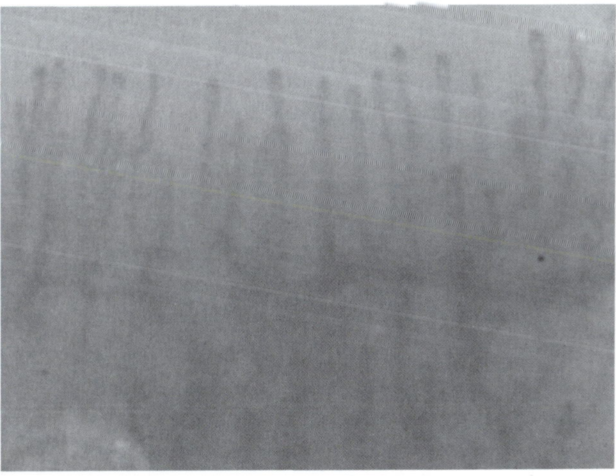

FIG. 1: Normal pattern of capillary vessels. ***(For color version, see Plate 1)***

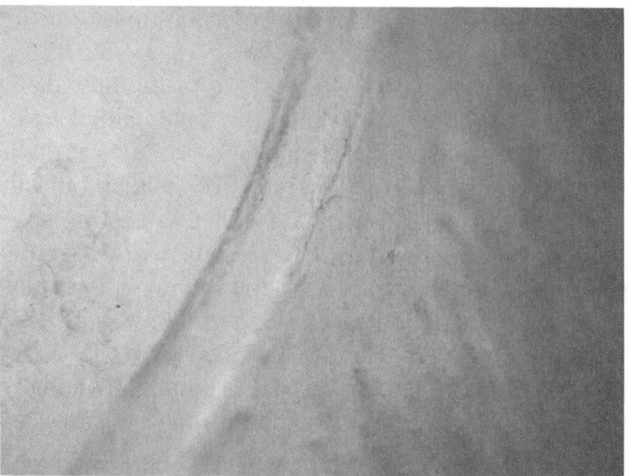

FIG. 2: Tortuous and enlarged capillaries in diabetes. ***(For color version, see Plate 1)***

Studies have evaluated the morphology and density of nailfold capillaries in patients with T1DM and T2DM and in healthy controls by means of videocapillaroscopy.[68-70]

The capillaries were more enlarged and tortuous in diabetes (**Fig. 2**). Nodular apical elongation is seen in long duration of diabetes, especially in the presence of clinical complications in T2DM.[71]

"Shoal of fish" appearance and "elephant nose" appearance of the capillary: Where the diameter increases more than five times.

Ischemic capillary response changes are seen in diabetes. There is no significantly different maximum area in increments, but takes longer to reach reperfusion.[72]

Nailfold videocapillaroscopy is a simple noninvasive procedure, which has acquired a diagnostic and prognostic role.

The cutaneous microvascular function can also be noninvasively examined using provocation protocols such as hyperemic responses to iontophoresis of acetylcholine and sodium nitroprusside, local heating, and vascular occlusion.

STUDIES OF SKIN VASCULATURE IN FOOT AMONG SUBJECTS WITH DIABETES

A pilot study was carried out on the microvascular perfusion of soles of the feet (n = 16 with diabetes; n = 23 with controls). Employing laser Doppler flowmetry following noninvasive provocation and power spectral densities was calculated using wavelet transform. Subjects with diabetes showed lower PSD_{ENDO1} (power spectral densities corresponding to endothelial NO-independent metabolic activities) and PSD_{ENDO2} compared to control, suggesting peripheral endothelial dysfunction in diabetes.[73] This method can identify early microvascular changes before the onset of diabetic ulcers, which can be predicted by edge detection methods.[74]

Infrared thermography has also been employed to identify the foot in subjects with diabetes mellitus. It can visualize the spatial and temporal patterns of surface temperature by capturing infrared energy that is radiated from the skin. It does not image the structure, but only the radiated energy. The advantages of infrared thermography consist in being carried out even with poor illumination over a wider area in the absence of any harmful radiation.[75] The study was carried out in 62 subjects with diabetes without active foot involvement and 20 controls. Using neural network analysis, it was possible to classify outputs from test image in identifying a foot without complication with a probability of 87.4%.

A related study investigated how reliable infrared thermography was in determining temperature of the foot skin; additionally, it also evaluated the relation of blood flow and skin temperatures in persons with T2DM. In a cohort of 85 subjects with T2DM, it was observed that the reliability of test-retest in foot skin temperature was high.[76]

CONCLUSION

Endothelial dysfunction disturbs the body homeostasis. This causes many pathophysiological conditions including diabetes. For prevention of vascular complications associated with all forms of diabetes mellitus, it becomes essential to manage endothelial dysfunction. NVC is one of the best diagnostic noninvasive imaging techniques to evaluate microcirculation and identify microvascular involvement in diabetes. Recent studies indicate that the skin and kidney microvascular functions may be affected independently in diabetes mellitus.[65]

Simultaneous decrease of hyperglycemia and insulin resistance is essential to mitigate the adverse effects leading to diabetic vasculopathy. Control of risk factors causing inflammation and oxidative stress and therapy that target intracellular mechanisms underlying metabolic changes becomes the keystone of management of diabetes mellitus.

REFERENCES

1. Bommer C, Sagalova V, Heesemann E, Manne-Goehler J, Atun R, Bärnighausen T, et al. Global Economic Burden of Diabetes in Adults: Projections From 2015 to 2030. Diabetes Care. 2018;41:963-70.
2. Cho NH,, Shaw JE, Karuranga S, Huang Y, da Rocha Fernandes JD, Ohlrogge AW, et al. IDF Diabetes Atlas: Global estimates of diabetes prevalence for 2017 and projections for 2045. Diab Res Clin Pract. 2018;138:271-81.
3. Zheng Y, Ley SH, Hu FB. Global aetiology and epidemiology of type 2 diabetes mellitus and its complications. Nat Rev Endocrinol. 2018;14:88-98.
4. Contreras F. Diabetes and hypertension: physiopathology and therapeutics. J Hum Hypertens. 2000;14:S26 31.

5. Vallance P. Importance of asymmetrical dimethylarginine in cardiovascular risk. Lancet. 2001;358: 2096-7.
6. Bonetti PO, Lerman LO, Lerman A. Endothelial dysfunction: a marker of atherosclerotic risk. Arterioscler Thromb Vasc Biol. 2003;23:168-75.
7. Chen G, Suzuki H, Weston AH. Acetylcholine releases endothelium-derived hyperpolarizing factor and EDRF from rat blood vessels. Br J Pharmacol. 1985;95:1165-74.
8. Palmer RM, Ferrige AG, Moncada S. Nitric oxide release accounts for the biological activity of endothelium-derived relaxing factor. Nature. 1987;327:524-6.
9. Ignarro LJ, Buga GM, Wood KS, Byrns RE, Chaudhuri G. Endothelium-derived relaxing factor produced and released from artery and vein is nitric oxide. Proc Natl Acad Sci U S A. 1987;84:9265-9.
10. Félétou M. The Endothelium: Part 1: Multiple Functions of the Endothelial Cells—Focus on Endothelium-derived Vasoactive Mediators. San Rafael (CA): Morgan & Claypool Life Sciences; 2011.
11. Romano C, Costa M, Messina M, Bertini M. Videocapillaroscopy in diabetes. Diabetes Res Open J. 2015;1:e3-6.
12. Vallance P, Chan N. Endothelial function and nitric oxide: clinical relevance. Heart. 2001;85:342-50.
13. Boulanger C, Luscher TF. Release of endothelin from the porcine aorta: inhibition by endothelium-derived nitric oxide. J Clin Invest. 1990;85:587-90.
14. Datta B, Tufnell-Barrett T, Bleasdale RA, Jones CJ, Beeton I, Paul V, et al. Red blood cell nitric oxide as an endocrine vasoregulator: a potential role in congestive heart failure. Circulation. 2004;109:1339-42.
15. Oemar BS, Tschudi MR, Godoy N, Brovkovich V, Malinski T, Luscher TF. Reduced endothelial nitric oxide synthase expression and production in human atherosclerosis. Circulation. 1998;97:2494-8.
16. Sena CM, Nunes E, Louro T, Proença T, Fernandes R, Boarder MR, et al. Effects of alpha-lipoic acid on endothelial function in aged diabetic and high-fat fed rats. Br J Pharmacol. 2008;153:894-906.
17. Muniyappa R, Montagnani M, Koh KK, Quon MJ. Cardiovascular actions of insulin. Endocrine. 2007;28:463-91.
18. Wheatcroft SB, Williams IL, Shah AM, Kearney MT. Pathophysiological implications of insulin resistance on vascular endothelial function. Diabet Med. 2003;20:255-68.
19. Cleland SJ, Petrie JR, Small M, Elliott HL, Connell JM. Insulin action is associated with endothelial function in hypertension and type 2 diabetes. Hypertension. 2000;35:507-11.
20. Vincent MA, Barrett EJ, Lindner JR, Clark MG, Rattigan S. Inhibiting NOS blocks microvascular recruitment and blunts muscle glucose uptake in response to insulin. Am J Physiol Endocrinol Metab. 2003;285:E123-9.
21. Taddei S, Ghiadoni L, Virdis A, Versari D, Salvetti A. Mechanisms of endothelial dysfunction: clinical significance and preventive non-pharmacological therapeutic strategies. Curr Pharm. 2003;9: 2385-402.
22. Laughlin MH, Newcomer SC, Bender SB. Importance of hemodynamic forces as signals for exercise-induced changes in endothelial cell phenotype. J Appl Physiol. 2008;104:588-600.
23. Cade WT. Diabetes-related microvascular and macrovascular diseases in the physical therapy setting. Phys Ther. 2008;88:322-35.
24. Addabbo F, Montagnani M, Goligorsky MS. Mitochondria and reactive oxygen species. Hypertension. 2009;53:885-92.
25. Hirose A, Tanikawa T, Mori H, Okada Y, Tanaka Y. Advanced glycation end products increase endothelial permeability through the RAGE/Rho signaling pathway, FEBS Lett. 2010;584:61-6.
26. Singh DK, Winocour P, Farrington K. Endothelial cell dysfunction, medial arterial calcification and osteoprotegerin in diabetes. Br J Diabetes Vasc Dis. 2010;10:71-7.
27. Highlander P, Shaw GP. Current pharmacotherapeutic concepts for the treatment of cardiovascular disease in diabetics. Therap Adv Cardiovasc Dis. 2010;4:43-54.
28. Beckman JA, Creager MA, Libby P. Diabetes and atherosclerosis: epidemiology, pathophysiology, and management. JAMA. 2002;15:2570-81.
29. Nesto RW. Correlation between cardiovascular disease and diabetes mellitus: current concepts. Am J Med. 2004;116:11S-22.
30. Riccardo C, Stella B, Terri JA. Linking diabetes and atherosclerosis. Exp Rev Endocrinol Metab. 2009;4:603-24.

31. Ceriello A. Point: postprandial glucose levels are a clinically important treatment target. Diabetes Care. 2010;33:1905-7.
32. Grassi D, Desideri G, Necozione S, Ruggieri F, Blumberg JB, Stornello M, et al. Protective effects of flavanol-rich dark chocolate on endothelial function and wave reflection during acute hyperglycemia. Hypertension. 2021;60:827-32.
33. Skyler JS, Bergenstal R, Bonow RO, Buse J, Deedwania P, Gale EAM, et al. Intensive glycemic control and the prevention of cardiovascular events: implications of the ACCORD, ADVANCE, and VA diabetes trials: a position statement of the American Diabetes Association and a scientific statement of the American College of Cardiology Foundation and the American Heart Association. Circulation. 2009;119:351-7.
34. Brownlee M. Biochemistry and molecular cell biology of diabetic complications. Nature. 2001;414:813-20.
35. Brownlee M. The pathobiology of diabetes complications: a unifying mechanism. Diabetes. 2005;54:1615-25.
36. Potenza MA, Gagliardi S, Nacci C, Carratu MR, Montagnani M. Endothelial dysfunction in diabetes: from mechanisms to therapeutic targets. Curr Med Chem. 2009;16:94-112.
37. Reaven GM. Banting lecture 1988. Role of insulin resistance in human disease. Diabetes. 1988;37:1595-607.
38. Natali A, Toschi E, Baldeweg S, Ciociaro D, Favilla S, Saccà L, et al. Clustering of insulin resistance with vascular dysfunction and low-grade inflammation in type 2 diabetes. Diabetes. 2006;55:1133-40.
39. Kawashima S, Yokoyama M. Dysfunction of endothelial nitric oxide synthase and atherosclerosis. Arterioscler Thromb Vasc Biol. 2004;24:998-1005.
40. Dresner A, Laurent D, Marcucci M, Griffin ME, Dufour S, Cline GW, et al. Effects of freefatty acids on glucose transport and IRS-1-associated phosphatidylinositol 3-kinase activity. J Clin Invest. 1999;103:253-9.
41. Boden G, She P, Mozzoli M, Cheung P, Gumireddy K, Reddy P, et al. Free fatty acids produce insulin resistance and activate the proinflammatory nuclear factor-kappa B pathway in rat liver. Diabetes. 2005;54:3458-65.
42. Gao Z, Zhang X, Zuberi A, Hwang D, Quon MJ, Lefevre M, et al. Inhibition of insulin sensitivity by free fatty acids requires activation of multiple serine kinases in 3T3-L1 adipocytes. Mol Endocrinol. 2004;18:2024-34.
43. Jove M, Planavila A, Sanchez RM, Merlos M, Laguna JC, Vazquez-Carrera M. Palmitate induces tumor necrosis factor-alpha expression in C2C12 skeletal muscle cells by a mechanism involving protein kinase C and nuclear factor-kappa B activation. Endocrinology. 2006;147:552-61.
44. Du X, Edelstein D, Obici S, Higham N, Zou MH, Brownlee M. Insulin resistance reduces arterial prostacyclin synthase and eNOS activities by increasing endothelial fatty acid oxidation. J Clin Invest. 2006;116:1071-80.
45. Giacco F, Brownlee M. Oxidative stress and diabetic complications. Circ Res. 2010;107:1058-70.
46. Cai H, Harrison DG. Endothelial dysfunction in cardiovascular diseases: the role of oxidant stress. Circ Res. 2000;87:840-4.
47. Harrison D, Griendling KK, Landmesser U, Hornig B, Drexler H. Role of oxidative stress in atherosclerosis. Am J Cardiol. 2003;91:7A-11.
48. Li JM, Shah AM. Endothelial cell superoxide generation: regulation and relevance for cardiovascular pathophysiology. Am J Physiol Regul Integr Comp Physiol. 2004;287:R1014-30.
49. Leopold JA, Loscalzo J. Oxidative enzymopathies and vascular disease. Arterioscler Thromb Vasc Biol. 2005;25:1332-40.
50. Maulik N, Das DK. Emerging potential of thioredoxin and thioredoxin interacting proteins in various disease conditions. Biochim Biophys Acta. 2008;1780:1368-82.
51. Fennell JP, Brosnan MJ, Frater AJ, Hamilton CA, Alexander MY, Nicklin SA, et al. Adenovirus-mediated overexpression of extracellular superoxide dismutase improves endothelial dysfunction in a rat model of hypertension. Gene Ther. 2002;9:110-7.
52. Zanetti M, Sato J, Katusic ZS, O'Brien T. Gene transfer of superoxide dismutase isoforms reverses endothelial dysfunction in diabetic rabbit aorta. Am J Physiol Heart Circ Physiol. 2001;280:H2516-23.

53. Wan JB, Huang LL, Rong R, Tan R, Wang J, Kang JX. Endogenously decreasing tissue n–6/n–3 fatty acid ratio reduces atherosclerotic lesions in apolipoprotein E-deficient mice by inhibiting systemic and vascular inflammation. Arterioscler Thromb Vasc Biol. 2010;30:2487-94.
54. Versari D, Daghini E, Virdis A, Ghiadoni L, Taddei S. Endothelial dysfunction as a target for prevention of cardiovascular disease. Diabetes Care. 2009;32:S314-21.
55. Grover-Páez F, Zavalza-Gómez AB. Endothelial dysfunction and cardiovascular risk factors. Diabetes Res Clin Pract. 2009;84:1-10.
56. Bhatti S, Hakeem A, Cilingiroglu M. Lp-PLA(2) as a marker of cardiovascular diseases. Curr Atheroscler Rep. 2010;12:140-4.
57. Roustit M, Cracowski JL. Assessment of endothelial and neurovascular function in human skin microcirculation. Trends Pharmacol Sci. 2013;34:373-84.
58. Toda N, Imamura T, Okamura T. Alteration of nitric oxide-mediated blood flow regulation in diabetes mellitus. Pharmacol Ther. 2010;127:189-209.
59. Nguyen TT, Shaw JE, Robinson C, Shaw JE, Schie CH, Carrington AL, et al. Diabetic retinopathy is related to both endothelium-dependent and -independent responses of skin microvascular flow. Diabetes Care. 2011;34:1389-93.
60. Holowatz LA, Thompson-Torgerson CS, Kenney WL. The human cutaneous circulation as a model of generalized microvascular function. J Appl Physiol. 2008;105:370-2.
61. Yamamoto-Suganuma R, Aso Y. Relationship between post-occlusive forearm skin reactive hyperaemia and vascular disease in patients with type 2 diabetes—a novel index for detecting micro- and macrovascular dysfunction using laser Doppler flowmetry. Diabet Med. 2009;26:83-8.
62. Kruger A, Stewart J, Sahityani R. Laser Doppler flowmetry detection of endothelial dysfunction in end-stage renal disease patients: correlation with cardiovascular risk. Kidney Int. 2006;70:157-64.
63. Roustit M, Cracowski JL. Non-invasive assessment of skin microvascular function in humans: an insight into methods. Microcirculation. 2012;19:47-64.
64. Clough GF, Kuliga KZ, Chipperfield AJ. Flow motion dynamics of microvascular blood flow and oxygenation: evidence of adaptive changes in obesity and type 2 diabetes mellitus/insulin resistance. Microcirculation. 2017;24:12331.
65. Jonasson H, Bergstrand S, Nystrom FH, Länne T, Östgren CJ, Bjarnegrd N, et al. Skin microvascular endothelial dysfunction is associated with type 2 diabetes independently of microalbuminuria and arterial stiffness. Diab Vasc Dis Res. 2017;14:363-71.
66. Guzzo G, Senesi M, Giordano N, Montagnani M. LaCapillaroscopia in medicina, tecnica, indicazioni, utilità, limitieprospettive. Milano: Collana Medico Scientifica; 1996.
67. Cutolo M, Pizzorni C, Sulli A. Capillaroscopy. Best Pract Res Clin Rheumatol. 2005;19:437-2.
68. Cacioppo A. (2011). Studio morfologico del microcircolo orale nel paziente diabetico. [online] Available from https://core.ac.uk/download/pdf/53296765.pdf. [Last accessed June, 2021].
69. Gasser P, Berger W. Nailfold videomicroscopy and local cold test in type I diabetics. Angiology. 1992;43:395-400.
70. Pazos-Moura CC, Moura EG, Bouskela E, Torres-Filho IP, Breitenbach MM. Nailfold capillaroscopy in diabetes mellitus: morphological abnormalities and relationship with microangiopathy. Braz J Med Biol Res. 1987;20:777-80.
71. Trevisan G. Capillaroscopianel diabete mellito in pediatria. Milan: Microcircolazione Oggi; 1985.
72. Halfoun VL, Pires ML, Fernandes TJ, Victer F, Rodrigues KK, Tavares R. Videocapillaroscopy and diabetes mellitus: area of transverse segment in nailfold capillary loops reflects vascular reactivity. Diabetes Res Clin Pract. 2003;61:155-60.
73. Wang JJ, Su XH, Hung G, He HY, Tseng WK. Quantitative reduction in the dynamic endothelial function on foot microcirculation in patients with diabetes mellitus. In: Lin P (Ed). Future Trends in Biomedical and Health Informatics and Cybersecurity in Medical Devices. New York: Springer; 2020. pp. 281-7.
74. Nageswara Rao K, Srinivasa Rao P, Appa Rao A, Sridhar GR. Sobel edge detection method to identify and quantify the risk factors for diabetic foot ulcers. Int J Comp Sci Inform Technol. 2013;5: 39-46.

75. Gururajarao SB, Venkatappa U, Shivaram JM, Sikkandar Y, Almudi AA. Infrared thermography and soft computing for diabetic foot assessment. In: Dey N, Borra S, Ashmour A, Shi F (Eds). Machine Learning in Bio-signal Analysis and Diagnostic Imaging, 1st edition. New York: Elsevier; 2019.
76. Chatchawan U, Narkto P, Damri T, Yamauchi J. An exploration of the relationship between foot skin temperature and blood flow in type 2 diabetes mellitus patients: a cross-sectional study. J Phys Ther Sci. 2018;30:1359-63.

CHAPTER 9

Blood Pressure in Pregnancy and Future Cardiometabolic Risks

G Nagamani, G Lakshmi

ABSTRACT

Hypertensive disorders of pregnancy are common. It is important to know to what extent they lead to vascular disease later in life. Initial studies on evaluating such association were limited by a number of methodological issues. As a result, the suggestions that the future risk of hypertension, diabetes, cardiovasculur disease, cerebrovascular disease, and thromboembolism is increased could not be conclusively established. Despite the biological basis for a common pathogenesis, only recently have properly powered studies suggested an increased risk of later hypertension, type 2 diabetes mellitus, and hypercholesterolemia. Therefore, women with hypertension during pregnancy must be given lifestyle counseling to lower the risk of future risk factors and vascular disease.

Keywords: *Eclampsia, Placenta, Inflammation, Insulin resistance.*

INTRODUCTION

Hypertension is well-recognized to be associated with insulin resistance, type 2 diabetes mellitus (T2DM), and pathological processes in the vascular system. A number of names were given to hypertension observed in pregnancy. Some forms are believed to be specific to the pregnant state. Little attention was given to the association of hypertension in pregnancy to the future health of the mother. Scattered reports before the current diagnostic criteria of hypertension in pregnancy were proposed suggested that preeclampsia, a pregnancy-specific form of hypertension, presages future risk of coronary artery disease, cerebrovascular disease, and venous thrombosis.

Inflammation, seen in hypertension of pregnancy, can be mediated by an imbalance in the population of CD4+ T cells. The imbalance between regulatory T-cells and T-helper 17 cells could play a role in the pathogenesis of preeclampsia.[17]

A confluence of genetic, immune, and vasoactive factors is believed to ultimately lead to preeclampsia; they could, thus, be potential targets for management of preeclampsia.[18-20]

In a nutshell, during early pregnancy, abnormal placentation results in the secretion of antiangiogenic factors, which acting synergistically with obesity and insulin resistance, lead to endothelial dysfunction in the mother along with the clinical signs and symptoms.[21]

BACKGROUND FOR PROPOSING AN ASSOCIATION BETWEEN PREECLAMPSIA AND FUTURE VASCULAR EVENTS

Analyzing the pathogenesis of preeclampsia shows a background of common pathogenetic factors with insulin resistance, diabetes mellitus, and vasculopathy. Factors common to insulin resistance are observed in women predisposed to hypertension of pregnancy such as gestational diabetes, polycystic ovary syndrome, and obesity, besides overlapping metabolic risk factors such as dyslipidemia.[22-24] Studies at biochemical identification of preeclampsia using gel electrophoresis showed differences in expression of protein abundance. These were involved in metabolism of lipids, activation of complement system, and coagulation.[25]

METABOLIC SYNDROME AND PREECLAMPSIA

It is evident that preeclampsia is associated with risk factors that come under the umbrella of *metabolic syndrome* [viz., obesity, hypertriglyceridemia, low high-density lipoprotein (HDL) cholesterol, and elevated fasting plasma glucose level]. Jeyabalan et al. proposed a multitude of connections between preeclampsia and individual components of metabolic syndrome.[26] The components of metabolic syndrome, operating through inflammation, are antecedents to both preeclampsia and cardiovascular disease. Preeclampsia occurs when poor placentation and hypoxia are accompanied by debris from trophoblasts and antiangiogenic factors enter the maternal circulation; these in turn activate maternal neutrophils and widespread inflammatory response in the mother. Obese women tend to be in a "subinflammatory" state even before they conceive; deficiency of the vasodilator nitric oxide could be at the interface of placenta and the mother.

Preeclampsia does not result merely from biochemical reactions. They are modified by other factors such as lifestyle, psychological stress, physical exercise, and dietary habits.

CAVEATS IN ASSESSING ASSOCIATION STUDIES

There have been many studies to evaluate the risk of future morbidity in women who have had preeclampsia. The *chief bottleneck is in the definition of exposure*.[27] Some of the earlier studies were small, retrospective in nature, with varying inclusion criteria in terms of definition of the condition, the parity, and other maternal variables.

PREECLAMPSIA AND HYPERTENSION IN LATER LIFE

Early studies on preeclampsia did not observe an increased risk of future hypertension[27] in contrast to more recent studies. Wilson et al. reported a relative risk between 2 and 4 when assessed by both questionnaire and physical measurement.[28] Women were chosen from the Aberdeen Maternity and Neonatal Databank who had preeclampsia during their first singleton pregnancy (n = 1,199). Outcomes were assessed by a combination of questionnaires, clinical assessment, and mortality data. There was significant positive association between preeclampsia, gestational hypertension, and onset of hypertension later in life.[27] Some of the earlier studies also showed a similar association.[29-31] These studies suffered from limitations of small sample sizes and association of only systolic blood pressure.[31] More recent prospective studies, although in relatively modest sample sizes (between 179 and 406), reported that preeclampsia, especially if recurrent, increased the risk of chronic hypertension.[32,33] Studies from Asia showed similar observations about future risk of recurrent hypertension and endothelial dysfunction.[34,35]

PREECLAMPSIA AND LARGE VESSEL DISEASE

Large cohorts were studied for the possible risk of future ischemic heart disease and cerebrovascular disease. A retrospective analysis (n = 129,920 women having first births) showed that the risk of hospitalization or death was twice in women with preeclampsia.[36] These findings from Scotland were reproduced in a larger cohort from Denmark (600,000 births).[37] The risk of death due to cardiovascular disease was higher in women with preeclampsia and preterm delivery. However, the role of genetics or lifestyle could not be assessed separately.[37]

A prospective cohort study of 1,400 general practitioners throughout the United Kingdom (original cohort @23,000) showed that nulliparous women who had preeclampsia had a trend toward increased occurrence of cerebrovascular disease, peripheral vascular disease, hypertension, ischemic heart disease, and thromboembolism.[38]

RECENT OBSERVATIONAL COHORT STUDY AND META-ANALYSIS

A recent large observational cohort study was performed to assess whether hypertension in pregnancy was related to cardiovascular risk factors in mothers. The subjects comprised parous women from the Nurses' Health Study II (n = 58,671) who did not have cardiovascular disease or any risk factors at baseline.[39] Self-reported diagnosis of hypertension, hypercholesterolemia, and T2DM was recorded from their first childbirth during a mean follow-up ranging from 25 to 32 years. Despite having similar lifestyle and demographic features as controls who were normotensive during pregnancy, women with hypertensive disorders were more likely to develop chronic hypertension (33.3%), T2DM (6.4%), and hypercholesterolemia (55.6%) at the end of the study period. The risks persisted even after adjustment for age, ethnicity, and parental education. This study is the first to report of such association after accounting for multiple confounders and also with the longest follow-up period.

Another interesting observation was that recurrent hypertensive disorders of pregnancy were associated with the highest rate of later hypertension, T2DM, and hypercholesterolemia.[39]

Ventura et al. published a meta-analysis of the effects of preeclampsia and eclampsia on the metabolic and biochemical outcomes in mothers later in life.[40] Prospective retrospective and prospective observational studies on singleton pregnancy published until November 2018 were included. The studies evaluated the effect of preeclampsia and eclampsia on biochemical outcomes and of metabolic outcomes after delivery. About 41 cohorts were studied comprising 3,300 women with preeclampsia/eclampsia and 13,967 women as controls who were normotensive. The postpartum follow-up ranged from 3 months to 32 years. In case clarification or supplemental information was required, the authors were contacted. Studies were reported principally from Europe and North America along with other regions of the world.

The baseline clinical and demographics were similar between arms of each study. Employing the Newcastle-Ottawa Scale (NOS) for assessment of quality, 40 out of the 41 studies were identified as high quality.

Systolic blood pressure was significantly higher in women with previous diagnosis of preeclampsia/eclampsia in 38 studies; diastolic blood pressure was higher in 37 studies. Heterogeneity was observed across studies. About 12 studies showed a higher prevalence of hypertension in women with preeclampsia/eclampsia.

Body mass index was higher in the study group in 34 studies, waist circumference was higher in 12 studies, and waist-hip ratio was higher in 10 studies. Body weight was more in 10 studies. Heterogeneity was low-to-moderate.

About 29 studies showed higher total cholesterol levels in study subjects, 29 studies showed low HDL cholesterol, and 24 studies showed higher low-density lipoprotein (LDL) cholesterol. About 28 studies reported higher triglycerides in the study group. Heterogeneity was low to high.

Serum glucose was higher in 25 studies. Serum insulin was higher in 14 studies. In 14 studies, Homeostatic Model Assessment of Insulin Resistance (HOMA-IR) index was higher in subjects.

In summary, this meta-analysis reported that hypertension and altered metabolic abnormalities occurred before the diagnosis of severe complications in women with preeclampsia/eclampsia. Abnormalities persisted even after the end of pregnancy. Therefore, these women should be educated, carefully monitored, and treated for obesity, dyslipidemia, dysglycemia, and hypertension on follow-up.

Is there any basis for such associations?

It is still not clear whether hypertension during pregnancy induces accelerated endothelial injury leading to cardiovascular disease or if it only unmasks cardiovascular risk though what has been termed the "stress test of pregnancy".[37]

Despite the lack of a clear mechanistic understanding, there is evidence that women who have hypertension during pregnancy are at increased risk of macrovascular disease later in life.

Common cardiovascular risk factors are associated with preeclampsia. Dyslipidemia, increased blood pressure, being overweight, and having family history of diabetes were all shown to be associated with preeclampsia. Similarly, during the course of pregnancy, women with preeclampsia have relative hypertriglyceridemia, hypercholesterolemia, and gestational diabetes mellitus. In addition, the uterine arteries demonstrate increased resistance and subnormal endothelial response. Impaired endothelial function may persist after delivery. It must be emphasized, however, that all these are only correlational and do not imply cause and effect.[41]

PREVENTIVE MANAGEMENT FOLLOWING PREECLAMPSIA

Therefore, preventive measures are best begun before the adverse effects are manifest. Lifestyle interventions have a broad role in preventing obesity, insulin resistance, T2DM, dyslipidemia, hypertension, coronary artery disease, and cerebrovascular disease, besides preserving and improving cognitive function. Considering that women who had preeclampsia already have predisposing factors leading to atherosclerosis, prevention can begin even before conception, viz., reduction of body weight,[26] particularly visceral obesity. Weight loss during pregnancy is not advisable. Weight loss measures are no different and consist of restricting calorie intake to attain a net negative energy balance, which is the chief method of losing weight. Lost weight maintenance can be attempted by continuing to be compliant with diet, topping up with physical exercise.

CONCLUSION

Similar to hypertension in the pregnant state, hypertension during pregnancy, even when transient, is associated with adverse cardiometabolic outcomes later in life. Common underlying risk factors exist including gestational diabetes mellitus, polycystic ovary syndrome, obesity and dyslipidemia; these are also influenced by modifiable lifestyle habits. Therefore, women with manifest hypertension during pregnancy, whether transient or permanent, must be counselled about preventive measures. They must be carefully followed up to prevent, identify and treat any adverse effects in future.

REFERENCES

1. American College of Obstetricians and Gynecologists, Task Force on Hypertension in Pregnancy. Hypertension in pregnancy. Report of the American College of Obstetricians and Gynecologists' Task Force on Hypertension in Pregnancy. Obstet Gynecol. 2013;122:1122-31.
2. Abalos E, Cuesta C, Grosso AL, Chou D, Say L. Global and regional estimates of preeclampsia and eclampsia: a systematic review. Eur J Obstet Gynecol Reprod Biol. 2013;170:1-7.
3. Sanjay G, Girija W. Preeclampsia-eclampsia. J Obst Gynecol India. 2014;64:4-13.
4. Ward K, Taylor RN. Genetic factors in the etiology of preeclampsia/eclampsia. In: Taylor RN, Roberts JM, Cunningham FG, Lindheimer MD (Eds). Cheley's Hypertensive Disorders in Pregnancy. Amsterdam: Elsevier; 2015. pp. 57-80.
5. Palei AC, Spradley FT, Warrington JP, George EM, Granger JP. Pathophysiology of hypertension in pre-eclampsia: a lesson in integrative physiology. Acta Physiol (Oxf). 2013;208:224-33.
6. Heimrath J, Czekanski A, Krawczenko A, Dus D. The role of endothelium in the pathogenesis of pregnancy-induced hypertension. Postepy Hig Med Dosw. 2007;61:48-57.
7. Pedersen M, Stayner L, Slama R, Sorensen M, Figueras F, Nieuwenhuijsen MJ, et al. Ambient air pollution and pregnancy-induced hypertensive disorders: a systematic review and meta-analysis. Hypertension. 2014;64:494-500.
8. O'Donovan G, Cadena-Gaitán C. Air pollution and diabetes: it's time to get active! Lancet Planet Health. 2018;2:e287-8.
9. Bowe B, Xie Y, Li T, Yan Y, Xian H, Al-Aly Z. The 2016 global and national burden of diabetes mellitus attributable to PM 2.5 air pollution. Lancet Planet Health. 2018;2:e301-12.
10. Subramaniam V. Seasonal variation in the incidence of preeclampsia and eclampsia in tropical climatic conditions. BMC Womens Health. 2007;7:18.
11. Nagamani G, Sundararaman PG, Sridhar GR. Visible signs of insulin resistance: opportunities lost. Int J Diabetes Dev Ctries. 2014;34:177-9.
12. Qin JZ, Pang LH, Li M, Fan X, Huang RD, Chen HY. Obstetric complications in women with polycystic ovary syndrome: a systematic review and meta-analysis. Reprod Biol Endocrinol. 2013;11:56.
13. Narasimha A, Vasudeva DS. Spectrum of changes in placenta in toxemia of pregnancy. Indian J Pathol Microbiol. 2011;54:15-20.
14. Furuya M, Ishida J, Aoki I, Fukamizu A. Pathophysiology of placentation abnormalities in pregnancy-induced hypertension. Vasc Health Risk Manag. 2008;4:1301-13.
15. George EM, Granger JP. Endothelin: key mediator of hypertension in preeclampsia. Am J Hypertens. 2011;24:964-9.

16. Shah DA, Khalil RA. Bioactive factors in uteroplacental and systemic circulation link placental ischemia to generalized vascular dysfunction in hypertensive pregnancy and preeclampsia. Biochem Pharmacol. 2015;95:211-26.
17. LaMarca B, Cornelius DC, Harmon AC, Amaral LM, Cunningham MW, Faulkner JL, et al. Identifying immune mechanisms mediating the hypertension during preeclampsia. Am J Physiol Regul Integr Comp Physiol. 2016;311:R1-9.
18. Ali SM, Khalil RA. Genetic, immune and vasoactive factors in the vascular dysfunction associated with hypertension in pregnancy. Expert Opin Ther Targets. 2015;19:1495-515.
19. Sowmya S, Ramaiah A, Nallari P, Jyothy A, Venkateshwari A. Role of IL-6-174(G/C) promoter polymorphism in the etiology of early-onset preeclampsia. Inflamm Res. 2015;64:433-9.
20. Nakayama T, Yamamoto T. Comparison between essential hypertension and pregnancy-induced hypertension: a genetic perspective. Endocr J. 2009;56:921-34.
21. Rana S, Karumanchi SA. Pathophysiology of preeclampsia. In: Polin RA, Abman SH, Rowitch DH, Benitz WE, Fox WW (Eds). Fetal and Neonatal Physiology. Philadelphia: Elsevier; 2017. pp. 1724-3.
22. Niromanesh S, Shirazi M, Dastgerdy E, Sharbaf FR, Shirazi M, Khazaeipour Z. Association of hypertriglyceridaemia with pre-eclampsia, preterm birth, gestational diabetes and uterine artery pulsatility index. Natl Med J India. 2012;25:265-7.
23. Ray JG, Diamond P, Singh G, Bell CM. Brief overview of maternal triglycerides as a risk factor for preeclampsia. BJOG. 2006;113:379-86.
24. Solomon CG, Seely EW. Brief review: hypertension in pregnancy: a manifestation of the insulin resistance syndrome? Hypertension. 2001;37:232-9.
25. Atkinson KR, Blumenstein M, Black MA, Hu SH, Kasabov N, Taolor RS, et al. An altered pattern of circulating apolipoprotein E3 isoforms is implicated in preeclampsia. J Lipid Res. 2009;50:71-80.
26. Jeyabalan A, Hubel CA, Roberts JM. Hypertensive disorders. In: Taylor RN, Roberts JM, Cunningham FG, Lindheimer MD (Eds). Chesley's Hypertensive Disorders in Pregnancy. Amsterdam: Academic Press; 2015. pp. 133-60.
27. Smith GCS. Long-term implications of pre-eclampsia for maternal health. In: Lyall F, Belfort M (Eds). Pre-eclampsia: Etiology and Clinical Practice. New York: Cambridge University Press; 2007. pp. 232-9.
28. Wilson BJ, Watson MS, Prescott GJ, Sunderland S, Campbell DM, Hannaford P, et al. Hypertensive diseases of pregnancy and risk of hypertension and stroke in later life: results from cohort study. BMJ. 2003;326:845-51.
29. Adams EM, Macgillivray I. Long-term effect of preeclampsia on blood-pressure. Lancet. 1961;2:1373-5.
30. Singh MM, Macgillivray I, Mahaffy RG. A study of the long-term effects of pre-eclampsia on blood pressure and renal function. BJOG. 1874;81:903-6.
31. Carleton H, Forsythe A, Flores R. Remote prognosis of preeclampsia in women 25 years old and younger. Am J Obstet Gynecol. 1988;159:156-60.
32. Sibai BM, El-Nazer AE, Gonzalez-Ruiz A. Severe preeclampsia-eclampsia in young primigravid women: subsequent pregnancy outcome and remote prognosis. Am J Obstet Gynecol. 1986;155: 1011-6.
33. Sibai BM, Sarinoglu C, Mercer BM. Eclampsia. VII. Pregnancy outcome after eclampsia and long-term prognosis. Am J Obstet Gynecol. 1992;168:1757-61.
34. Urooj H, Jabeen M, Ashfaq S, Sultan S, Irfan SM. Prevalence of recurrence of pre-eclampsia and its association with raised body mass index in multiparous women. J Soc Obstet Gynecol Pak. 2017;7: 206-10.
35. Fatma J, Karoli R, Siddiqui Z, Gupta HP, Chandra A, Pandey M. Cardio-metabolic risk profile in women with previous history of pre-eclampsia. J Assoc Physicians India. 2017;65:23-7.
36. Smith GC, Pell JP, Walsh D. Pregnancy complications and maternal risk of ischemic heart disease: a retrospective cohort study of 129,290 births. Lancet. 2001;357:2002-6.
37. Irgens HU, Reisaeter L, Irgens LM, Lie RT. Long-term mortality of mothers and fathers after pre-eclampsia: population-based cohort study. BMJ. 2001;323:1213-7.
38. Hannaford P, Ferry S, Hirsch S. Cardiovascular sequelae of toxemia of pregnancy. Heart. 1997;77: 154-8.

39. Stuart JJ, Tanz LJ, Missmer SA, Rimm EB, Spiegelman D, James-Todd TM, et al. Hypertensive disorders of pregnancy and maternal cardiovascular disease risk factor development. Ann Intern Med. 2018;169:224-32.
40. Ventura VA, Li Y, Pasupuleti V, Roman YM, Hernandez AV, López FRP. Effects of preeclampsia and eclampsia on maternal metabolic and biochemical outcomes in later life: a systematic review and meta-analysis. Metabolism Clin Exp. 2020;102:154012.
41. Rich-Edwards JW, Ness RA, Roberts JM. Epidemiology of pregnancy-related hypertension. In: Taylor RN, Roberts JM, Cunningham FG, Lindheimer MD (Eds). Chesley's Hypertensive Disorders in Pregnancy. Amsterdam: Academic Press; 2015. pp. 37-55.

CHAPTER 10

Recent Trends in Managing Male Sexual Dysfunction in Diabetes

Deepak K Jumani

ABSTRACT

Diabetes is increasing in prevalence and diabetic sexual dysfunction is the biggest sexual health tsunami. The most common sexual dysfunctions in men with diabetes are erectile dysfunction (ED), early ejaculation, and low desire. In women having diabetes, common sexual disorders include hypoactive sexual desire and depression.

The penis remains in a constant flaccid state due to generalized cavernosal vasoconstriction because of raised advanced glycated end products, activation of RhoA/Rho kinase activity, and reduced endothelial nitric oxide synthase (eNOS) and nitric oxide (NO) in the smooth muscle cells of the corpora cavernosa. Control of hyperglycemia is essential to prevent or postpone vascular complications. Metformin, which is often the first oral agent of choice, improves endothelial function, a significant cause of male sexual dysfunction. Sodium-glucose cotransporter-2 (SGLT-2) inhibitors used along with metformin, besides their well-known benefits, provide physiological erections. Insulin pump therapy has improved sexual functions in men to the tune of 83%.

To increase the blood flow in the penile vasculature and to achieve erections, phosphodiesterase type 5 (PDE5) inhibitors are the ideal choice. The available PDE5 inhibitors include sildenafil 25, 50, and 100 mg, tadalafil 2.5, 5, 10, and 20 mg, vardenafil 10 and 20 mg, udenafil 100 mg, and avanafil 100 and 200 mg.

Phosphodiesterase type 5 inhibitors vary in their onset and duration of actions and in the side effects. PDE5 inhibitors are erectogenic drugs and do not increase the desire. The recent trend is to give low dose of tadalafil 5 mg to every diabetic if he is not on nitrates.

Testosterone replacement therapy is given with caution when indicated, with monitoring prostate-specific antigen (PSA). Given TRT (testosterone replacement therapy) with caution for 2 years, remission of diabetes, reduction of insulin resistance, improvement in the symptoms of hypogonadism and improvement in sexual dysfunction was observed.

Phytoneutraceuticals such as L-arginine and fenugreek which are safe, have shown promising results in increasing the desire and sexual functions both in males and females.

Counseling on nutrition, exercise, mental health, and lifestyle measures continue to be the most important mainstay for the treatment of sexual dysfunctions in diabetes.

Keywords: *Endothelial dysfunction, Nitric oxide, PDE5 inhibitors, Rho-associated protein kinase.*

INTRODUCTION

Currently, India has over 75 million people with diabetes. A patient dies of diabetes and two develop diabetes[1] every second of the hour. ED is a distressing and common complication of diabetes, especially in men.[2] ED, as a marker of endothelial dysfunction, is a sentinel marker of myocardial ischemia.[3,4] This epidemiological transition is largely because of the increase in the prevalence of cardiovascular diseases (CVDs) and CVD risk factors in India.[5] China and India have the distinction of being diabetes capitals of the world.[2] If ED is the earliest complication of diabetes in men, they form the ED capital of the world as well.

Erectile dysfunction affects the individual resulting in low self-esteem and depression; it also affects his partner and can impact on the relationships leading to unhappiness, marital discord, and even divorces.[6] ED, defined as consistent inability to have an erection firm enough for sexual intercourse, has a prevalence between 20 and 85 in men with diabetes. Among men with ED, those with diabetes are likely to have experienced the problem as much as 10–15 years earlier than men without diabetes.[7,8]

Endothelial function expressed by the brachial artery flow-mediated dilation (FMD) was impaired in young ED patients. ED may be the first clinical sign of endothelial dysfunction and can serve as a preclinical marker for CVDs. Traditional cardiovascular risk factors and metabolic disorders may be the underlying pathogenesis of ED in young patients as in the elderly. Our study highlights endothelial function measurement and Homeostasis Model Assessment (HOMA)-index calculation as important methods to improve our ability of predicting and treating ED as well as secondary CVD early for young men under the age of 40 years.[9]

The proposed mechanisms of ED in diabetic patients[10] include elevated advanced glycation end-products, increased levels of oxygen-free radicals, impaired nitric oxide (NO) synthesis, increased endothelin B receptor-binding sites and upregulated RhoA/Rho-kinase pathway, neuropathic damage, and impaired cyclic guanosine monophosphate (cGMP)-dependent protein kinase-1.

PATHOPHYSIOLOGY OF ERECTILE DYSFUNCTION IN DIABETES

The dynamics of erection in men depend on a coordinated function of neurologically mediated arterial inflow, relaxation of the corpora spongiosa smooth muscles to allow the blood to flow in the penile vasculature, and finally venous obstruction which allows the blood to remain in the penile vasculature and let the penis remain erect. Disturbances in any of the three result in ED.

The endothelium, the innermost single layer of the vascular bed, considered to be the brain of the vascular system, has an important role in vascular homeostasis. It secretes mediators such as NO, prostacyclin, and endothelin that regulate vascular tone, platelet activity, and coagulation factors but also influence vascular inflammation and cell migration. The vascular endothelium in the penile vasculature produces endothelial nitric oxide synthase (eNOS) and the neuronal tissues produce neuronal nitric oxide synthase (nNOS), both these synthases transport the NO in the corpora spongiosa smooth muscle and convert the guanosine triphosphate into cGMP, with the help of an enzyme guanylate cyclase. This cyclic guanosine monophosphate (GMP) relaxes the smooth muscle and allows the blood to flow in the penis. cGMP also potentiates protein kinase G which inhibits calcium conduction and opens up potassium ion channels which further relax the smooth muscles. The cGMP soon hydrolyzes into GMP with the help of an enzyme, phosphodiesterase 5 (PDE5), which is present in the penile smooth muscles and the smooth muscle contracts and leads to detumescence (**Fig. 1**).

So, for a good erection one needs to have a good functional endothelium which produces adequate amount of eNOS and also nNOS, and NO, which initiates the erectogenic mechanism. In addition, there should be adequate

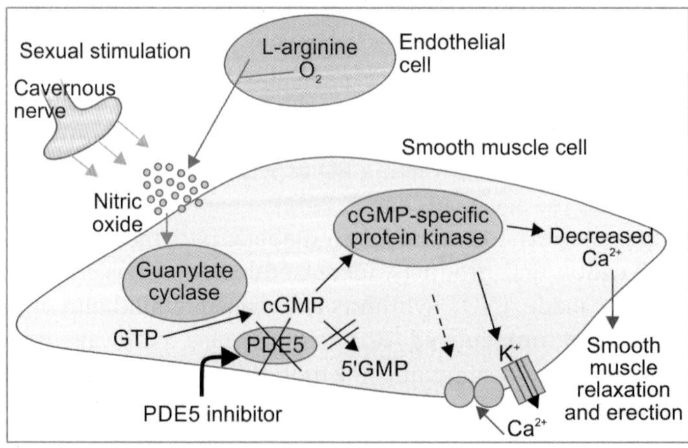

FIG. 1: Pathophysiology of erectile dysfunction.

guanylate cyclase activators and stimulators, cGMP in the more bioavailable form to keep the penile smooth muscle in a relaxed state, and something to block the phosphodiesterase type 5 (PDE5) like PDE5 inhibitors to sustain erection.

Rho-A/Rho-kinase pathway[11] is the key pathway which inhibits relaxation of the penile smooth muscle vasculature. Rho-associated protein kinase (ROCK) is a kinase which induces the formation of stress fibers and focal adhesions by phosphorylating myosin light chain. Due to this phosphorylation, the actin binding of myosin II and contractility increases. Protein kinase C and ROCK are involved in regulating calcium ion intake and these calcium ions in turn stimulate a myosin light chain kinase forcing contraction. So, inhibition of these pathways will help in relaxation of the cavernous smooth muscle and produce sustained erection.

MANAGEMENT OF ERECTILE DYSFUNCTION IN DIABETES

Control of hyperglycemia and other comorbid conditions such as hypertension and dyslipidemia, quitting smoking, reducing intake of alcohol or any other substance of abuse, reducing anxiety, and stresses is mandatory for initiating the treatment of ED in men. There has been a tremendous breakthrough in managing ED in diabetics.

In 1998, Food and Drug Administration (FDA) approved sildenafil citrate as a PDE5 inhibitor for treatment of ED, which marked the beginning of a new era in the treatment of ED. With three effective and safe PDE5 inhibitors, sildenafil, tadalafil, and vardenafil, clinicians have multiple choices for treating patients with ED of all severities and etiologies. However, there are 30–40% nonresponders. The possible strategies to these nonresponders are a challenge. A proper counseling, switching over to alternate PDE5 inhibitors, chronic use of the PDE5 inhibitors or alternate measures were then adopted. Chronic use of PDE5 inhibitors especially tadalafil in low dose of 2.5, 5, or 10 mg has proved to be having a favorable pharmacokinetic profile and good therapeutic option with better compliance.

The newer formulations which emerged were oral dispersible vardenafil, which proved to be >44% efficacious, with less side reactions.

A newer agent, udenafil, increases the cGMP concentration, but cost is a constraint for widespread use. A novel molecule recently introduced in our Indian market, so avanafil. This is available in the dose of 100 mg/200 mg, it has a fastest onset of action—15–20 minutes, and has a half-life of 5 hours. It also has less PDE6 and PDE11 inhibition due to which patients do not get myalgia or visual side effects. Another advantage of this molecule is that it can be given with caution to patients who are on nitrates. As all nitrates have a short half-life, if a patient is advised to skip his nitrate and wishes to take avanafil which eventually shall be washed out in his body within 5 hours, he can enjoy a satisfying intercourse. It was effective in men with diabetes.

If oral therapy is ineffective, local injection of intracavernous papaverine and chlorpromazine is recommended. This needs to be supported with proper counseling for the possibility of priapism. Low-intensity extracorporeal shock wave therapy, which is noninvasive, showed promising results in mild-to-moderate vasculogenic ED. If all these fail, penile implants can be inserted by surgical means.

Newer Agents

There are three new molecules soon to enter the Indian market which are mentioned below:

- *SLx-2101*[12] (Surface Logic, Inc.) is an oral, selective, fast-onset, PDE5I, which exhibits excellent potency in both ex vivo and in vivo experiments and a long-lasting duration (at least 36–48 hours at all doses studied). The active metabolite SLx-2081 is responsible for this extended duration of the PDE inhibition
- *Mirodenafil*[12] is a pyridopyrimidine compound marketed in South Korea for the treatment of ED. A phase III study demonstrated a mean 7.6- and 11.6-point improvement in International Index of Erectile Function-Erectile Function (IIEF-EF) domain score in the group receiving 50 and 100 mg of mirodenafil, respectively, versus a 3.4-point increase in the placebo group. Due to the modification in its structure, mirodenafil has got a 10-fold higher PDE5 selectivity than sildenafil. Pharmacokinetic data showed a shorter half-life than the other currently available PDE5Is, with this property representing an advantage in terms of lower incidence of common side effects.
- *Lodenafil carbonate*[12] (Helleva®) 80 mg once a day 2 hours before the sexual act. This has been proven to be very effective in patients with diabetes in Brazil.

Orally dissolving films of sildenafil and tadalafil are available, which have a more rapid onset of action and fewer side effects compared to oral formulations.

NOVEL MOLECULAR TARGETS[13] FOR TREATMENT OF ERECTILE DYSFUNCTION IN DIABETES

- Platelets and microparticles
- Myeloperoxidase
- Heme oxygenase-1
- Sonic hedgehog
- Galanin
- Stromal vascular fraction
- Vascular endothelial growth factor (VEGF)
- Nanoparticles[14]
- Pigment epithelium-derived factor (PEDF)[15]

Rho-kinase inhibitors are a recent addition with great promise. Rho-kinase phosphorylates and inhibits the regulatory subunit of myosin phosphatase within smooth muscle cells, which maintains phosphorylation of myosin filaments and contractile tone within the smooth muscle. Inhibition of the calcium sensitization pathway with Rho-kinase inhibitors acts without targeting the NO/sGC (soluble guanylate cyclase)/cGMP pathway.

Sonic Hedgehog

Sonic hedgehog[13] using aligned peptide amphiphile nanofibers plays a significant role in peripheral nerve regeneration and has clinical potential to be used as a regenerative therapy for the cavernous nerve (CN) regeneration.

Lastly gene therapy and stem cell therapy act by enhancing the NO production or NO-mediated signaling pathways, K^+ channel activity of the SMCC [N-succinimidyl 4-(maleimidomethyl)cyclohexanecarboxylate].

Mesenchymal stem cells along with VEGF lack robust data for their safety and long-term effects.

Nanotechnology[14]

Primarily this technology applies to topical delivery of drugs for on demand erectile function, injectable gels into the penis to prevent morphology changes postprostatectomy, hydrogels to promote CN regeneration/neuro-protection, and encapsulation of drugs to increase erectile function (primarily of PDE5i).

Phytochemicals have evolved as novel therapies in the treatment of erectile dysfunction in diabetes.

Modern phytochemicals have developed from traditional herbs. Protodioscin is a phytochemical agent derived from *Tribulus terrestris* L plant, which improves sexual desire and enhance erection via the conversion of protodioscin to DHEA (dehydroepiandrosterone). Many other herbal plants such as ginseng, pycnogenol, eurycoma longifolia, pimpinella pruacen, muira puama, ginkgo biloba, and yohimbe have been tried.

A combination of L-arginine which is a NO donor along with phyto-chemicals such as fenugreek in saponized forms is an alternative to PDE5 inhibitors, because PDE5 are misused and have side effects. This combination of L-arginine and fenugreek is useful to both males and females in treatment of most of sexual dysfunctions.

RECENT TRENDS IN MANAGEMENT OF SEXUAL DYSFUNCTIONS IN MEN WITH DIABETES

Counseling and lifestyle management form the first and most important need in management of sexual dysfunction. Advice about diet and nutrition, quitting smoking, alcohol or any other substance of abuse, reduction of stress, and regular exercise is now included in the process of care for management of ED.

Amongst the oral hypoglycemic agents (OHAs), two drugs which are a boon to every diabetic for restoring their sexual functions to normal are metformin and sodium-glucose cotransporter-2 (SGLT-2) inhibitors.

METFORMIN

Arteriogenic ED[12] is caused by (1) endothelium-dependent vasodilatory impairment, (2) sympathetic nerve activity elevation, and (3) atherosclerotic luminal narrowing—all of which have been linked to insulin resistance. Metformin, an insulin sensitizer modulates multiple metabolic pathways that affect vascular function and consequently erectile function. Metformin may enhance endothelium-dependent vasodilatation through improved flow-mediated vasodilation as well as increased transcription of NO synthase in erectile tissues. It could also regulate sympathetic tone reflected by blood pressure and heart rate attenuation thereby improving erectile function.

SODIUM-GLUCOSE COTRANSPORTER-2

Sodium-glucose cotransporter-2 inhibitors[13] improve glycemic control in type 2 diabetes mellitus (T2DM) patients and have cardioprotective effects.[14] A link between SGLT-2 inhibition and improved macro- and microvascular endothelial functions may involve the role of SLGT-2 in the regulation of endothelial physiology. SGLT-2 inhibitors, by reducing hyperglycemia and body weight, reduce oxidative stress and improve endothelial function. When used along with metformin, it results physiological erections by positive effects on vasculogenic ED, potentially avoiding the need for PDE5 inhibitors.

PHOSPHODIESTERASE TYPE 5 INHIBITORS

Amongst all the five PDE5 inhibitors, currently available are sildenafil, tadalafil, vardenafil, udenafil, and avanafil. The best choice appears to be tadalafil in a low dose of 2.5 or 5 or 10 mg on chronic basis.[15] In men with diabetes and ED, once-daily tadalafil 2.5 and 5 mg was efficacious and well-tolerated, suggesting this may be an alternative to on-demand treatment for some men, eliminating the need to plan sex within a limited timeframe. No study drug-related serious adverse events were observed.[16-19] Treatment-emergent adverse events observed in ≥5% of the patients during the first year of either open-label extension were dyspepsia, headache, back pain, and influenza. No clinically meaningful abnormalities associated with tadalafil were observed for electrocardiograms or clinical laboratory measures. Mean IIEF domain scores improved from baseline to the conclusions of the 1- and 2-year open-label extensions, respectively: –EF, +10.4 and +10.8; –IS, +4.0

and +3.7; and -OS, +3.0 and +3.2. At the conclusion of the 2-year open-label extension, 95.7 and 92.1% of the patients reported positive responses to GAQ1 and GAQ2, respectively. Treatment with tadalafil significantly improved all primary efficacy variables, regardless of baseline glycated hemoglobin (HbA1c) level.[17]

COUNSELING AND LIFESTYLE MODIFICATION

Counseling and lifestyle modification (LSM) form the mainstay of treatment for management of ED. With intensive lifestyle interventions which included (10% fat whole foods vegetarian diet, aerobic exercise, stress management training, smoking cessation, and group psychosocial support), there was reversal of coronary artery disease (CAD)[20] for 5 years.

USE OF TESTOSTERONE REPLACEMENT THERAPY

Men with functional hypogonadism experienced remission of T2DM[21] when treated with injectable testosterone undecanoate. 2-year treatment with testosterone therapy resulted in normalized testosterone levels, improved glycemia, endothelial functions, lipids and insulin sensitivity, and quelled the symptoms of hypogonadism such as ED, low libido thus potentiating reduction of cardiovascular risk in obese men with functional hypogonadism and T2DM.

CONCLUSION

Erectile dysfunction is one of the most common complications of diabetes in men. The causes of ED are mainly psychogenic, vasculogenic, neurogenic, hormonogenic, and iatrogenic. The deadly quartet of noncommunicable diseases which include diabetes, hypertension, dyslipidemia, and obesity are surely affected with ED. Points to ponder is that if ED is considered as a symptom, then these patients need pharmacotherapy like low-dose short course of testosterone with caution and monitoring of prostatic-specific antigen. But if ED is considered as a disease, our aim should be to cure it which is possible with regenerative cell-based therapies which include stem cells, gene therapy, etc. and phytoneutraceuticals such as L-arginine, fenugreek, and other herbal compounds. Sexual dysfunction is not an option for a diabetic, it is how gracefully we handle the process and how lucky we are as the process handles us. We have the expertise and scientific wisdom for managing sexual dysfunction and so several million lives can be saved. We must act now.

Strategies to make ED as correctile dysfunction are control of hyperglycemia with metformin and SGLT-2 inhibitors, low-dose PDE5 inhibitors such as tadalafil 2.5 mg or 5 mg on chronic dosing. Statins such as rosuvastatin can be a life saver.

Lastly counseling for nutritional intervention and lifestyle modification forms the mainstay of treatment for improvement of sexual dysfunctions in diabetes. Needless to say, that with counseling, LSM, metformin, SGLT-2 inhibitors, ED in diabetes is a correctile dysfunction and if so, sex has no expiry date.

REFERENCES

1. IDF Atlas 2019. [online] Available from: https://diabetesatlas.org/. [Last accessed January 2022].
2. Ramachandran A, Snehalatha C, Shetty AS, Nanditha A. Trends in prevalence of diabetes in Asian countries. World J Diabetes. 2012;3(6):110-7.
3. Guay AT. ED2: erectile dysfunction = endothelial dysfunction. Endocrinol Metab Clin North Am. 2007;36(2):453-63.
4. Miner MM, Kuritzky L. Erectile dysfunction: a sentinel marker for cardiovascular disease in primary care. Cleve Clin J Med. 2007:74 Suppl 3:S30-7.
5. Abdul-Aziz AA, Desikan P, Prabhakaran D, Schroeder LF. Tackling the Burden of Cardiovascular Diseases in India. Circ Cardiovasc Qual Outcomes. 2019;12(4):e005195.
6. Hawton K. The prevalence and effects of sexual problems. In: Sex Therapy: A Practical Guide, 1st edition. Oxford: Oxford University Press; 1985. pp. 43-55.
7. Kouidrat Y, Pizzol D, Cosco T, Thompson T, Solmi M, Bertoldo B, et al. High prevalence of erectile dysfunction in diabetes: a systematic review and meta-analysis of 145 studies. Diabet Med. 2017;34(9):1185-92.
8. De Angelis L, Marfella M, Siniscalchi M, Napoo F, Marino L, Giugliano F, et al. Erectile and endothelial dysfunction in Type II diabetes: a possible link. Diabetologia. 2001;44(9):1155-60.
9. Yao F, Liu L, Zhang Y, Huang Y, Liu D, Lin H, et al. Erectile dysfunction may be the first clinical sign of insulin resistance and endothelial dysfunction in young men. Clin Res Cardiol. 2013;102(9):645-51.
10. Thorve VS, Kshirsagar AD, Vyawahare NS, Joshi VS, Ingale KG, Mohite RJ. Diabetes-induced erectile dysfunction: epidemiology, pathophysiology and management. J Diab Complications. 2011;25(2):129-36.
11. Bivalacqua TJ, Champion HC, Usta MF, Cellek S, Chitaley K, Webb RC, et al. RhoA/Rho-kinase suppresses endothelial nitric oxide synthase in the penis: A mechanism for diabetes-associated erectile dysfunction. Proc Natl Acad Sci U S A. 2004;101(24):9121-6.
12. Leonardi R, Alemanni M. The management of erectile dysfunction: innovations and future perspectives. Arch Ital Urol Androl. 2011;83(1):60-2.
13. Stallmann-Jorgensen I, Webb RC. Emerging molecular targets for treatment of erectile dysfunction: vascular and regenerative therapies on the horizon. Curr Drug Targets. 2015;16(5):427-41.
14. Wang AY, Podlasek CA. Role of nanotechnology in erectile dysfunction treatment. J Sex Med. 2017;14(1):36-43.
15. Che D, Fang Z, Yan L, Du J, Li F, Xie J, et al. Elevated pigment epithelium-derived factor induces diabetic erectile dysfunction via interruption of the Akt/Hsp90β/eNOS complex. Diabetologia 2020;9(63): 1857-71.
16. Patel JP, Lee EH, Mena CI, Walker CN. Effects of metformin on endothelial health and erectile dysfunction. Transl Androl Urol. 2017;6(3):556-65.
17. Ugusman A, Kumar J, Aminuddin A. Endothelial function and dysfunction: Impact of sodium-glucose cotransporter 2 inhibitors. Pharmacol Ther. 2021;224:107832.
18. Lopaschuk GD, Verma S. Mechanisms of cardiovascular benefits of sodium glucose co-transporter 2 (SGLT2) inhibitors: A state-of-the-art review. JACC Basic Transl Sci. 2020;5(6):632-44.
19. Hatzichristou D, Gambla M, Rubio-Aurioles E, Buvat J, Brock GB, Spera G, et al. Efficacy of tadalafil once daily in men with diabetes mellitus and erectile dysfunction. Diabet Med. 2008;25(2):138-46.
20. Porst H, Rajfer J, Casabé A, Feldman R, Ralph D, Vieiralves LF, et al. Long-term safety and efficacy of tadalafil 5 mg dosed once daily in men with erectile dysfunction. J Sex Med. 2008;5(9):2160-9.
21. Sáenz de Tejada I, Anglin G, Knight JR, Emmick JT. Effects of tadalafil on erectile dysfunction in men with diabetes. Diabetes Care. 2002;25(12):2159-64.

CHAPTER 11

Artificial Intelligence in Diabetic Retinopathy

Bhavana Sosale, Aravind Ramachandra Sosale

ABSTRACT

Diabetic retinopathy is a leading cause of preventable blindness. Advances in machine learning have enabled the development of artificial intelligence algorithms that can aid in the diagnosis of diabetic retinopathy. Cloud based and offline algorithms provide an immediate diagnosis of diabetic retinopathy. These technologies overcome several barriers to screening and are scalable solutions for the developed and developing world. Access to the algorithms and fundus cameras are some of the limitations associated with these technologies. This chapter summarizes the various machine learning algorithms available today. Deep learning algorithms allow screening of diabetic retinopathy to be widely employed to identify, treat, and prevent visual loss.

Keywords: *Screening, Diabetic retinopathy, Offline AI, Smartphone-based AI.*

INTRODUCTION

Diabetic retinopathy (DR) is a common preventable cause of blindness. The prevalence of DR in India at the time of diagnosis of diabetes is 5–6% and in those with diabetes of >5 years the prevalence is 35%.[1-3] One in three individuals with diabetes have DR and one in ten have sight-threatening diabetic retinopathy (STDR).[4] It is, thus, prudent to screen everyone with diabetes for DR to ensure early referral for preventing blindness.

With >73 million individuals with diabetes in India, the burden of manual screening is enormous for ophthalmologists to take on by themselves.[5] Other challenges to conventional screening include lack of access to ophthalmologists and loss to follow-up when patients are referred from primary care to the ophthalmologist. To screen and prevent blindness at the community level, a paradigm shift to move screening from the ophthalmologist to the primary care physician is necessary. Artificial intelligence (AI) algorithms can help address these operational challenges. AI can help aid in DR screening by involving nonophthalmologist doctors or other trained healthcare workers to screen for DR.

Advances in machine learning (ML) have led to the development of AI algorithms that can detect retinal disease. Several companies such as Google, Eyenuk, IDX, and Remidio Innovative Solutions have been working on detection of DR using AI. IDx-DR is currently the only AI algorithm approved by the Food and Drug Administration (FDA) for DR screening.

ARTIFICIAL INTELLIGENCE ALGORITHMS FOR DIABETIC RETINOPATHY SCREENING

Artificial intelligence algorithms are currently trained and developed to identify referable diabetic retinopathy (RDR). RDR is defined as disease more than moderate nonproliferative diabetic retinopathy (NPDR) or the presence of diabetic macular edema (DME).

Artificial intelligence algorithms for DR screening are deep learning algorithms based on convolutional neural networks (CNNs). CNNs self-learn and have the ability to also identify subtle changes on a fundus photograph. Large datasets of retinal images obtained from teleophthalmology networks or hospital medical records are divided into a development set and a validation set. The algorithms are developed by feeding large amounts of data (training data) into the algorithm to train it to identify patterns of disease (e.g., microaneurysms, hemorrhages, or neovascularization). The algorithms separate images without RDR (combined no DR and mild NPDR) and images with RDR. A part of the development set is used as the “tune set” to optimize model.[6]

Artificial intelligence algorithms are developed with the aim of maximizing the ability of the AI to identify all cases of RDR and maximizing its ability to rule out DR. This translates to the ability of an algorithm in achieving a high sensitivity for RDR and a high specificity for all grades of DR optimizing them for screening.

Artificial intelligence algorithms have multiple neural networks for different tasks. Images postprocessing are initially analyzed by a quality control algorithm and those that pass the quality check are then analyzed for signs of DR. Images, which fail the quality control, are flagged to alert the operator to recapture the image or refer to the ophthalmologist. Most algorithms provide a binary diagnosis of DR or no DR and some have the ability to provide a diagnosis of STDR. In order to train algorithms to grade DR, a greater number of images with adequate representation in each grade is necessary.[6] Many algorithms are currently being trained to grade DR and DME.

Algorithms, once trained, are validated internally (validation set) and in external data sets. Validation studies are necessary to evaluate if the performance of the AI can be reproducible in a new set of images previously unseen by the AI. Validation studies assess the performance of the AI by evaluating the sensitivity, specificity, and the area under the curve (AUC).[6] The sensitivity is a measure that evaluates the ability of a new diagnostic test to correctly identify all individuals with disease. The specificity is a measure that evaluates the ability of the new diagnostic test to correctly identify as healthy, everyone without disease. The AUC is a graphical representation of the trade-off between sensitivity and specificity.

The performance of AI algorithms is linked to several factors. It is dependent on the number of images used for training, the quality of the ground truth, the quality of the images, and the camera used to capture the images. If algorithms are trained on images from only one fundus cameras, it may not be able to possible to reproduce the performance of the AI, when images from a different camera are captured in the real world. It is, thus, essential for the training dataset to include images (mydriatic and nonmydriatic) from a wide range of cameras. This would help to improve the robustness of the algorithms' performance across all images captured in the real world.[6]

Most AI algorithms are "cloud based". This means that the analysis and reporting take place on an online server. Retinal images captured at the point of screening are uploaded into the software and within a certain turnaround time, a report is generated. Limitations include the need for internet in order for these algorithms to provide an immediate diagnosis. The Medios AI is the only algorithm that works "offline" integrated into the Remidio Fundus on Phone (FOP) camera (**Fig. 1**). This term "offline" refers to the fact that the

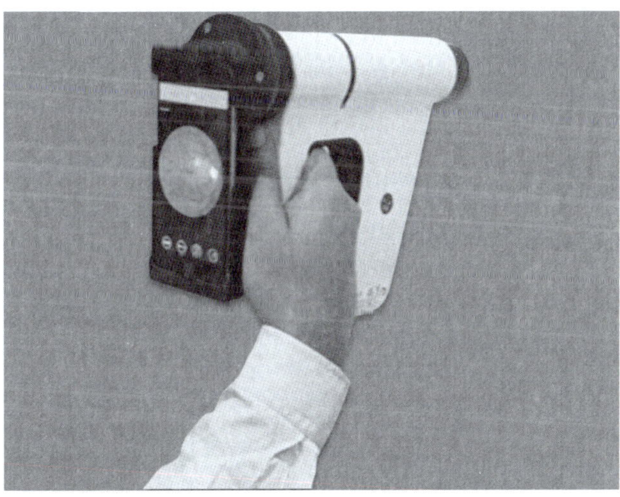

(AI: artificial intelligence; FOP: Fundus on Phone)

FIG. 1: The Remidio FOP with the offline Medios AI. ***(For color version, see Plate 2)***

inferencing of the AI takes place on the smartphone, i.e., the iPhone. The processing abilities of the iPhone and multiple libraries that enable building of deep learning applications enable the Medios algorithm to complete "offline" all the tasks that an online cloud-based algorithm would perform. Offline AI has the advantage of aiding in uninterrupted DR screening in countries with limited resources without continuous internet or electricity.[7,8] In addition, this is the only AI algorithm available for screening in India today.

GROUND TRUTH

The diagnosis of the AI is only as good as the ground truth that it is trained with and validated against. Deep learning systems (DLSs) learn and identify areas of pathology on the images they are trained with. It is, thus, apparent that the output of the AI is directly dependent on the labeling of the images in the training dataset. Since AI algorithms are also validated against the diagnosis of ophthalmologists, the performance in validation studies is also dependent on labeling of the "ground truth".

Studies on interobserver variability have taught us that there is variability among ophthalmologists in DR grading. Intergrader variability is assessed by measuring the "kappa" statistic. Cohen's kappa of >0.59 is considered moderate and >0.79 is considered strong and >0.9 is considered almost perfect.[9] When assessing the interobserver variability for different grades of DR, a quadratic weighted kappa is often calculated with greater penalties levied when diagnosis (or grade) is off by a greater degree.

While grading is based on the International Clinical Diabetic Retinopathy Severity (ICDRS) score, there are several images which fall into "gray zones" or appear to be in-between two classes.[10] There is always a potential for misclassification when the diagnosis of a single grader is used. Differences in diagnosis are also attributed to various factors such as the fundus camera used to capture the image, image transfer software, image resolution, image color, magnification, artifacts, image viewer, and training or experience of the reader. Missed microaneurysms, artifacts, and misclassification of hemorrhages have been identified as common causes of discordance.

The methods to reduce intergrader variability include having a senior arbitrator, considering a majority diagnosis or adjudication until a consensus is reached. Most studies have compared DR screening algorithms to a majority diagnosis of ophthalmologists. A study by Krause et al. demonstrated an increase in the performance of a DR screening algorithm if adjudication of images is performed, compared to an individual or majority diagnosis.[11] While adjudication currently appears to be the best possible method to reduce intergrader variability, it is time-consuming, expensive, and not practical when grading a large number of images. For large retrospective studies evaluating AI algorithms in greater than lac individuals, even a single grader diagnosis from a reading center has been considered for ground truth.[12] While this may not be ideal, it is comparable to DR screening in the real world by a single ophthalmologist or grader.

PERFORMANCE OF ARTIFICIAL INTELLIGENCE ALGORITHMS

Artificial intelligence algorithms such as IDx-DR, EyeArt, Google AI, and Medios have been validated in retrospective studies using datasets and in prospective studies. Both types of studies demonstrate the performance of the AI with images captured in the real world and images not previously seen by the AI. Such studies further reiterate the ability of the AI in identifying RDR and STDR when fed with images from individuals with DR. **Table 1** summarizes the performance of AI algorithms in the detection of RDR.

TABLE 1 Performance of AI algorithms in the diagnosis of referable diabetic retinopathy.

	AI software	Camera	Images	Sensitivity	Specificity
FDA cutoff for superiority[13]	–	–	–	85%	82.5%
SMART study by Sosale et al.[8]	Medios AI	Remidio FOP	Nonmydriatic	93%	92.5%
Sosale et al.[7]	Medios AI	Remidio FOP	Mydriatic	98.8%	86.7%
Natarajan et al.[14]	Medios AI	Remidio FOP	Mydriatic	100%	88.4%
Rajalakshmi et al.[15]	EyeArt	Remidio FOP	Mydriatic	99.3%	68.8%
Bhaskaranand M et al.[12]	EyeArt	Desktop cameras	Mydriatic and nonmydriatic	91%	91%
IDx[13]	IDx-DR	Topcon	Mydriatic and nonmydriatic	87.2%	90.7%
Gulshan et al.[16]	Google AI	• Topcon • 3nethra • Forus	Nonmydriatic	Site 1—88.9% Site 2—92.1%	Site 1—92.2% Site 2—95.2%
Ting et al.[17]	–	• Zeiss • Topcon • Cannon	–	90.5%	91.6%

(AI: artificial intelligence; FDA: Food and Drug Administration; FOP: Fundus on Phone)

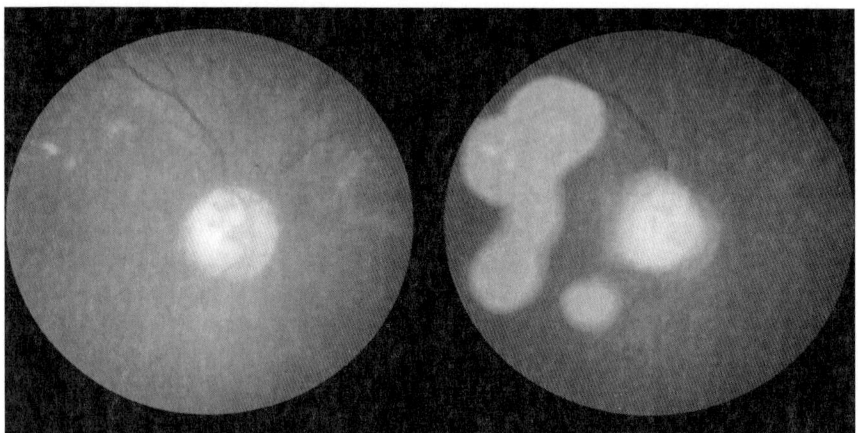

FIG. 2: A report generated by the Medios artificial intelligence (AI) in an individual with diabetic retinopathy. ***(For color version, see Plate 2)***

Result: Signs of retinopathy are detected. Examples of lesions are highlighted.

Most studies have used images captured from desktop high-end cameras, while some have used images from low cost smartphone cameras. These algorithms have been validated using both mydriatic and nonmydriatic images with no significant degradation in performance observed even with nonmydriatic images. This is noteworthy as most DR screening programs have protocols that necessitate the use of nonmydriatic imaging.

In addition to detection of RDR, the performance of the AI in detecting STDR has also been evaluated (**Fig. 2**). The sensitivity and specificity of EyeArt to detect STDR were observed to be 99.1% and 80.4% in the study by Rajalakshmi et al.[15] The sensitivity of the Medios AI in the detection of STDR was found to be between 98.7 and 100% in different studies.[7,8,14] The DLS used in the study by Ting et al. also reported a sensitivity of 100% for STDR.[17]

A recent effort to grade DR and DME was published by Ruamviboonsuk et al. using 25,326 images from a nationwide screening program in Thailand. The DLS had a sensitivity and specificity of 0.96 and 0.95 to detect moderate or worse NPDR. It performed better than individual grader in detecting severe or worse NPDR, PDR, and DME with an AUC of 0.99. Across all grades, the DLS reduced the false-negative rate by 23% and increased the false-positive rates by 2% compared to individual graders.[18]

Most validation studies use retinal images that need to pass a certain quality check (deemed gradable by the grader) and by the AI. However, in the real world, it is likely that all images captured may not meet the same standards. Speculation on whether AI algorithms can perform similar to that seen in validation studies is often a concern. A few studies help us address this issue and have explored the use of "not so ideal" images or images deemed unfit by the AI. Natarajan et al. reported no drop in sensitivity of RDR with an increase in false-positive results with the Medios AI. These sensitivity analyses have concluded that use of images which fail the inbuilt AI quality control system does not lead to concerns with patient safety as all individuals with RDR are identified by the AI. A slightly higher referral rate could perhaps add to healthcare costs without undermining safety. Currently, operators operating most AI systems are trained to recommend "referral" if images are flagged "unscreenable" or if the images fail quality check.

BENEFITS AND LIMITATIONS OF ARTIFICIAL INTELLIGENCE ALGORITHMS

Artificial intelligence algorithms provide an immediate diagnosis at the point-of-care. They can aid primary care physicians and health workers in ensuring timely referral in those with RDR. Some AI algorithms that use class activation mapping can also highlight areas of lesions in the reports.[14,19] This increases the confidence in the decision of the AI when a report of "referral" is generated and increases the referrals to the specialists when DR is detected. Heat maps improve acceptance for clinical use for both doctors and individuals with diabetes.

Artificial intelligence can help screen the millions with diabetes without access to ophthalmologists. Indigenous AI like the Medios AI on the Remidio FOP can be used for screening even in areas without electricity or internet.

Most AI algorithms run on images captured from desktop cameras, which may not be feasible financially and practically for large scale screening. IDx-DR, EyeArt, and Google AI are also not available in India and other developing countries. The Remidio FOP with the Medios AI, the only AI available in India, can overcome these logistic challenges of cost and portability.

Artificial intelligence algorithms trained and validated against a majority or adjudicated diagnosis that can help overcome barriers associated with teleophthalmology such as access and intergrader variability. With an increasing number of algorithms performing better than individual ophthalmologists, technology can help reduce variability in reporting, minimize subjective bias and provide a more consistent diagnosis.

Artificial intelligence algorithms, currently in use, can provide a binary diagnosis of referral or no referral. Further work into grading of DR is necessary. This can assist primary care physicians and patients get a better understanding of disease severity and triaging for timely referral.

All AI algorithms have a false-negative and false-positive rate. The FDA mandated limit for sensitivity and specificity for RDR is 85% and 82.5%. While the sensitivity and specificity of the algorithms in use are high, they can never approach 100% accuracy rates. While this may be acceptable for screening, it is important to have clear cut, cutoff values for sensitivity and specificity for STDR from the regulatory bodies.

Artificial intelligence algorithms for DR detection cannot replace a comprehensive eye examination. Greater research and development into integrating algorithms for detection of DR, glaucoma, and other retinal disorders into one algorithm can aid in providing better comprehensive care.

FUTURE OF ARTIFICIAL INTELLIGENCE AND DIABETIC RETINOPATHY SCREENING

We are in the era of the AI revolution. AI-related research is on the rise and the technology is promising. However, in many fields, the work on AI appears to be limited to research.

If addressed to solve existing problems, technology integrated into medical practice has the potential to changes the way we practice medicine and touch lives.

Diabetic retinopathy is an example of one of the few conditions in medicine where the use of AI is not limited to research and publications. It is one of the few conditions where AI algorithms can be implemented in everyday practice. DR screening technologies will never be a threat to replace doctors. AI will instead serve as decision support system or as a physician assist technology to enable screening, triage, and timely referrals in areas without access to ophthalmologists. With time, it is likely that we will have a better understanding of how AI algorithms can be integrated into the workflow and aid in decision-making.

Advancements to look forward include grading of retinopathy, detection of DME, and expansion of AI into identifying systemic links to cardiovascular disease and renal disease. The day this is achieved, the eye will truly be a window into our physical and mental health.

CONCLUSION

As treating physicians, the onus is on us to screen our patients with diabetes for DR. If we do not embrace and integrate DR screening algorithms into clinical care, our patients are likely to go blind.[20]

REFERENCES

1. Gadkari S, Maskati Q, Nayak B. Prevalence of diabetic retinopathy in India: The All India Ophthalmological Society Diabetic Retinopathy Eye Screening Study 2014. Indian J Ophthalmol. 2016;64:38-44.
2. Sosale A, Prasanna KM, Sadikot SM, Nigam A, Bajaj S, Zargar AH, et al. Chronic complications in newly diagnosed patients with type 2 diabetes mellitus in India. Indian J Endocrinol Metab. 2014;18:355-60.
3. Sosale B, Sosale AR, Mohan AR, Kumar PM, Saboo B, Kandula S. Cardiovascular risk factors, micro and macrovascular complications at diagnosis in patients with young onset T2 diabetes in India: CINDI 2. Indian J Endocrinol Metab. 2016;20:114-8.
4. Yau J, Rogers S, Kawasaki R, Lamoureux E, Kowalski J, Bek T, et al. Global Prevalence and Major Risk Factors of Diabetic Retinopathy. Diabetes Care. 2012;35:556-64.

5. International Diabetes Federation (IDF). (2017). IDF Diabetes Atlas Across the Globe. [online] Available from http://www.diabetesatlas.org/across-the-globe.html. [Last accessed December, 2020].
6. Raman R, Srinivasan S, Virmani S, Sivaprasad S, Rao C, Rajalakshmi R. Fundus photograph-based deep learning algorithms in detecting diabetic retinopathy. Eye. 2018;33:97-109.
7. Sosale B, Sosale AR, Murthy H, Sengupta S, Naveenam M. Medios—an offline, smartphone-based artificial intelligence algorithm for the diagnosis of diabetic retinopathy. Indian J Ophthalmol. 2020;68:391-5.
8. Sosale B, Aravind SR, Murthy H, Narayana S, Sharma S, Gowda SG, et al. Simple, Mobile-based Artificial Intelligence Algorithm in the detection of Diabetic Retinopathy (SMART) Study. BMJ Open Diabetes Res Care. 2020;8:e000892.
9. McHugh ML. Interrater reliability: the kappa statistic. Biochem Med (Zagreb). 2012;22:276-82.
10. Wilkinson C, Ferris F, Klein R, Lee P, Agardh C, Davis M, et al. Proposed international clinical diabetic retinopathy and diabetic macular edema disease severity scales. Ophthalmology. 2003;110:1677-82.
11. Krause J, Gulshan V, Rahimy E, Karth P, Widner K, Corrado G, et al. Grader Variability and the Importance of Reference Standards for Evaluating Machine Learning Models for Diabetic Retinopathy. Ophthalmology. 2018;125:1264-72.
12. Bhaskaranand M, Ramachandra C, Bhat S, Cuadros J, Nittala M, Sadda S, et al. The Value of Automated Diabetic Retinopathy Screening with the EyeArt System: A Study of More Than 100,000 Consecutive Encounters from People with Diabetes. Diabetes Technol Ther. 2019;21:635-43.
13. Abràmoff MD, Lavin PT, Birch M, Shah N, Folk JC. Pivotal trial of an autonomous AI-based diagnostic system for detection of diabetic retinopathy in primary care offices. NPJ Digit Med. 2018;39:1.
14. Natarajan S, Jain A, Krishnan R, Rogye A, Sivaprasad S. Diagnostic Accuracy of Community-Based Diabetic Retinopathy Screening With an Offline Artificial Intelligence System on a Smartphone. JAMA Ophthalmol. 2019;137:1182-8.
15. Rajalakshmi R, Subashini R, Anjana R, Mohan V. Automated diabetic retinopathy detection in smartphone-based fundus photography using artificial intelligence. Eye. 2018;32:1138-44.
16. Gulshan V, Rajan R, Widner K, Wu D, Wubbels P, Rhodes T, et al. Performance of a Deep-Learning Algorithm vs Manual Grading for Detecting Diabetic Retinopathy in India. JAMA Ophthalmol. 2019;137:987-93.
17. Ting D, Cheung C, Lim G, Tan G, Quang N, Gan A, et al. Development and Validation of a Deep Learning System for Diabetic Retinopathy and Related Eye Diseases Using Retinal Images From Multiethnic Populations With Diabetes. JAMA. 2017;318:2211-23.
18. Ruamviboonsuk P, Krause J, Chotcomwongse P, Sayres R, Raman R, Widner K, et al. Deep learning versus human graders for classifying diabetic retinopathy severity in a nationwide screening program. NPJ Digit Med. 2019;2:25.
19. Raman R, Srinivasan S, Virmani S, Sivaprasad S, Rao C, Rajalakshmi R. Fundus photograph-based deep learning algorithms in detecting diabetic retinopathy. Eye. 2018;33:97-109
20. Sosale AR. Screening for diabetic retinopathy—is the use of artificial intelligence and cost-effective fundus imaging the answer? Int J Diabetes Dev Ctries. 2019;39:1-3.

CHAPTER 12

Teleconsultation in Diabetes Care

Jothydev Kesavadev, Sreelakshmi R, Gopika Krishnan, Arun Shankar

ABSTRACT

Teleconsultation has become the mainstay of treatment for lifestyle disorders, especially with the emergence of Coronavirus disease 2019 (COVID-19). The chapter sheds light on the evolution of telemedicine, components, and studies that underline the benefit of telemedicine in diabetes management and care. There are mentions on the architecture of telemedicine with "Diabetes Tele Management System®" as a model, research output of the attained glycemic goals and the challenges in running such a system. An overview of the guidelines published by the Medical Council of India for the healthier and legalized practice of telemedicine in India is also described.

Keywords: *Telemedicine, DTMS®, RMP, EMR, First consult, Follow-up consult.*

INTRODUCTION

The burgeoning chronic lifestyle diseases, associated comorbidities, and treatment burden have ushered the use of technologies to redesign the global healthcare system for better care. Combined technologies led to the fusion of a 150-year-old telecommunication technology with new information technology, the telemedicine.

EVOLUTION OF TELEMEDICINE TO MAINSTREAM HEALTH CARE

The first telemedicine consultation began with the invention of telephone by Alexander Graham Bell, documented in the *Lancet* on 29th November, 1879: a doctor diagnosed the disease of a child at night over the telephone.[1] The National Aeronautics and Space Administration (NASA) has played a pivotal role in the initial stages of telemedicine, starting[2] in the early 1960s. During the period from 1972 to 1975, the NASA involved in the Space Technology Applied to Rural Papago Advanced Health Care (STARPAHC) delivered medical care to the Papago Indian Reservation intending to provide health care to astronauts in space.[3] Since then, many countries followed the technology for the treatment and prevention of various ailments including lifestyle disorders such as diabetes. In India, the Medical Council of India on 25th March 2020, published the telemedicine practice guidelines—amendment to the Indian Medical Council Regulations 2002 in view of the outbreak of Coronavirus disease 2019 (COVID-19) pandemic.

How to Define Telemedicine?

Telemedicine, a combination of two words *Tele*, a Greek word meaning "distance" and *mederi*, a Latin word meaning "to heal" in its simplest form, can be defined as the use of telecommunication technology in the treatment of diseases when distances part the healthcare providers and the patients.[4]

DEFINITION OF TELEMEDICINE BY THE WORLD HEALTH ORGANIZATION

The World Health Organization (WHO) defines telemedicine as "the delivery of healthcare services, where distance is a critical factor, by all healthcare professionals using information and communication technologies for the exchange of valid information for diagnosis, treatment and prevention of disease and injuries, research and evaluation, and for the continuing education of healthcare providers, all in the interests of advancing the health of individuals and their communities."

TELEMEDICINE SYSTEM

The telemedicine system can be described as an interface between hardware, software, and a communication channel that connects two geographical locations for teleconsultation.[4]

TELEMEDICINE FOR DIABETES CARE

Diabetes is a chronic noncommunicable disease which requires regular consultations for treatment and counseling. According to the International Diabetes Federation (IDF), in 2019, about 463 million people are living with diabetes. Among these, about 79% of adults with diabetes are from low- and middle-income countries. It is evident that novel technologies are needed to reduce the burden of diabetes care.

Effective treatment of diabetes requires a personalized approach in restyling the lifestyle of patients and motivating them to adapt to the therapy for optimal outcome. The major challenges in treating diabetes are maintaining drug adherence, monitoring diet, exercise, and self-management of glucose instructions. The prime objective will be to maintain the blood glucose in the prescribed target level and be in the specified duration of time-in-range (TIR), which can be more easily achieved with a telemedicine-based frequent follow-up program rather than in-person visits. To widen the existing measures of therapy, telemedicine shows a promising future for the short-term and long-term management of diabetes with better outcomes. Also, telemedicine is believed to modify the traditional health care in diabetes by complementing effective solutions to the prevailing gaps and limitations.

The treatment of diabetes in patients aims to achieve normoglycemia with an appropriate balance between diet, physical activity, and insulin dosages. The treatment of diabetes being complex, costly, and time-consuming, the introduction of various applications of information technology into diabetes care can result in the delivery of cost-effective treatment along with other benefits.

There are two main approaches to telemedicine consultations: (1) The doctor-centric approach; and (2) The patient-centric approach. In a doctor-centric approach, telemedicine helps doctors in maintaining a patient database, statistical analysis of data, interpretation programs for representation, etc. In a patient-centric approach, the system can be used by patients for the collection, storage, and retrieval of the data such as from glucose monitoring devices.[5,6]

The integrated system of telemedicine in diabetes management and care was first addressed by the DIACRONO system implemented in 1987, which has a portable microcomputer, data collection facilities, and decision-making systems for the evaluation and interpretation of the glucose monitoring data, but the system faced many limitations with the microcomputer, hardware, software, and in decision-making. Further advancements in telemedicine for diabetes care reached the status of advising patients over the telephone on insulin doses, diet, exercise, etc., after the interpretation of data by a healthcare provider.[7] For instance, the telemedicine application which stressed on the dietary aspects of patients with diabetes was the Diabeto project with educational programs related to the diet.[8] The SESAM-DIABETE was a sophisticated approach using the French videotext telecommunication which provided patients access from their dwelling place and advices on diet and nutrition, physical activity, ketonuria, hypoglycemia, and hyperglycemia.[9] The projects 'Guardian Angel' and 'HumaLink' also are advanced forms of teleconsultation systems that support patients for the proper management of diabetes.[10] The DIABTel program developed in the later stages of the developmental approach covered many of the limitations of the earlier teleconsultation ventures and provided an integrated platform for doctors and patients for the exchange of data and timely advices to improve the various levels of diabetes care.[11]

The implementation of the Diabetes Control and Complications Trial (DCCT) had contributed to an increased glucose profile data of patients with diabetes. The DCCT demonstrated the advantages both for doctors in monitoring data for decision-making and for patients in blood glucose monitoring and adjusting insulin doses when the data was transferred to the doctors.

In the past, telemedicine technology was limited mostly to type 1 diabetes mellitus (T1DM) patients. Concepts such as "user modeling" and "context awareness"[12] in telemedicine technology, wearable computers, personal digital assistants,[13] laptops,[14] mobile phone platforms, automated dialog systems, etc., promoted the implementation of telemedicine in the management of type 2 diabetes mellitus (T2DM) as well. With telemedicine practices, there has been a paradigm shift from visit-by-visit systems to day-by-day systems that satisfied both the physician and patient requirements.[15] Though the concept of telemedicine is more than a century old, we have probably never explored the many benefits of this technology to patient care, education, research, administration, and public health.[16]

According to Klonoff et al., for a telemedicine system to be functional, it requires five major components: (1) An accurate data collection procedure, (2) An electronic medical record to incorporate and remotely transmit data, (3) A set of protocols for distant data analysis, (4) Different communication tools which allow effective communication between patients and healthcare providers, and (5) A system that provides feedback on the data.[17]

As a telemedicine prototype for the comprehensive management of diabetes from the author's real-time experience of more than two decades, a brief description of some of the advantages of the telemedicine program, the Diabetes Tele Management System (DTMS®), originally introduced at Jothydev's Diabetes Research Centre at Trivandrum South India in 1998, with a proven history of successful applications at various levels of diabetes management and care, has been included.[15]

ARCHITECTURE OF THE DIABETES TELE MANAGEMENT SYSTEM®

The DTMS® has five major components such as: (1) A customized software which includes electronic medical records (EMR) with different user interfaces, (2) A decision support system provided by the multidisciplinary team, (3) Telecommunication with the help of telephones, e-mails, and internet using a secure website, (4) Telemedicine enabled customized empowerment, education, and troubleshooting, and (5) Ensuring multidrug compliance in diabetes by linking DTMS® with diabetes pharmacy.[15] In DTMS®, titration of insulin and oral drug dosage is based on several patient-specific characteristics such as glycated hemoglobin (HbA1c), blood pressure, low-density lipoprotein (LDL), etc., and not on any fixed algorithm.

TABLE 1 Parameters showing the individual characterization for therapeutic goals.

Patient characteristics	Disease characteristics
• Age of the patient	• Type of diabetes
• Level of education and motivation	• Duration of diabetes
• Presence of caregiver at home/staying alone	• Baseline glycated hemoglobin value
• Socioeconomic status	• Previous history of serious hypoglycemic episodes
• Continuous glucose monitoring data, if available	• Comorbid illness

Education modules on insulin injection technique, diet, exercise, use of a glucometer, hypoglycemia, and compliance to medications are administered to the patient *via* DTMS®. Blood glucose are reported over several months to years and are stored in the database for further reference. DTMS® has been found advantageous in many aspects of diabetes management such as, frequently titrating the doses of medications, drastically reducing the number of hospital visits, providing cost-effective treatment, and suggestions on lifestyle-tuning measures that ultimately aid them to achieve their customized goals of therapy.

The uniqueness of DTMS® is the individualization of therapeutic goals based on the following parameters that is given in **Table 1**.[15]

CLINICAL EVIDENCES FOR THE FEASIBILITY OF TELEDIABETES FROM ACROSS THE WORLD

Across the world, there has been the practice of telemedicine that contributes to the betterment of diabetes therapy with varying numbers and characteristics of chosen patient cohort. For instance, the PLATEDIAN (Telemedicine on Metabolic Control in Type 1 Diabetes Mellitus Andalusian Patients) study conducted on 388 T1DM patients to assess the impact of telemedicine visit using the platform 'Diabetic' compared to face-to-face visits on clinical outcomes, patient's health-related quality of life (HRQoL), and physician's satisfaction reported that the use of telemedicine platforms provide similar efficacy and safety outcomes as face-to-face visits.[18] Another study which evaluated how patients perceive telehealth for the management of T2DM showed that the patients viewed and considered telehealth as a potential tool to upgrade their quality of life.[19] A study conducted on subjects with T1DM who used an automated Diabetes Interactive Diary (DID) to calibrate the individual's appropriate insulin dose for each meal, which got published in 2013, revealed that the feasibility and comparability of using the DID in terms of the outcome is equivalent to in-person traditional carbohydrate counting and also in reducing moderate/severe hypoglycemia risks.[20] A German observational study conducted among overweight or obese children and adolescents to determine the acceptance and effectiveness of a sophisticated mobile motion sensor device and a digital camera integrated into a mobile phone revealed that utilization of the system resulted in significant weight reduction among the cohort.[21] Another observational study on 117 patients with T1DM or T2DM from US also reported satisfactory results in its primary outcome measure as change in glucose level and reinforced the feasibility of incorporating a telediabetes system into existing diabetes management programs.[22] The US telephone-based self-management telediabetes program which was unique in terms of focusing on safety issues and adverse event characteristics, including detection alerts, preventability, enhancing potential, and primary care provider awareness of such events had observed that telephone surveillance had facilitated self-management support program for the detection of adverse events.[23] A study on pediatric patients with T1DM a mean age of 12 years, which investigated the feasibility of making scheduled telephone calls from a "pediatric diabetes educator" on a bimonthly basis reported that the telemedicine is a better supportive aid for diabetes care.[24] All these studies provide evidence to the use of telemedicine for the effective management of diabetes at various levels.

TELEMEDICINE IN DIABETES MANAGEMENT DURING CORONAVIRUS DISEASE 2019

Coronavirus disease 2019 has revolutionized the widespread implementation and application of telemedicine in various fields of medicine. Even though telemedicine was practiced for several decades, it was due to COVID-19, there is resurgence in the use of telemedicine, especially in lifestyle illnesses.

Diabetes has emerged as one of the major risk factors for increased mortality in COVID-19 patients and treatment modalities, therefore, should adhere to achieve better glycemic control in patients with diabetes. In diabetes, we require frequent change of dosages to titrate the dose of medication and frequent visits to hospitals either to meet the doctors or the nurses, which is possible with telemedicine and is not possible with in-person visits. Telemedicine also has the provision for exchange of messages or brief communications *via* audio/video which is convenient for both physicians and patients during the COVID-19 period where there are restrictions on in-person hospital visits and difficulty in face-to-face consultations. Various platforms such as Zoom for Telehealth, AMC Health, Doxy.me, etc., and specialized programs such as the DTMS® for treating diabetes can be made use of to avail telemedicine consultations.

Scientific studies provide evidence to the merits of telemedicine consultation for diabetes during COVID-19. A cross-sectional study, which analyzed the effectiveness of telephone-based advice which focused on glycemic control, emotional control, and behavioral status in elderly patients with T2DM (aged ≥60 years) revealed that telemedicine can improve glycemic control and anxiety in patients during COVID-19.[25] A study from a tertiary care center in India that utilized telemedicine for diabetes management in patients (n = 103) showed that diabetes care can be efficiently delivered through telemedicine platforms.[26] Studies also discuss the evidences and guidelines regarding the use of telemedicine in diabetes management.[27] A study which investigated telemedicine feasibility and effectiveness in managing insulin dosage and new-onset diabetes education in T1DM adult patients on multiple daily insulin injections and pediatric patients on insulin pump and use continuous glucose monitoring (CGM) with commercially available analysis software (Dexcom CLARITY and Glooko) for generating ambulatory glucose profiles and summary reports for interpretation showed that it is safe and effective to use telemedicine for new-onset T1DM training and education for both pediatric and adult patients and their families.[28] A report by Antonio Ceriello opined that lessons learnt from COVID-19 crisis has prompted the healthcare industry to adopt telemedicine as the tool for managing diabetes and associated comorbidities where in-person consultations became difficult and to be carried forward as an effective method of treatment delivery in any disaster outbreak.[29] These studies provide insights into the significant contribution of telemedicine in diabetes management.

Analysis, management, and storage of patient data pose yet another challenge to healthcare professionals. Innovations in information technology had revolutionized the transformation from paper documents to EMR. The utilization of EMR paved the way to capture biographical, clinical, and biochemical data at a particular instance and on follow-up.[30,31]

PRECEDENCE OF TELEMEDICINE IN DIABETES CARE

Impact on Glycemic Control

Telemedicine ensures achievement of treatment targets of glycemia in motivated patients adhering to the instructions of the telemedicine program. Research studies on patients who are utilizing telemedicine programs such as the DTMS® had reported that frequent telemedicine follow-ups based on self-monitoring of blood glucose (SMBG) enable slow and steady titration of drug dose and reducing the risk of hypoglycemia or significantly low instances of serious hypoglycemia.[32]

Reducing Microvascular and Macrovascular Complications

The long duration of diabetes is associated with the development of micro- and macrovascular complications which eventually lead to retinopathy, leg ulcers, and increased cardiovascular morbidities and mortalities. Telemedicine-based care through programs like DTMS® had aided in the sustainability of the glycemic goals in subjects translating to the prevention of vascular complications in about 93.5% of the T2D subjects.[33]

Cost-effectiveness of Telemedicine in Diabetes

The treatment of diabetes through telemedicine was found to be cost-effective as the patients can avail it with the minimal requirement of a land phone/cell phone. Telemedicine is found to be effective in patients to save time and money and can also take advantage of the treatment at the comfort of the patient's home/office. In this aspect, a retrospective study on the cost-effectiveness of telemedicine program, DTMS® analyzed in T2DM patients with a 6-month follow-up data, revealed that telemedicine for the management of diabetes is cost-effective and safe.[34]

Ensuring Multidrug Compliance

Loss of multidrug compliance in the long term is one of the major reasons for the development of complications in diabetes. Virtual communications via programs such as DTMS® ensure compliance to drugs for the treatment of glycemia and associated comorbidities.

CHALLENGES WITH TELEMEDICINE CONSULTATIONS

- Communication errors, inefficiency to respond to questions, unavailability of the physician to attend the phone, etc., can cause discomfort to patients in teleconsultation.
- Even the slightest error in communication during a telemedicine consultation can result in serious consequences. Therefore, extensive and continuous training, and supervision of a multidisciplinary team are required to ensure quality and expert delivery of service to patients. Multiple checks on the existing drugs and their dosage by the telemedicine team should be considered a must.
- Alternative funding resources and mode of payment are to be sought in case patients are not willing to pay extra for the teleconsultation.
- One-to-one and group patient education programs should include benefits and cost-effectiveness of telemedicine in diabetes in short and long term to gain the confidence of the patients in teleconsultation.

- Teleconsultation still lacks a universally recommended telemedicine protocol, or consensus guidelines to implement recommendations for telemedicine in diabetes customized to geographical and clinic-specific variables.

Considering the merits and demerits of telemedicine (**Table 2**), the merits outweigh the demerits and even if there are a couple of demerits, we can easily explore solutions to overcome those since telemedicine in diabetes invariably reduces long-term complications and the enormous cost burden incurred by diabetes.

TABLE 2 Merits and demerits of telemedicine.

Merits	Demerits
More chances of achieving glycated hemoglobin (HbA1c) goals	Face-to-face consultations are not possible
Proven to be effective in the prevention of hypoglycemia	Proper physical examination is a challenge in telemedicine
Cost-effective, safe, and time-saving	Telemedicine is not adopted by many doctors due to unfamiliarity with use of technologies In India, patients are not being familiar with technological advances, probably are not considering teleconsultation as real consultation
Exchange of data and necessary advice is possible via audio/video/text messages	Cannot perform investigations in hospitals as it requires patient visits directly to hospitals
Reduces frequent in-hospital visits	Quality of patients in terms of education and skill in using the technology is essential in teleconsultation
Ensures long-term multidrug compliance for treatment of glycemia and other comorbidities	Errors in communication, inefficiency to respond to queries, and absence of doctors during consultations cause discomfort to patients
Provides better adherence to exercise and dietetic recommendations	Teleconsultation still lacks a universally accepted telemedicine protocol or consensus guidelines for its implementation customized to geographic and clinic-specific variables
Proven to reduce short-term and long-term complications of diabetes	Requires extensive, continuous training and supervision of the healthcare team to ensure quality and expert delivery of services to patients as even a slight error may result in serious adverse outcomes
Reduce microvascular and macrovascular complications	Funding for telemedicine is a challenge in many areas
Applicable to patients with type 1 and type 2 diabetes mellitus	Revenue of hospital pose challenge to many big hospitals and small clinics to implement telemedicine

TELEMEDICINE PRACTICE IN INDIA

The Medical Council of India had recently published guidelines for the practice of telemedicine in India in par with the COVID-19 outbreak and includes the important aspects of initiating a telemedicine practice in the country.

- *Registered Medical Practitioner (RMP)*: A RMP is entitled to provide telemedicine consultation to patients from any part of India. RMPs using telemedicine shall uphold the same professional and ethical norms and standards as applicable to traditional in-person care within the intrinsic limitations of telemedicine.
- *Telemedicine applications*: The guidelines classify telemedicine applications into four basic types: (1) According to the mode of communication, (2) Timing of the information transmitted, (3) The purpose of the consultation, and (4) The interaction between the individuals involved—be it RMP-to-patient/caregiver or RMP-to-RMP.
  - *According to the mode of communication*: Telemedicine consultations can be either through video using telemedicine facility apps, video on chat platforms, Skype/FaceTime, etc., or through audio using phone, Voice over Internet Protocol (VoIP), apps, etc., or text based using the telemedicine chat-based applications such as specialized telemedicine smartphone apps, websites, other internet-based systems, etc., and general messaging/text/chat platforms such as WhatsApp, Google Hangouts, Facebook Messenger, etc., or asynchronous methods such as email/fax, etc.
  - *According to timing of information transmitted*: For real-time video/audio/text interactions, the RMPs can use either video/audio/text for the exchange of relevant information for diagnosis, medication, health education, and counseling. For asynchronous exchange of relevant information such as the transmission of summary of patient complaints and supplementary data including images, laboratory reports, and/or radiological investigations between stakeholders can be forwarded to different parties at any point of time and thereafter accessed as per convenience or need.
  - *According to the purpose of the consultation*: The guidelines clearly differentiate the two main concepts of telemedicine, the first consult and follow-up consult. As for a nonemergency consult, the first consult is the one that is initiated by the patient with any RMP for diagnosis/treatment/health education/counseling and the follow-up consult is the one which patients may use the service for follow-up consultation on his ongoing treatment with the same RMP who prescribed the treatment in an earlier in-person consult.
  - *According to the individuals involved*: According to the individuals involved, the telemedicine services may be utilized to connect patient to RMP, caregiver to RMP, RMP-to-RMP, and health worker to RMP.

In addition to the aforementioned aspects, the guidelines spell out the seven elements which should be always taken into consideration before initiating a telemedicine consultation (**Table 3**).

In the case of prescribing medicines *via* telemedicine consultation (**Table 4**), the RMP shall provide a photo, scan, digital copy of a signed

TABLE 3 Seven elements of telemedicine.

Elements of telemedicine	Definitions/Concepts
Context	Telemedicine should be appropriate and sufficient as per the context
Identification of Registered Medical Practitioner (RMP) and patient	RMP and the patient should reveal their identities. Every RMP shall display the registration number on prescriptions, website, etc.
Mode of communication	Multiple technologies such as video, audio, or text can be used to deliver telemedicine consultations
Patient consent	Patient consent is necessary for any telemedicine consultation which can be of implicit if initiated by the patient or of explicit if initiated by a health worker, RMP, or a caregiver
Patient evaluation	Collect and maintain sufficient medical information about patient such as history/examination, findings/investigation, reports/past records, etc., to exercise proper clinical judgment
Type of consultation	Properly demarcate the two types of patient consultations, which are the first consult and the follow-up consult
Patient management	RMP may proceed with a professional judgment to provide health education as appropriate in the case and/or provide counseling related to specific clinical condition and/or prescribe medicines according to the patient's condition

TABLE 4 Prescribing medicines via telemedicine consultations.

Classification of medicines	Description
List O	Medicines used for common conditions and are often available "over-the-counter" such as paracetamol, oral rehydration solution (ORS), cough lozenges, etc.
List A	Medications which can be prescribed during the first consult which is a video consultation, refill, and in case of follow-up
List B	Medications which are prescribed for a patient who is undergoing follow-up consultation in addition to those which have been prescribed during in-person consult for the same medical condition
Prohibited list of medicines	Schedule X of Drugs and Cosmetics Act and Rules or any narcotic and psychotropic substance listed in the Narcotic Drugs and Psychotropic Substances Act, 1985

prescription, or e-prescription to the patient *via* email or any messaging platform. The components of an e-prescription include the name, qualification, register number, address, contact details including e-mail and phone number of the RMP, date of consultation, details of the patient, descriptions on chief complaints, medical history, examination and laboratory findings, suggested investigations, special instructions, if any, and the signature and stamp of the RMP.

CONCLUSION

The implementation of telemedicine in treating various ailments has been a better choice for long-term management of lifestyle diseases such as diabetes. It offers new means for the practitioners and patients to communicate through web-based platforms such as e-mail, interactive chats, or videoconferences, thereby increasing the convenience level for the patient by reducing the number of visits required for in-patient consultations. The concept of telemedicine with applications that covers diverse scope, including computer-assisted diagnosis, online databases, and tools to ensure standards of care, safety, and more number of consultations to guide patients to reach therapeutic goals in the home and hospice care environments, thus serves as a potential treatment mode for the effective diabetes management and care.

REFERENCES

1. Aronson SH. The Lancet on the telephone 1876-1975. Med Hist. 1977;21(1):69-87.
2. Atmosphere US. Superintendent of Documents. Washington: US Government Printing Office; 1962.
3. Brown N. A brief history of telemedicine. Telemed Inform Exch. 1995;105(4):833-5.
4. Dasgupta A, Deb S. Telemedicine; a new horizon in public health in India. Indian J Community Med. 2008;33(1):3-8.
5. Lehmann ED, Deutsch T. Application of computers in diabetes care—a review. I. Computers for data collection and interpretation. Med Inform (Lond). 1995;20(4):281-302.
6. Lehmann ED, Deutsch T. Application of computers in diabetes care—a review. II. Computers for decision support and education. Med Inform (Lond). 1995;20(4):303-29.
7. Gómez-Aguilera EJ, del Pozo F, Serrano RM. (1987). Diacrono: a new portable microcomputer system for diabetes management. [online] Available from http://www.gbt.tfo.upm.es/pubsrv/index.php/publications/show/4. [Last accessed December, 2020].
8. Turnin MCG, Beddok RH, Clottes JP, Martini PF, Abadie RG, Buisson JC, et al. Telematic expert system Diabeto: New Tool for Diet Self-Monitoring for Diabetic Patients. Diabetes Care. 1992;15(2):204-12.
9. Levy M, Ferrand P, Chirat V. SESAM-DIABETE: an expert system for insulin-requiring diabetic patient education. Comput Biomed Res. 1989;22(5):442-53.
10. Albisser AM, Harris RI, Sakkal S, Parson ID, En Chao SC. Diabetes intervention in the information age. Med Inform (Lond). 1996;21(4):297-316.
11. Gómez EJ, del Pozo F, Hernando ME. Telemedicine for diabetes care: the DIABTel approach towards diabetes telecare. Med Inform (Lond). 2009;21(4):283-95.
12. Bellazzi R. Telemedicine and diabetes management: current challenges and future research directions. J Diabetes Sci Technol. 2008;2(1):98-104.

13. García-Sáez G, Hernando ME, Martínez-Sarriegui I, Rigla M, Torralba V, Brugués E, et al. Architecture of a wireless personal assistant for telemedical diabetes care. Int J Med Inform. 2009;78(6):391-403.
14. Boren SA, Puchbauer AM, Williams F. Computerized prompting and feedback of diabetes care: a review of the literature. J Diabetes Sci Technol. 2009;3(4):944-50.
15. Kesavadev J, Saboo B, Shankar A, Krishnan G, Jothydev S. Telemedicine for diabetes care: An Indian perspective—feasibility and efficacy. Indian J Endocrinol Metab. 2015;19(6):764-9.
16. Ganapathy K. Telemedicine and neurosciences. Neurol India. 2018;66(3):642-51.
17. Klonoff DC, True MW. The missing element of telemedicine for diabetes: decision support software. J Diabetes Sci Technol. 2009;3(5):996-1001.
18. de Adana MS, Alhambra-Expósito MR, Muñoz-Garach A, Gonzalez-Molero I, Colomo N, Torres-Barea I, et al. Randomized Study to Evaluate the Impact of Telemedicine Care in Patients With Type 1 Diabetes With Multiple Doses of Insulin and Suboptimal HbA1c in Andalusia (Spain): PLATEDIAN Study. Diabetes Care. 2020;43(2):337-42.
19. Lee PA, Greenfield G, Pappas Y. Patients' perception of using telehealth for type 2 diabetes management: a phenomenological study. BMC Health Serv Res. 2018;18(1):549.
20. Rossi MC, Nicolucci A, Lucisano G, Pellegrini F, Di Bartolo P, Miselli V, et al. Impact of the "Diabetes Interactive Diary" telemedicine system on metabolic control, risk of hypoglycemia, and quality of life: a randomized clinical trial in type 1 diabetes. Diabetes Technol Ther. 2013;15(8):670-9.
21. Schiel R, Kaps A, Bieber G. Electronic health technology for the assessment of physical activity and eating habits in children and adolescents with overweight and obesity IDA. Appetite. 2012;58(2):432-7.
22. Klug C, Bonin K, Bultemeier N, Rozenfeld Y, Vasquez RS, Johnson M, et al. Integrating telehealth technology into a clinical pharmacy telephonic diabetes management program. J Diabetes Sci Technol. 2011;5(5):1238-45.
23. Sarkar U, Handley MA, Gupta R, Tang A, Murphy E, Seligman HK, et al. Use of an interactive, telephone-based self-management support program to identify adverse events among ambulatory diabetes patients. J Gen Intern Med. 2008;23(4):459-65.
24. Nunn E, King B, Smart C, Anderson D. A randomized controlled trial of telephone calls to young patients with poorly controlled type 1 diabetes. Pediatr Diabetes. 2006;7(5):254-9.
25. Fatyga E, Dzięgielewska-Gęsiak S, Wierzgoń A, Stołtny D, Muc-Wierzgoń M. The coronavirus disease 2019 pandemic: telemedicine in elderly patients with type 2 diabetes. Pol Arch Intern Med. 2020;130(5): 452-4.
26. Joshi R, Atal S, Fatima Z, Balakrishnan S, Sharma S, Joshi A. Diabetes care during COVID-19 lockdown at a tertiary care centre in India. Diabetes Res Clin Pract. 2020;166:108316.
27. Ghosh A, Gupta R, Misra A. Telemedicine for diabetes care in India during COVID-19 pandemic and national lockdown period: guidelines for physicians. Diabetes Metab Syndr. 2020;14(4):273-6.
28. Garg SK, Rodbard D, Hirsch IB, Forlenza GP. Managing New-Onset Type 1 Diabetes During the COVID-19 Pandemic: Challenges and Opportunities. Diabetes Technol Ther. 2020;22(6):431-9.
29. Ceriello A. "Diabetes as a case study of chronic disease management": Eight years later. The opportunity learned from the COVID-19 pandemic. Diabetes Res Clin Pract. 2020;167:108384.
30. Sridhar G, Rao AA, Muraleedharan M, Kumar RJ, Yarabati V. Electronic medical records and hospital management systems for management of diabetes. Diabetes Metab Syndr. 2009;3(1):55-9.
31. Sridhar G, Murali G. Computerization of data in diabetes centers. Int J Diabetes Dev. 2011;31(2):48-50.
32. Kesavadev J, Rasheed SA, Nair DR. Achieving Desirable Glycemic Targets without the risks of Hypoglycemia using a Teletitration Programme. Diabetes. 2007;56:421.
33. Kesavadev J, Shankar A, David A, Krishnan G, Na A, Sanal G, et al. Are Complications Preventable with Periodic Education via Telemedicine? A Study of 414 Compliant T2DM Patients Followed Up for 19 Years. Diabetes. 2018;67(Suppl 1):685-P.
34. Kesavadev J, Shankar A, Pillai PBS, Krishnan G, Jothydev S. Cost-Effective Use of Telemedicine and Self-Monitoring of Blood Glucose via Diabetes Tele Management System (DTMS) to Achieve Target Glycosylated Hemoglobin Values Without Serious Symptomatic Hypoglycemia in 1,000 Subjects with Type 2 Diabetes Mellitus—A Retrospective Study. Diabetes Technol Ther. 2012;14(9):772-6.

CHAPTER 13

Can Artificial Intelligence Help Prevent Hypoglycemia?

GR Sridhar, G Lakshmi

ABSTRACT

Risk of hypoglycemia is the stumbling block in achieving normoglycemia with current antidiabetic medications. The risk can be mitigated by regulating timing and amount of diet to match with the dose of medications. Considering the number of variables involved, efforts to avoid hypoglycemic events. Machine learning and artificial intelligence (AI) can help to predict and warn about imminent hypoglycemic episodes, giving time to abort an attack. Most studies employing AI are still in the early phases, but one can expect rapid progress to bridge the gap from concept to clinical practice. AI methods commonly depend on large sets of data obtained from continuous glucose monitoring in insulin-treated subjects with type 1 diabetes mellitus to predict nocturnal hypoglycemia. Other studies are trying to identify postprandial hypoglycemia in type 2 diabetes mellitus, using fewer values of glucose obtained by home glucose monitoring. Advances in wearable smartwatch technologies can make them more widely applicable.

Keywords: *Machine learning, Continuous glucose monitoring, Prediction, Type 1 diabetes mellitus.*

INTRODUCTION

Glucose levels in healthy persons are exquisitely kept in a narrow "normal" range by many checks and balances, of which insulin is a key player. Diabetes is characterized by elevated levels of blood glucose among other metabolic abnormalities. Hyperglycemia in diabetes is essentially due to a relative or absolute lack of insulin. To correct the imbalance, in type 2 diabetes mellitus (T2DM), drugs are used to either improve the action of available of insulin or to stimulate the secretion of insulin. Over time, the effectiveness of oral drugs wanes and insulin is often necessary for glycemic control.

SPECTRE OF HYPOGLYCEMIA

Actions of oral drugs and insulin are not governed by the physiological feedback of glucose homeostasis, making hypoglycemia the single most important limitation in achieving euglycemia.[1,2] Endocrine and diabetes societies around the world seized with the issue of preventing hypoglycemia.[3] One faces a dilemma: Does one let glucose levels hover high and run the risk of future vascular complications or does one aim to get glucose levels down to the "normal" range and run the immediate risk of hypoglycemia. Often, it is a compromise between the two, with a via media position arrived among the treating physician, the patient and her family after a discussion of the pros and cons as well as the methods needed to achieve it.

CURRENT METHODS TO PREVENT HYPOGLYCEMIA

The aim of treatment is to bring the glucose level to as normal a range as possible while minimizing the risk of hypoglycemia. This is achieved by balancing the amount of food and time that is eaten, the dose and time of antidiabetic drugs, and by regulating the physical activity.

The situation is more distressing in children, who often have type 1 diabetes mellitus (T1DM) because they need multiple doses of insulin injection: Swings of hypo- and hyperglycemia are common, leading to anxiety from hypoglycemic episodes. The current standard of care in children with T1DM is insulin given as multiple doses or as an insulin infusion pump.

Even the use of pumps requires a regulation of diet and physical exercise as well as adjusting the rate of insulin infusion based on frequently measured glucose levels to match the carbohydrate content in the food. These are difficult to reconcile; carbohydrate counting requires adequate training and education; any errors lead to incorrect insulin dose.

The use of closed loop insulin infusion systems addresses some of these issues. There are two methods: The first system involves infusion of only insulin and the second involves infusion of insulin (to lower high glucose levels) and glucagon (to increase glucose levels when they fall too low). Infusion of insulin alone requires meal-time boluses, which again depend on assessing nutrition intake with its attendant drawbacks. Two hormone pumps expensive and not widely available. Besides continuous glucose monitoring (CGM), it is not used routinely due to issues of cost and availability.

ARTIFICIAL INTELLIGENCE

Multiple glucose measurements, either by capillary method or by CGM, provide a large number of data points. With the large amount of data, artificial intelligence (AI) can be employed to analyze them and provide warning or advice.

What is artificial intelligence?

Artificial intelligence uses computer algorithms to do the work one associates with the intelligence of a human. Generally, AI incorporates a spectrum of learning processes such as deep learning, machine learning (ML), and natural language process.[4] In consonance with its scope, AI has been defined as "the use of computers for automated decision-making to perform tasks that normally require human intelligence".[5]

Artificial intelligence is not a new tool like an innovative equipment or a drug; rather, it is the technology that is needed for large quantities of data to be processed, often beyond the ability of the human brain.[6] Therefore, the concept of AI is not to imitate the intelligence of humans, but to "explore the ability to build intelligent artifacts".[7] In summary, AI does not aim at imitating humans, but seeks to be inspired by them.[8]

Use of Artificial Intelligence in Diabetes

There has been a surge of publications on the use of AI in diabetes mellitus; the steep upward curve has begun in the last decade due to the availability of data and the ability to analyze them. Contreras and Vehi studied publications from the PubMed database between the years 2010 and 2018. From a review of 141 papers included in the analysis, the broad methods aimed: (a) to discover information, (b) to learn to use the information so gained, and (c) finally to learn using the information or to extract the summary to be put to use.[9] The clinical areas covered: Blood glucose control strategies: (a) blood glucose prediction, (b) detection of adverse glycemic events, (c) insulin bolus calculators and advisory systems, (d) risk and patient personalization, (e) detection of meals, exercise, and faults, and (f) lifestyle and daily-life support in diabetes management.[9]

The bulk of studies, mostly published after 2015, were carried out on predicting glycemic excursions. The holy grail of diabetes mellitus has been the development of an "artificial pancreas" to mimic normal physiology. The components consist of a sensor of glucose levels, an algorithm, and a device to infuse insulin to safely achieve normoglycemia. A number of studies related to algorithms in artificial pancreas estimate the dose of insulin. These mainly comprised of fuzzy logic, neural networks, and reinforcement learning, which reduced hypoglycemic episodes.

Efforts are onto predict glycemic excursions to improve treatment outcomes. There are challenges because of a number of physiological variables involved such as rate of absorption of insulin, food intake and lag in measuring glucose in the interstitial fluid.

The following are representative studies that were carried out to identify, prevent, or treat hypoglycemia. Most were conducted in subjects with T1DM, who require insulin for glycemic control, with the attendant risk of serious hypoglycemia. Recent studies are looking at excursions in adults with T2DM as well.

NOCTURNAL AND POSTPRANDIAL HYPOGLYCEMIA

Pharmacological target of normoglycemia is laudable for its ability to prevent vascular complications of diabetes; yet, there are serious risks involving hypoglycemia. Hypoglycemia at night-time is more common in subjects of T1DM is serious, but is more feasible to predict. The first and most obvious one is generally food is not eaten after going to bed or is insulin injected; then, there is no physical activity unlike daytime activities, which can change the need and rate of absorption of insulin. On the other hand, nocturnal hypoglycemia may occur over a longer time span (viz., the duration of sleep), which could handicap predictive methods.[10] Therefore, there are methods to predict nocturnal hypoglycemia.

OVERVIEW OF THE STEPS INVOLVED IN MACHINE LEARNING METHODOLOGY

The process of ML begins with cleaning of data on which analyzes are to be carried out, followed by the identification of various influencers. Next, training and test data are prepared and run. The final stage consists of optimizing the performance of ML architecture.[11]

PREDICTING NOCTURNAL HYPOGLYCEMIA FROM CONTINUOUS GLUCOSE MONITORING

The Novo Nordisk trial (onset 5 trial), which was originally a parallel group which had a run in period of 4 weeks, followed by treatment period of 16 weeks. Treatment consisted of comparing Fiasp® and NovoRapid® insulins efficacy and safety when given by infusion subcutaneously. Blinded CGM was performed three times of 2 weeks. Data used in this study was extracted from three periods from 472 subjects.

The study employed ML methods to predict nocturnal hypoglycemia. The aim was to provide a warning, built into the CGM devices, when hypoglycemic episode could occur at night; however, since the alarm disturbs sleep, the prediction method was constructed so that a warning of potential hypoglycemia was provided before bedtime in the evening itself. That would then allow the subject to adjust the insulin infusion rate and/or ingestion of complex carbohydrates to avoid hypoglycemia. Training period consisted of 3 days of monitoring, beginning in the evening. This proof-of-concept study identify nocturnal hypoglycemia with a sensitivity of 75% and specificity of 70% [receiver operating characteristic-area under the curve (ROC-AUC): 0.79].[10] Further improvements are necessary before it can be widely used.

INTEGRATION OF DIFFERENT MACHINE LEARNING METHODS TO PREVENT HYPOGLYCEMIA

Continuous delivery of insulin by pump is the best available option to achieve near normal glucose levels with less risk of hypoglycemia.[12] However, the device and monitoring systems are out of reach for many due to their expense. Therefore, Vehi et al. employed four ML methods as decision support tools to predict and thereby prevent hypoglycemic events in T1DM.[13] The different approaches included grammatical evolution to predict blood glucose levels, identification of postprandial hypoglycemic events using support vector machines, overnight hypoglycemic episodes by artificial neural networks, and finally data mining to describe different scenarios of managing diabetes. In all, they comprised an exploratory analysis of targeted datasets from glucose sensor or capillary values and fitness tracker band, which provided basic information. This was followed by data cleaning to fix structural errors such as suspicious pump values, data outliers, and missing values. The final feature engineering phase was constructed to provide additional value to the dataset.

Predictive modeling algorithms learn patterns from the data that is fed to them, while ignoring randomness or information that is irrelevant. The limitation of such methods is their ability to only perform well in the training set but poorly on unrelated new data due to overfitting. The core system for management was able to achieve continuous prediction (1 h), postprandial prediction (4 h), nocturnal prediction (6 h), and daily profile classification (24 h).[12] This improves patient safety and prediction horizon can be selected for each module depending on the requirement. The chief advantage of this integrated predictive modeling system is the potential ability to be used for both continuous subcutaneous insulin infusion users and multiple daily insulin injection users.

PREDICTING POSTPRANDIAL HYPOGLYCEMIA

Current closed loop systems require carbohydrate counting in their meal for appropriate mealtime insulin. Carbohydrate counting is complex; errors can lead to wrong information being fed thereby resulting in wrong insulin dose. Therefore, ML methods were employed to predict postprandial hypoglycemia by an easy-to-use computationally efficient ML algorithm. Unique data driven features were employed for prediction.[14]

The data were extracted from the records of 411 patients undergoing CGM who recorded at least one hypoglycemic episode (<70 mg/dL). In the feature extraction stage, the glucose trends were analyzed to identify meaningful features for postprandial hypoglycemia, which were used to define mealtime hypoglycemia risk (time window 35 min to 4 h following a meal). The following ML models were used: Random forest, support vector machine using linear function, support vector machine using radial basis function, and a K-nearest neighbor.[14] The performance was assessed by AUC of a ROC curve, sensitivity, specificity, and F1 score.

Eventually, 3-day CGM datasets ($n = 107$) from 104 subjects were analyzed, equally divided between T1DM ($n = 52$) and T2DM ($n = 52$). The random forest method had the best predictive ability, while employing a few CGM data and simple announcements at meal, which makes it easy to use.

A longer horizon for predicting hypoglycemia gives more time to take preventive actions; however, there is a trade-off between the prediction time frame and the model accuracy. A decision must be made on the model based on the subject's need. A 30-minute horizon for prediction hits the sweet spot between allowing time to take preventive action and the accuracy of prediction. The method can be employed in stand-alone real-time CGM devices.

This model must be followed by a prospective study using a longer time frame to identify the risk of hypoglycemia. Even though the subject must decide on the time of meal intake, it is less cumbersome and less prone to error than carbohydrate counting and entering the insulin dose that is required by the existing methods.[14]

WEARABLE DEVICES TO DETECT AND WARN OF HYPOGLYCEMIA

Maritsch et al. have developed a proof-of-concept model with smartphone sensors to predict hypoglycemia,[15] this could substitute though not replace the more expensive and accurate closed-loop artificial pancreas system. It was based on heart rate variability in response to sudden physiological changes and its correlation with hypoglycemia.[16] They demonstrated hypoglycemia prediction from heart rate variability using a smartwatch.[15] Li et al. developed a personalized blood glucose prediction model for individuals.[17] They plan to employ a synthesis of group as well as patient-based analysis for prediction. Access to devices based on internet of things (IoT) is likely to make prediction models accurate and more widely available.[18]

DATA ASSIMILATION FOR GLUCOSE FORECASTING IN TYPE 2 DIABETES MELLITUS

Most published studies are limited to insulin use in T1DM, with access to large number of glucose data; there is less information on subjects with T2DM on basal insulin or oral antidiabetic drugs. Albers et al. employed data assimilation methods to predict glycemic excursions based on nutritional intake.[19] They have used glucose data points commonly found in real-life situations using self-monitoring practices.

SUMMARY

Deep learning and artificial neural network methods are being increasingly applied to predict the risk of hypoglycemia in both insulin-treated subjects and in those using oral agents. It is expected that technology will rapidly mature to help subjects using oral antidiabetic agents or basal insulin and with fewer glucose values. Innovative methods where ML is meshed with indirect evidence of hypoglycemia using smartwatch sensors provide an exciting new avenue for greater access using widely available sensor methodologies.

REFERENCES

1. UK Hypoglycaemia Study Group. Risk of hypoglycaemia in types 1 and 2 diabetes: effects of treatment modalities and their duration. Diabetologia. 2007;50:1140-7.
2. American Diabetes Association. Glycemic Targets: Standards of Medical Care in Diabetes—2021. Diabetes Care. 2021;44:S73-S84.
3. Seaquist ER, Anderson J, Childs B, Cryer P, Samuel Dagogo-Jack S, Fish L, et al. Hypoglycemia and diabetes: a report of a workgroup of the American Diabetes Association and the Endocrine Society. Diabetes Care. 2013;36:1384-95.
4. He J, Baxter SL, Xu J, Xu J, Zhou X, Zhang K. The practical implementation of artificial intelligence technologies in medicine. Nat Med. 2019;25:30-6.
5. USAID. (2019). Artificial Intelligence in Global Health: Defining a Collective Path Forward. [online] Available from https://www.usaid.gov/cii/ai-in-global-health. [Last accessed February, 2021].
6. Rajkomar A, Dean J, Kohane I. Machine Learning in Medicine. N Engl J Med. 2019;380:1347-58.
7. Pereira LM, Lopes AB. Machine ethics. In: Lorenzo M (Ed). Studies in Applied Philosophy, Epistemology and Rational Ethics. Switzerland: Springer; 2020.
8. Sridhar GR, Lakshmi G. Artificial intelligence in medicine: diabetes as a model. In: Srinivasa KG, Siddesh GM, Manisekhar SR (Eds). Artificial Intelligence for Information Management: A Healthcare Perspective, 1st edition. Singapore: Springer; 2021; pp 283-305.
9. Contreras I, Vehi J. Artificial Intelligence for Diabetes Management and Decision Support: Literature Review. J Med Internet Res. 2018;20:e10775.
10. Jensen MH, Dethlefsen C, Vestergaard P, Hejlesen O. Prediction of nocturnal hypoglycemia from continuous glucose monitoring data in people with type 1 diabetes: a proof of concept study. J Diab Sci Technol. 2020;14:250-6.
11. Sudharsan B, Peeples M, Shoma M. Hypoglycemia prediction using machine learning models for patients with type 2 diabetes. J Diabetes Sci Technol. 2015;9:86-90.
12. Brown SA, Kovatchev BP, Raghinaru D, Lum JW, Buckingham BA, Kudva YC, et al. Six-month randomized, multicenter trial of closed-loop control in type 1 diabetes. N Engl J Med. 2019;381:1707-17.
13. Vehi J, Contreras I, Oviedo S, Biagi L, Bertachi A. Prediction and prevention of hypoglycaemic events in type-1 diabetic patients using machine learning. Health Informatics J. 2020;26:703-18.
14. Seo W, Lee YB, Lee S, Jin SM, Park SM. A machine-learning approach to predict postprandial hypoglycemia. BMC Med Inform Decis Mak. 2019;19:210.
15. Maritsch M, Lehman V, Kraus M, Kowatsch T, Stettler C, Wortmann F, et al. (2020). Towards Wearable based Hypoglycemia Detection and Warning in Diabetes. [online] Available from https://www.alexandria.unisg.ch/259515/1/Martisch%20et%20al%202020%20Wearable-based%20Hypoglycemia%20Detection%20and%20Warning.pdf. [Last accessed February, 2021].
16. Schächinger H, Port J, Brody S, Linder L, Wilhelm FH, Huber PR, et al. Increased high-frequency heart rate variability during insulin-induced hypoglycaemia in healthy humans. Clin Sci. 2004;106:583-8.
17. Li J, Fernando C. Smartphone-based personalized blood glucose prediction. ICT Express. 2016;2:150-4.
18. Rodríguez-Rodríguez I, Rodríguez JV, Chatzigiannakis I, Izquierdo MAZ. On the possibility of predicting glycaemia 'on the fly' with constrained IoT devices in type 1 diabetes mellitus patients. Sensors (Basel). 2019;19:4538.
19. Albers DJ, Levine M, Gluckman B, Ginsberg H, Hripcask G, Mamykina L. Personalized glucose forecasting for type 2 diabetes using data assimilation. PLoS Comput Biol. 2017;13:e1005232.

CHAPTER 14

Mindful Meditation in Metabolic Syndrome and Diabetes

K Madhu, S Aruna Sri, GR Sridhar

ABSTRACT

Mindfulness meditation is based on the practice of Buddhist meditation, which has been adapted to suit Western cultures. It seeks to passively focus one's attention to the present moment, and to discriminate thoughts and emotions with positive effects from those with adverse effects. It is often administered in a group-format, with the learners committing to practice at home in the intervening periods. A number of biochemical, physiological, and psychological pathways are being uncovered for the beneficial effects in conditions such as diabetes and its complications, hypertension, depression, and cardiac disease, among others. One must be aware of the limitations of the practice, which however, offers cost-effective solutions to many conditions when employed judiciously.

Keywords: *Buddhist meditation, Self-awareness, Nonjudgmental, stress, Autonomic nervous system, Hypothalamo-pituitary-adrenal axis, Complementary medical system, and Health systems.*

INTRODUCTION

"Mindfulness" refers to a specific condition of psychological consciousness, an exercise which encourages this consciousness, an approach toward processing information and a personality trait.[1-4]

The concept arose from Buddhism contemplative traditions, which were integrated to meditation. It aims to ensure that the individual becomes aware of changed cognition and emotion in oneself, increase self-acceptance and result in lowering stress.[5] Mindfulness is well-defined as "moment-by-moment awareness"[2] or as "a state of psychological freedom that occurs when attention remains quiet and limber, without attachment to any particular point of view".[6]

Mindfulness is regarded as a particular condition and not a quality and this might be accomplished by practicing specific activities such as meditation which is different from them. The significant aspect of mindfulness is to observe, accept and gain an ease with pressures, worry, and discomfort as also equally distressing emotions such as anxiety, irritation, frustration, feelings of worthlessness, and uncertainty. Such transformation requires adoption of new perspectives and new ways of coping with change.

People resist to experience stress and negative emotions to cope with such conditions. At times resistance is needed. The ability to say "No" helps a person from being overburdened and body's immune system is made to counter attack external invaders. When we are matured physiologically, our psychological immune system also develops to protect from intrusive or aggressive dynamisms, possible harmful conditions, and toxic relationships by comprising a sequence of bouncing restrictions and doorways. Apparently, the absence of a network of resistances would make people susceptible to oppression, delicate and noticeable.

The problem arises when people do not know when or how to let down the boundaries. That is when the resistance stops being a useful filtering device, and becomes a barrier.

The management of intrusive thoughts and anxiety, relaxation of the mind and the body, a change in the perception of the situation and an adoption of healthier ways of dealing with one's life can be accomplished by practicing certain proven mind/body techniques.

CONCEPT OF MINDFULNESS

Kabat-Zinn, the founder of the Stress Reduction Clinic at the Center for Mindfulness at UMass Memorial Medical Center in Worcester was the first to offer the course in mindful meditation.[7]

The origin of mindful meditation is mainly from the Buddhist tradition which promotes better consciousness, insight, and enables individuals to live every second completely in the present. Unlike other practices of meditation, mindfulness encourages a focus on disturbing thoughts, feelings, and biological distress.

An 8-week program of mindfulness-based stress reduction (MBSR) intended to help people acquire healthier self-care and cultivate a healthy life by managing different "stressors" or distress which were preventing them from living life to the fullest. To participate in the MBSR course the participants are required to consider important issues. Firstly, they should make a personal commitment to MBSR meditation practice for 45–60 days daily for 6 days a week for 8 weeks.

Secondly, the participants are required to make a personal commitment to practice mindfulness in daily living (informal mindfulness practice). This includes the conscious act of remembering and bringing attention to the present moment and simple activities throughout the day. Thirdly, the practice stipulates that any desire to use MBSR to reach a certain objective (e.g., relaxation, pain relief, inner peace) should be kept aside as it will allow them to fully experience a primary part of the program, which is "non-doing" or "non-striving." Lastly, the participants should approach the practice with an attitude of kindness, compassion, gentleness, openness, and inquisitiveness toward self and others. The participants should just observe, developing a deeper awareness.

The MBSR program has been developed to complement the treatment of physical and psychological health ailments. In this program mindful meditation is used to relieve anxiety, depression, skin infections, blood pressure, diabetes mellitus, pain, and immune system dysfunctions. The structured practice of mindfulness resulted in clinically significant and progressive changes in both psychological and physical illnesses.[8-10]

APPLICATION OF MINDFULNESS IN HEALTH

The MBSR program emphasizes thorough practice and training in mindfulness meditation and its application into daily life encounters. Adding this practice to standard cardiac recovery treatments resulted in reduced mortality (41%), relapse (46%), disease, emotional distress, triglycerides, hypertension, weight, and blood sugar levels.[11,12] In individuals with coronary artery disease, exercise-induced myocardial ischemia was reduced by practicing mindfulness mediation only.[12,13]

This training also helped in a better management of hypertension when compared to medication and other lifestyle changes such as salt control, weight management, and improved workout.[14-16]

There is published evidence for decreasing mood disturbances and stress,[17] for a period of at least 6 months.[18] Similarly, survival time and stress in malignancies were improved.[19-21]

Practicing mindfulness meditation reduced pain, mood fluctuations, anxiety, and depression. Usage of pain management drugs was lessened and improved daily activities and self-esteem were observed. These differences were noticeable and there were no such changes found in the traditional pain clinic comparison group.[22] All these improvements were sustained till a 4-year follow-up.[22]

Poorly managed type 1 diabetes mellitus (T1DM) individuals' sugar levels were lowered noticeably in mindful meditation trained individuals.[7] Mindfulness training helped in lowering headaches, symptoms of anxiety, emotional suffering, and mild depression[23] and these changes lasted for 3 years.[24] Along with cognitive therapy mindfulness training skills resulted in marked reduction in the relapse of major depression episodes in individuals treated for depression.[25] Relaxation training helped in reducing the frequency of asthma attacks, nonadherence to treatment and improved psychological health and over all well-being.[26] The marked progress has been shown in quality-of-life and efficiency in individuals, with decreased physical and psychological symptoms.[27]

Kabat-Zinn emphasized the significance of mindfulness that mindfulness trained individuals are able to manage their lives better, can see stressful situations as opportunities and have a better sense of meaning in life.[28]

Mindfulness meditation encourages self-consciousness that individual aware of the thoughts and interpret them, possibly respond to them but not acknowledged with "me". As individuals activate to soothe the mind, self-awareness can be encouraged profoundly, as a consequence they understand who they are actually.

The precise physiological consequences and different mechanisms of mindfulness meditation such as focused attention, relaxed self-observation of one's present experience, and kind-hearted compassion practice were investigated by mindfulness researchers by developed neurological technologies.[29-30]

BIOPSYCHOLOGICAL BASIS OF MINDFULNESS

Mindfulness interventions in populations experiencing high stress operate at many levels: Attention monitoring skills and acceptance skills act at the brain stress resilience pathways to upregulate regulatory pathway and downregulate reactive pathways. Psychologically, there is improvement of emotion regulation by decreasing distress and rumination, as well as psychosocial resources such as positive emotions. These in turn lead to lessened stress reactivity acting through lowering of sympathetic nervous activity and hypothalamo-pituitary-adrenal axis reactivity. Simultaneous behavior changes occur in the form of reduced stress-related negative health behaviors and improved coping skills.[31]

Recent studies looked at changes in brain morphometry following mindfulness meditation, which revealed changes in brain cortical thickness, gray matter volume, pointing to involvement of brain networks, rather than isolated brain regions.[32] Particular changes were observed in the frontopolar cortex, sensory cortices, insula, hippocampus, anterior cingulated cortex, midcingulate cortex, orbitofrontal cortex, and superior longitudinal fasciculus, and corpus callosum. These regions are involved in meta-awareness, body awareness, memory, emotion regulation, and communication among the brain hemispheres.

Future research can uncover the neurophysiological methods of meditation and the advantages of enduring practice on the brain. Studying neuroplasticity may enlighten the association among duration and quality of meditation exercise, phases of progression in meditators, and treatment outcomes. Further exploration is required for more knowledge about the advantages of meditation practice attained over time which can lead to an improved evidence of the usage of MBSR.

Though mindfulness meditation is not recognized as a standard health procedure, health experts should recommend this practice to individuals with chronic diseases so as to better manage the complications resulting from chronic diseases.

MINDFULNESS IN CLINICAL SCENARIOS: DIABETES, METABOLIC SYNDROME, AND CORONARY ARTERY DISEASE

Diabetes distress refers to "negative emotions in response to living with diabetes".[33] It is associated with frustration, hopelessness, anger guilt, and fearfulness, without clinical depression and anxiety.[34] All these lead to poor self-management of diabetes and resultant unsatisfactory glycemic control. Mindfulness therapy has been employed as an intervention in the management of diabetes distress.

Guo et al. performed a meta-analysis on the effects of mindfulness therapy on diabetes distress.[34] Eight studies comprising 649 participants were analyzed. They concluded that the process may be employed as part of management choice in reducing diabetes distress. Mindfulness therapy was best delivered as a group format and led to improvement of distress when adults with diabetes have high baselines scores, when structured training was associated with practice at home, for long-term outcomes.[34]

Painful diabetic neuropathy is a debilitating and often recalcitrant long-term complication of diabetes mellitus. A number of methods are used to manage it, but residual symptoms persist. Mindfulness meditation was tried in a group of elderly women with diabetes having chronic pain due to neuropathy. Pain was assessed by the Brief Pain Inventory modified for painful diabetic peripheral neuropathy.[35] Although mindful meditation did not completely eliminate the pain, it helped them to obtain skills to a productive life consisting of lesser discomfort. It could reduce the need for medicines to relieve pain, and thereby the risk of addiction.

Insulin resistance in adolescents, if often a harbinger of type 2 diabetes mellitus (T2DM). Shomaker et al. assessed the effect of mindfulness-based intervention on clinical outcomes among adolescents who were at risk for T2DM (viz., having symptoms of depression and family history of T2DM).[36] A randomized controlled trial outcome at the end of 1 year showed that compared to cognitive behavior therapy, six-session mindfulness-based intervention led to greater lowering in scale for depression. The authors proposed that reduced depression could have improved behavioral risk factors such as sleep, activity, and food habits that could lead to diabetes mellitus.[36] This was a small pilot study, requiring replication.

Elevated blood pressure is a key component of metabolic syndrome. Pharmacological agents alone are often ineffective in normalizing blood pressure, besides the harm of side effects. Earlier studies have shown that decreasing stress lowers response of sympathetic nervous system to stress, and thereby lowers blood pressure. In a systematic review and meta-analysis on the effect of mindfulness interventions to reduce blood pressure, Intarakamhang et al. concluded that mindfulness interventions could be a useful and effective means to assist lowering blood pressure in subjects with noncommunicable diseases.[5]

Effects of mindfulness meditation on vascular function: Aging and hypertension result in vascular dysfunction and hardening of the arteries, both risk factors for cardiovascular disorders. Operative factors involve a chronic low-grade inflammatory condition. Amarasekera and Chang reviewed the effect of Buddhist meditation, on which mindfulness meditation is based, on vascular endothelial function and on blood pressure.[37] Out of 407 relevant articles, five met the selection criteria for review. The studies showed that meditation had the potential of lowering levels of stress, increase mindfulness, and improve vascular function. The beneficial effects could be mediated via action on psychological stress and on inflammation. By reducing depressive mood, cardiovascular risk factors are alleviated.[37] Further studies must be done employing randomized design on large sample sizes including diverse ethnic groups.

Scientific Statement by American Heart Association (AHA) on mind-heart-body connection: The AHA recently published a statement titled "psychological health, well-being, and the mind-heart-body connection".[38] Mindfulness-based interventions were shown to reduce psychological stresses and improve healthy lifestyle. A meta-analysis of the effects of mindfulness-based interventions on psychological and physiological measures in adults with cardiovascular disease (CVD) showed favorable effects, although the authors cautioned that further studies with longer follow-up periods are required to investigate if they improve disease outcomes.[39]

PRINCIPLES OF INTEGRATING MINDFULNESS IN CLINICAL CARE

Integration of mindfulness in individual therapy: Generally, mindfulness-based interventions are offered in group-based format. Applying the principles to individual, rather than group-based therapy needs attention to specific aspects. There are as yet, few empirical studies in this area. The challenges include among others, unskilled attempts to integrate mindfulness into individual therapy, use in a disintegrated way without a broader perspective and a lack of background knowledge.[40] The following recommendations were offered: (1) Therapists should practice personal mindfulness themselves; (2) Consider various aspects before integrating mindfulness practice into individual therapy such as practicing oneself and evidence of mindfulness being an appropriate intervention for the individual subject; and (3) Integration of mindfulness into a coherent whole. Finally, therapists offering such treatment must bring compassion into practice of mindfulness.[40]

Applicability of mindfulness medication into the health system: Ajari recently elaborated on the nature of mindfulness meditation and what it can offer, in the context of the African continent.[41] An interesting distinction has been made between mindfulness, which was likened to strength or flexibility, and mindfulness practices as running or going to the gym.

As a measure of caution, potential negative consequences of mindfulness meditation were described. They include resurfacing of suppressed bad memories, disorientation, boredom, or derealization following such practices; uncommon perhaps, but one must be aware of the potential. Paradoxically, some may experience anxiety and panic as a result of relaxation.[41]

There are limitations in the methods employed among published studies: Well, known are small sample size, attrition during the study, lack of randomization, and an absence of psychological theories on which the studies were based.

Finally, the limitations of mindfulness meditation must also be considered such as lack of objective measures to assess outcomes, to assess the trainers themselves and a disparity in language between them and the learners. Interpersonal differences in populations and coexisting psychological and psychiatric disorders may result in mindfulness mediation being ineffective.

Despite these caveats, the major strength for incorporating mindfulness meditation into the healthcare system is its ease of adaptation, which is as relevant for India as it is for the African continent. It is comparatively inexpensive, easy, and can be offered to groups of subjects. One must be aware of the need for training local trainers and the potential of uncertified workers hijacking and hyping or otherwise misusing the practice.[41]

CONCLUSION

Mindfulness meditation is a resource that enables individuals to observe their own life and the world around them from a novel view point. Mindfulness meditation provides individuals the opportunity to identify those behaviors which contribute to their own distress and this can help them choose to make a change.

REFERENCES

1. Brown KW, Ryan RM, Creswell JD. Mindfulness: Theoretical foundations and evidence for its salutary effects. Psychol Enq. 2007;18:211-37.
2. Germer C, Siegel R, Fulton P. (Eds.). Mindfulness and Psychotherapy. New York: Guilford Press; 2005.
3. Kostanski M, Hassed C. Mindfulness as a concept and a process. Aust Psychol. 2008;43:15-21.
4. Siegel DJ. The Mindful Brain: Reflection and Attunement in the Cultivation of Well-being. New York: Norton & Company; 2007.
5. Intarakamhang U, Macaskill A, Prastittichok P. Mindfulness interventions reduce blood pressure in patients with non-communicable diseases: a systematic review and meta-analysis. Heliyon. 2020;6:e03834.
6. Martin JR. Mindfulness: A proposed common factor. J Psychother Integr. 1997;7:291-312.
7. Kabat-Zinn J. Full Catastrophe Living: Using the Wisdom of Your Body and Mind to Face Stress, Pain, and Illness. New York, NY: Delacorte; 1990.
8. Kaplan KH, Goldenberg DL, Galvin-Nadeau M. The impact of a meditation-based stress reduction program on fibromyalgia. Gen Hosp Psychiatry. 1993;15:284-9.
9. Goldenberg DL, Kaplan KH, Nadeau MG, Brodeur C, Smith S, Schmid CH. A controlled study of a stress-reduction, cognitive-behavioral treatment in fibromyalgia: a randomized controlled trial. J Musculoskel Pain. 1994;2:53-66.
10. Weissbecker I, Salmon P, Studts JL, Floyd AR, Dedert EA, Septon SE. Mindfulness-Based Stress Reduction and sense of coherence among women with fibromyalgia. J Clin Psychol Med Settings. 2002;9:297-307.
11. Linden W, Stossel C, Maurice J. Psychosocial interventions for patients with coronary artery disease. Arch Intern Med. 1996;156:745-52.
12. Zamarra JW, Schneider RH, Besseghini I, Robinson DK, Salerno JW. Usefulness of the Transcendental Meditation program in the treatment of patients with coronary artery disease. Am J Cardiol. 1996;78: 77-80.
13. Ornish DM, Scherwitz LW, Doody RS, Kesten D, McLanahan SM, Brown SE, et al. Effects of stress management training and dietary changes in treating ischemic heart disease. JAMA. 1983;249:54-9.
14. Schneider RH, Staggers F, Alexander C, Sheppard W, Rainforth M, Kondwani K, et al. A randomized controlled trial of stress reduction for hypertension in older African Americans. Hypertension. 1995;26;820-7.
15. Linden W, Chambers L. Clinical effectiveness of non-drug treatment for hypertension: a meta-analysis. Ann Behav Med. 1994;16:35-45.
16. Alexander CN, Robinson P, Rainforth M. Treating alcohol, nicotine and drug abuse through Transcendental Meditation: a review and statistical meta-analysis. Alcohol Treat Q. 1994;11:13-87.
17. Speca M, Carlson LE, Goodey E, Angen M. A randomized, wait-list controlled clinical trial: the effect of a mindfulness meditation-based stress reduction program on mood and symptoms of stress in cancer outpatients. Psychosom Med. 2000;62:613-22.
18. Carlson LE, Ursuliak Z, Goodey E, Angen M, Speca M. The effects of a mindfulness meditation-based stress reduction program on mood and symptoms of stress in cancer outpatients: 6-month follow up. Support Care Cancer. 2001;9:112-23.
19. Fawzy FI, Fawzy NW, Hyun CS, Elashoff R, Guthrie D, Fahey JL, et al. Malignant melanoma. Effects of an early structured psychiatric intervention, coping, and affective state on recurrence and survival 6 years later. Arch Gen Psychiatry. 1993;50:681-9.
20. Spiegel D, Bloom JR. Group therapy and hypnosis reduce metastatic breast carcinoma pain. Psychosom Med. 1983;45:333-9.
21. Bridge LR, Benson P, Pietroni PC, Priest RG. Relaxation and imagery in the treatment of breast cancer. Br Med J. 1988;297:1169-72.

22. Kabat-Zinn J. An outpatient program in behavioral medicine for chronic pain patients based on the practice of mindfulness meditation: theoretical considerations and preliminary results. Gen Hosp Psychiatry. 1982;4:33-47.
23. Kabat-Zinn J, Massion AO, Kristeller J, Peterson LG, Fletcher KE, Pbert L, et al. Effectiveness of a meditation-based stress reduction program in the treatment of anxiety disorders. Am J Psychiatry. 1992;49:936-43.
24. Miller JJ, Fletcher K, Kabat-Zinn J. Three-year follow-up and clinical implications of a mindfulness meditation-based stress reduction intervention in the treatment of anxiety disorders. Gen Hosp Psychiatry. 1995;17:192-200.
25. Teasdale JD, Segal ZV, Williams JM, Ridgeway VA, Soulsby JM, Lau MA. Prevention of relapse/recurrence in major depression by mindfulness-based cognitive therapy. J Consult Clin Psychol. 2000;68:615-23.
26. Devine EC. Meta-analysis of the effects of psychoeducational care in adults with asthma. Res Nurs Health. 1996;19:367-76.
27. Reibel DK, Greeson JM, Brainard GC, Rosenzweig S. Mindfulness-based stress reduction and health-related quality of life in a heterogeneous patient population. Gen Hosp Psychiatry. 2001;23:183-92.
28. Kabat-Zinn J. Mindfulness-based interventions in context: Past, present, and future. Clin Psychol Sci Pract. 2003;10:144-56.
29. Lutz A, Slagter HA, Dunne JD, Davidson RJ. Attention regulation and monitoring in meditation. Trends Cogn Sci. 2008;12:163-9.
30. Lutz A, Slagter HA, Rawlings NB, Francis AD, Greischar LL, Davidson RJ. Mental training enhances attentional stability: Neural and behavioral evidence. J Neurosci. 2009;29:13418-27.
31. Creswell JD, Lindsay EK, Villalba DK, Chin B. Mindfulness training and physical health: mechanisms and outcomes. Psychosom Med. 2019;81:224-32.
32. Tang YY, Holzel BK, Posner MI. The neuroscience of mindfulness meditation. Nat Rev Neurosci. 2015;16:213-25.
33. Fisher L, Polonsky WH, Hessler DM, Masharani U, Blumer I, Peters AL, et al. Understanding the sources of diabetes distress in adults with type 1 diabetes. J Diabetes Complications. 2015;29:572-7.
34. Guo J, Wang H, Luo J, Guo Y, Xie Y, Lei B, et al. Factors influencing the effect of mindfulness-based interventions on diabetes distress: a meta-analysis. BMJ Open Diab Res Care. 2019;7:e000757.
35. Hussain N, Said ASA. Mindfulness-based meditation versus progressive relaxation meditation: impact on chronic pain in older female patients with diabetic neuropathy. J Evid Based Integr Med. 2019;24:1-8.
36. Shomaker LB, Pivarunas B, Annameier SK, Gulley L, Quaglia J, Brown KW, et al. One-year follow-up of a randomized controlled trial piloting a mindfulness-based group intervention for adolescent insulin resistance. Front Psychol. 2019;10:1040.
37. Amarasekera AT, Chang D. Buddhist meditation for vascular function: a narrative review. Integr Med Res. 2019;8:252-6
38. Levine GN, Cohen BE, Mensah YC, Fleury J, Huffman JC, Khalid U, et al. Psychological health, well-being, and the mind-heart-body connection: A Scientific Statement From the American Heart Association. Circulation. 2021;143:(10):e763-83.
39. Scott-Sheldon LAJ, Gathright EC, Donahue ML, Balletto B, Feulner MM, DeCosta J, et al. Mindfulness-Based Interventions for Adults with Cardiovascular Disease: A Systematic Review and Meta-Analysis. Ann Behav Med. 2020;54:67-73.
40. Michalak J, Crane C, Germer CK, Gold E, Heidenreich T, Mander J, et al. Principles for a responsible integration of mindfulness in individual therapy. Mindfulness. 2019;10:799-811.
41. Ajari EE. Mindfulness meditation as a complementary health therapy: a useful import into Africa? Eur J Environ Public Health. 2020;4:em0048.

A Tribute and Remembrances

This has been a searing personal loss to all of us

Madhu responded to my messages, and I to his until two days before I received the news from Ashok

Our association goes back to 1983. Madhu had submitted his PhD dissertation; I was doing my MD

The last words I spoke to him were my acknowledgment to him for the work we had done together. It was for a Review article that was being published

That morning, I put him on hold, went in to get the proof and read out to him

At that time I thought it was I who did it.

I didn't realise it was God who made me do

My personal pain pales before the abyssal loss of his loving family

Madhu has been an affectionate, considerate and loving husband, and an even more doting father.

A fond brother to all his siblings; the affection was reciprocated in a measure more than equal

Madhu mentioned in passing that he and Dr Jeevan would have dinner together. Every day

Either one would have been shattered to have known of what happened to the other.

They left it to their families to bear the grief

Madhu's marriage, the birth of his two children, and his stellar professional career seem like they happened yesterday

These are tormenting days yet for all of us

When it harrowing having to refer Madhu in the past tense

By and by, it is our earnest desire and belief, that, like the daffodils in the Lake District, Madhu will fill our hearts by his balming memories.

Dr GR Sridhar

CHAPTER 15

Gelotology or Laughter Therapy as an Adjuvant Management of Diabetes

GR Sridhar, V Rama Kumar

ABSTRACT

Laughter can be divided into spontaneous, when triggered by a stimulus, and simulated when it is voluntarily triggered. The latter is not caused by humor or other specific stimuli. Laughter is an evolutionary phenomenon with roles in social interactions. Studies have shown that in particular, simulated laughter reduces stress, depression, and anxiety. Early reports show promise of laughter in improving clinical outcomes in a variety of conditions including diabetes mellitus. Mechanisms to elucidate the two are being worked out. In appropriate circumstances laughter yoga, humor and yoga are inexpensive, safe complementary management options to traditional treatments.

Keywords: *Humor, Laughter, Neuroendocrine axis, Prevention, Evolution, Duchenne laughter, Management, Questionnaire.*

INTRODUCTION

Gelotology refers to the study of laughter, assessing its ability to relieve bodily stress.[1,2] The use of humor and laughter has been increasingly employed to reduce physical pain, improve quality of life, and immune functions as a complementary method of treatment.[3] Among it's advantages are that it does not require significant money or time and in being easily implemented. The effect of humor is being studied on psychological outcomes such as stress, on physiological responses, and ultimately on health outcomes.[3]

Conceptually, *humor* refers to cognition, emotional responses, behavior, and social aspects in terms of psychological perspectives. *Laughter*, on the other hand, is the common expression of humour. Laughter has both physiological effects and positive psychological benefits.[3]

ORIGINS AND FUNCTIONS OF HUMOR AND LAUGHTER

Both humor and laughter were recognized by Charles Darwin as having evolutionary significance, although interest of biologists and psychologists has begun for the past 45 years or so.[4] Gervais and Wilson propose a balanced evolutionary perspective and many levels of analysis. Laughter is universal and observed in all cultures of the world. It forms one of the first social expressive sounds in humans, which begins between the ages of two and six months. It has been proposed that human beings are genetically wired to produce and perceive laughter.[4] Great ape play pant has been suggested to be homologous to human laughter. Humor is the most well-recognized stimulus for laughter, which essentially consists of incongruity and unexpectedness.

The name given to proximate causes of laughter is *Duchenne laughter*, which results from an unexpected and sudden change in events based on nonserious social incongruity. *Protohumor* refers to rough-and-tumble play, tickling, or physical mishaps seen in both apes and in infants, referring to origin from antiquity. Darwin described humor as a "tickling of the mind." It has been proposed that there is a laughter-coordinating center in the dorsal upper pons.

Evolution shaped laughter-evoking context by cultural norms and learning, viz., biology and culture.[4] Does laughter serve a social purpose? Spontaneous laughter is believed to smooth social interactions and promote feelings of positivity. Learned social laughter has been called strategic *non-Duchenne laughter*, which serves as a punctuation effect, employed as a metacommunicative marker. Different neural pathways were proposed for the generation of involuntary laughter and of consciously controlled laughter.

For the sake of classification, *Duchenne laughter* may be considered as humor driven and *non-Duchenne laughter* may be considered as conversational laughter. Laughter is a learned phenomenon which can be employed in different situations. Gradation between *Duchenne* and *non-Duchenne* laughter is often difficult to discern. Laughter should have originated and evolved by being either neutral or advantageous; benefits could have accrued at the level of the individual or the group.[4] It is proposed that laughter, particularly vocalized *Duchenne laughter*, preceded the development or, indeed evolved independently of language.

ASSESSMENT OF HUMOR AND LAUGHTER

Laughter and humor must be defined and quantified by means of psychological instruments to obtain comparable data across studies. Humour is difficult to measure in an individual. Earlier approaches consisted of appreciating humor, not encompassing the complex and multifaceted nature it is now known to be.[5] Self-reported scales were developed in order to conceptualize and measure sense of humor. Early scale was the *Situational Humor Response Questionnaire* and the shorter

Coping Humor Scale.[5] Reliability and validity of the instruments were established.

These questionnaires focused on the stress-modifying concept and showed that differences in the sense of humor mediated the effect of stressful life events and negative moods.[5] In other words, sense of humor may aid in coping by the way a stressful situation is considered. Those with high humor scores tended to be more stable over self-concepts over time. For a more nuanced ability to obtain the relation between humor scale and other measures of psychological well-being, the *Humor Styles Questionnaire* was developed.

The chief drawback of this approach was an inability to show causal relations among the variables that were studied. Social psychologists used experimental methods to overcome the limitation, but these were somewhat "artificial." A practical solution would be to employ both models to address the limitations of either.

In psychological terms, *humor* may be considered as part of a multifaceted psychological phenomenon comprising of *cognitive* elements, *emotional* components, and finally *social or interpersonal* aspects.[5] *Laughter* is seen as a "hard-wired nonverbal expression" of mirth.[5]

Finally, the *sense of humor* may be considered to be multifaceted, with studies in twins suggesting a heritable component in humor styles, making it difficult to substantially change humor styles.[5] Rather than teach people their ability to create humor, it is *more practical to teach the humor they already have in a more adaptive way*, as in positive psychology.

POSSIBLE PHYSIOLOGICAL PATHWAYS FOR THE BENEFICIAL EFFECTS OF LAUGHTER

Stress Hormones

Laughter could reduce stress and improve natural killer cell activity.[6] It was postulated to act at the general effects of stress, involving the sympathetic nervous system, the endocrine system, and the lymphatic system.[3,7] Berk et al. described the neurohormonal responses to mirthful laughter. In a pilot study involving 10 healthy men, five experimental subjects viewed a 60-minute video showing humorous content; the controls did not view the video. Serum levels of corticotropin, cortisol, beta-endorphin, 3,4-dihydrophenylacetic acid (DOPAC), epinephrine, norepinephrine, growth hormone, and prolactin were measured serially. Cortisol and DOPAC in the experimental group were reduced more rapidly from baseline than controls. Epinephrine levels in the experimental group were also lower. Laughter reduced the levels of cortisol, DOPAC, and epinephrine, suggesting that it could operate in reversing the stress hormone response.[8]

Psychoneuroimmune Response

Laughter could also moderate the immunoendocrine system. Forty college students were administered by Daily Hassles Scales and humor by Situational Humor Response Questionnaire and other subscale.[9] Immunoglobulin A (IgA) levels in saliva were used as a measure of immune function. When IgA was measured about 6 weeks apart, sense of humor did not appear to affect on salivary immune function, with at best a modest effect. Sense of humor was believed to be a buffer between the effects of daily hassles on IgA. However the early studies could not be replicated.[9]

To assess if exposure to a humorous situation could lead to enhanced immune response, pilot studies were carried out employing humor videos. Sense of humor scores was positively correlated with salivary IgA level *before* viewing the videos, which led to the conclusion that sense of humor may not have an effect on the physiological outcome. However, subjects had increased IgA levels after they watched the humorous video with its attendant laughter. In conclusion, there is no clear evidence for the interaction of humorous situation on salivary IgA.[9]

Other studies evaluated the NK cell cytotoxicity to measure functioning of the immune function. NK cells are lymphocytes described as non-B, non-T, or null cells and are capable of lysing tumor cells in vitro, while sparing normal cells. Preliminary evidence suggests that NK cell activity can have a role in preventing certain infections caused by virus. Japanese patients with cardiovascular disease were reported to have a positive correlation between NK cell activity and sense of humor scale; the correlational work suggested an association between general positive feelings and increased activity of NK cells.[9] When the ability of NK to lyse cells and the influence of humor was studied in subjects with cancer, coping humor scale correlated positively with NK cell number, but the results were equivocal.

A larger study involved 52 healthy adult men who viewed an hour long humor video. They had increased NK cell activity and immunoglobulin G (IgG) lasting for 12 hours.[10] Those who merely smiled on watching the humor video did not have favorable immune function changes, in contrast to those who laughed out a loud; immune enhancement was observed in the latter group. The improvement may be at least temporary and can be useful in cognitive-behavioral interventions, which were shown to be effective in management of diabetes mellitus. Further studies are clearly needed.

Other Physiological Effects of Laughter

Effects of laughter on blood pressure were studied. Mirthful laughter on exposure to 15-minute audio track with comic content over 14 episodes was followed by a gradual decrease of initial increase of blood pressure; a clear difference was observed between mirthful and stimulated laughter.[11] Other changes included elevated levels of IgA, IgG, IgM, and complement C3 along with surface markers such as CD3+DR+ and CD4-CD8 ratio.[10] Laughter could also act indirectly such as reduction in reactive oxygen species and increased free radical scavenging ability of the saliva. However, a direct mechanistic association has not been established.

Additional effects of laughter could involve arterial stiffness. Following a 30-minute comic video show, a group of 18 healthy subjects had a reduction in pulse wave velocity and augmentation index, both of which indicate arterial elasticity. In addition, brachial vasodilatation increased on watching a comedy video resulting in laughter. All these indicate a positive effect of laughter on endothelial function.

An interesting study assessed whether laughter could influence the expression of the gene coding for prorenin, a molecule known to play a role in the progression of diabetic nephropathy. After subjects with diabetes watched a comedy show, their levels of blood prorenin and expression of prorenin receptor gene were studied. Laughter reduced prorenin levels in those without nephropathy and upregulated prorenin receptor gene in those without nephropathy. No changes were observed in controls. It was proposed that laughter could have a beneficial effect in slowing the progression of nephropathy by acting through prorenin receptor gene and, thereby, reducing blood prorenin levels.[12]

In conclusion while mirthful laughter could have beneficial effects on endothelial vasoreactivity, one must consider the potential of its association with wild swings of blood pressure and, thereby, vascular accidents due to hemorrhage, although such occurrences were rarely reported.[13]

APPLICATION OF LAUGHTER AND HUMOR AS COMPLEMENTARY THERAPIES

There have been pioneering studies where laughter was used as therapy. Effect of laughter yoga alleviated psychological distress in subjects with coronary heart disease.[14] In a small study on noninsuln users of type 2 diabetes mellitus ($n = 19$) exposure to a comedy show together with many others coparticipants in the audience, postprandial glucose was lowered by 46 mg/dL following laughter.[15] Similarly, laughter modulated the renin-angiotensin system in diabetes and could be an adjunct treatment to preventing microvascular complications.[16] The frequency with which laughter is expressed per day is associated with lower prevalence of cardiovascular diseases.[17] However, other confounding factors such as depression may be contributing to the association. A recent study from southern India showed that laughter therapy could contribute to normalization of blood pressure in subjects with hypertension.[18]

PRACTICAL USE OF LAUGHTER AS THERAPY

Classification of Different Laughter Therapies

Therapies were classified based on the way laughter was induced, as mentioned in the primary study's methods section. Interventions were classified as "using humor," "not using humor," or "unknown." The classifications were classified as follows: an intervention was classified as "using humor" (spontaneous laughter), if some humorous stimulus was mentioned as being part of the therapy such as humor, jokes, or humorous videos. Interventions were classified "not using humor" (simulated laughter) if it was specifically mentioned that only laughter yoga (which is nonhumorous per definition) or nonhumorous laughter was used or when all elements of the interventions were clearly mentioned and none of them involved humor.

Principles of Laughter Yoga

Laughter yoga is a unique concept where anyone can laugh without relying on humor, jokes, or comedy; laughter is initiated as an exercise in groups, but it will turn into real laughter with eye contact and child-like playfulness. It was named laughter yoga because it uses laughter exercise and yogic breathing. Laughter yoga was started in 1995 at Bombay by a medical doctor Madan Kataria and his wife. There are currently thousands of laughter clubs in over 120 countries.

Laughter should be sustained at least for 10–15 minutes to get health benefits; natural laughter lasts for only few seconds. Because laughter yoga is done as an exercise, we can have prolonged laughter which brings beneficial physiological, hormonal, and psychological changes in body.

Laughter should be deep that is belly laughter using diaphragm to bring all the physiological benefits, which is possible in laughter yoga clubs. Laughter should be unconditional.

Steps in Laughter Yoga

Steps in laughter yoga include: (1) clapping, (2) breathing exercise, (3) child-like playfulness, and (4) laughter yoga exercises. The potential benefits of laughter yoga comprise not just health and emotion, but can cross over to include benefits in business, social interactions, and ability to laugh during times of adversity.

Laughing Qigong Program

Laughing Qigong Program (LQP) is a hybrid technique, which combines qigong techniques with stimulated laughter, focusing on mind-body connections. It has three components: (a) Chinese medicine or yin-yang theory; (b) qigong or relaxation, core strength, deep diaphragmatic breathing; and (c) positive psychology.[19] Similar to laughter yoga, the LQP passes through different stages of warmup at the beginning, generates "warmth" inside, transformation stage, and ends with cool-down stage. Belonging to a social group is integral to the LQP.[19]

INTEGRATION OF HUMOR IN HEALTHCARE RELATIONSHIP

Humor is not used in silos but must instead be integrated in relationship with the healthcare team. Sharing humor leads to a sense of being together, close, and friendly. It also promotes positive communication in therapy. A qualitative therapy among 88 health professionals from Portugal showed that humor was a useful tool in therapeutic relationship, but must be employed in patients with who they share a cordial relationship. Humor must be employed in moderation, with a careful consideration of the patient's sociocultural background. Used judiciously, humor has favorable on both professionals and patients.[20] Trust must first be established for humor to reap its positive health benefits.

CONCLUSION

There are many varieties of laughter and humor: Spontaneous, induced, associated with social interaction, relaxation, and gentle exercises. Laughter is inexpensive, simple, and can be used without significant expenditure in a cost-effective manner. It has positive effects on different psychological aspects such as depression, stress, and anxiety, across age groups, in addition to promising results on clinical and biochemical variables. Laughter therapy is currently used complementary to other regular treatments with few, if any contraindications.[21]

REFERENCES

1. Chang C, Tsai G, Hsieh CJ. Psychological, immunological and physiological effects of a Laughing Qigong Program (LQP) on adolescents. Complement Ther Med. 2013;21:660-8.
2. Ramakumar V, Rama Mohan MV, Vijaya Kumar G, Kalra S. Laughter therapy in diabetes. J Pak Med Assoc. 2021;71:1696-7.
3. Bennett MP, Lengacher CA. Humor and Laughter may Influence Health. I. History and Background. Evid Based Complement Alternat Med. 2006;3:61-3.
4. Gervais M, Wilson DS. The evolution and functions of laughter and humor: a synthetic approach. Q Rev Biol. 2005;80:395-430.
5. Martin R, Kuiper NA. Three Decades Investigating Humor and Laughter: An Interview with Professor Rod Martin. Eur J Psychol. 2016;12:498-512.
6. Strean WB. Laughter prescription. Can Fam Physician. 2009;55:965-7.
7. Selye H. The general adaptation syndrome and the diseases of adaptation. J Clin Endocrinol Metab. 1946;6:117-230.

8. Berk LS, Tan SA, Fry WF, Napier BJ, Lee JW, Hubbard RW, et al. Neuroendocrine and stress hormone changes during mirthful laughter. Am J Med Sci. 1989;298:390-6.
9. Bennett MP, Lengacher C. Humor and Laughter May Influence Health IV. Humor and Immune Function. Evid Based Complement Alternat Med. 2009;6:159-64.
10. Berk LS, Felten DL, Tan SA, Bittman BB, Westengard J. Modulation of neuroimmune parameters during the eustress of humor-associated mirthful laughter. Altern Ther Health Med. 2001;7:62-76.
11. Noureldein MH, Eid AA. Homeostatic effect of laughter on diabetic cardiovascular complications: the myth turned to fact. Diabetes Res Clin Pract. 2018;135:111-9.
12. Hayashi T, Urayama O, Hori M, Sakamoto S, Nasir UM, Iwanaga S, et al. Laughter modulates prorenin receptor gene expression in patients with type 2 diabetes. J Psychosom Res. 2007;62:703-6.
13. Miller M, Fry WF. The effect of mirthful laughter on the human cardiovascular system. Med Hypotheses. 2009;73:636-9.
14. Rouhi S, Etemadi S, Pooraghajan M. Laughter in Combination with Yoga Exercises: Changes in Psychological Distress and Quality of Life in Patients with Coronary Heart Disease (CHD). Open Psychol J. 2020;13:144-50.
15. Hayashi K, Hayashi T, Iwanaga S, Kawai K, Ishii H, Shoji S, et al. Laughter lowered the increase in postprandial blood glucose. Diabetes Care. 2003;26:1651-2.
16. Nasir UM, Iwanaga S, Nabi AH, Urayama O, Hayashi K, Hayashi T, et al. Laughter therapy modulates the parameters of renin-angiotensin system in patients with type 2 diabetes. Int J Mol Med. 2005;16: 1077-81.
17. Hayashi K, Kawachi I, Ohira T, Kondo K, Shirai K, Kondo N. Laughter is the Best Medicine? A Cross-Sectional Study of Cardiovascular Disease Among Older Japanese Adults. J Epidemiol. 2016;26: 546-52.
18. Josephine SP, Priya JJ. Effectiveness of laughter therapy on blood pressure among patients with hypertension. Asian J Pharmaceutical Clin Res. 2017;10:246-50.
19. Chang C, Tsai G, Hsieh CJ. Psychological, immunological and physiological effects of a Laughing Qigong Program (LQP) on adolescents. Complement Ther Med. 2013;21:660-8.
20. De almeida CV, Nunes C. Humor Is Important in Healthcare Relationship?—The Perceptions of Doctors and Nurses. Open Access Library J. 2020;7:e6372.
21. van der Wal CN, Kok RN. Laughter-inducing therapies: systematic review and meta-analysis. Soc Sci Med. 2019;232:473-88.

CHAPTER 16

Treat Metabolic Syndrome by Targeting Nerves to the Adipocyte

GR Sridhar, G Lakshmi

ABSTRACT

Adipocytes exist in various forms: White adipocytes are the most extensively found, playing a role in energy storage and in communicating with other cells through adipocytokines. Brown adipocytes are related to nonshivering thermogenesis; they are found in neonates, although recent studies showed small depots are found in adults. A subset of white adipocytes can transform themselves into thermogenic beige or brite adipocytes via sympathetic nervous system activation. Among agents that increase thermogenesis by conversion to beige adipocytes, mirabegron, a beta-3 adrenoceptor agonist, was effective in improving glucose homeostasis. These proof-of-concept studies deserve to be taken further whether mirabegron could be useful in the treatment of human obesity, metabolic syndrome, and type 2 diabetes mellitus.

Keywords: *Brown adipocytes, Beige adipocytes, Sympathetic nervous system, Beta-3 adrenergic agonists, Mirabegron, Cytokines, Nonshivering thermogenesis, PPAR-γ.*

BACKGROUND

The adipocyte is emerging as a renaissance cell: from being considered as an inert repository of energy storage, it is now a target for drugs acting on nerves regulating it, as potential treatment of obesity and type 2 diabetes mellitus (T2DM).

Adipose tissue comprises of adipocytes, preadipocytes, macrophages, endothelial cells, fibroblasts, and leukocytes. It not only stores energy, but is an endocrine organ secreting a variety of chemicals that regulate various aspects of metabolism.[1]

Bioactive factors released by the adipocytes, such as adipokines, enter the circulation and coordinate the activity of liver, muscle, brain, and pancreas.

A number of adipocyte cytokines have been identified such as leptin, visfatin, adiponectin, vaspin, apelin, hepcidin, chemerin, and omentin.[1]

Energy metabolism had its evolutionary origins where human genetic programming allowed survival through periods of hunger. During times of food availability, energy is stored as fat to enable survival when food is lacking.[2] Before edible animal fat was available, Hunter-gatherer communities had slower food transit in gut. When meat became available as food with controlled use of fire, high-energy diets allowed the development of greater muscle which improved the ability to hunt.

The principal role of adipose tissue is to store lipids to prevent lipotoxicity in tissues such as the heart and muscle; lipotoxicity disrupts membrane fluidity leading to release of lipidic mediators and oxygen metabolites followed by insulin resistance, inflammation, and apoptosis.[3] When there is positive energy, new adipocytes are produced leading to immune cell infiltration, angiogenesis, and hypertrophy of existing adipocytes.

TYPES OF ADIPOCYTES

Mammalian adipocytes exist in three classes: (1) *White*, (2) *Brown, and* (3) *Brite (or beige)*. They have different regions of origin, morphological features, and genes related to thermogenesis.[1]

White adipocytes vary in size between 25 and 200 µg. They have a lipid droplet, with few mitochondria, consistent with their role in storing triglycerides as energy. In general, fat deposited in the visceral tissues has an unfavorable metabolic outcome in contrast to fat in subcutaneous tissues. The property of visceral fat leading to metabolic syndrome and related vascular complications results from secretion of adipocytokines, proteins, lipids, and microribonucleic acids (miRNAs); they affect food intake, chronic inflammation, and insulin resistance.[2] Adiponectin and retinol-binding protein 4 have favorable metabolic effects; resistin has obesity effects, while nesfatin regulates appetite.

Visceral adipose tissue surrounds the abdominal organs and the heart. It is susceptible to apoptosis and contains many beta-adrenergic receptors. In addition, visceral fat has a direct connection to the liver through the portal vein. Essentially, the fat around the internal organs is metabolically active and is sensitive to weight loss.

Subcutaneous adipose tissue, on the contrary, tends to improve metabolic status and insulin signaling. Its accumulation may lower the risk of metabolic syndrome.[2] Subcutaneous adipose tissue is found principally in the gluteal, femoral, and abdominal regions.

The lipid metabolism in white adipose tissue is regulated at the levels of uptake of free fatty acids, lipid formation, and hydrolysis, which again are regulated by insulin, catecholamines, and cytokines. It is also regulated by the circadian rhythm in the central (suprachiasmatic nucleus of hypothalamus) and the peripheral clocks (e.g., BMAL1, CRY) by modulating fat synthesis, storage, and utilization.[2]

Brown adipocytes are multilocular and have abundant mitochondria; they dissipate stored energy as heat. Uncoupling protein 1 (UCP1), found on the inner membrane of the mitochondria, plays a role in uncoupling fuel oxidation from synthesis of adenosine triphosphate (ATP).[2] They occur predominantly in the abdomen (perirenal regions) of infants; similar tissue was identified in adult humans in the supraclavicular regions and in the lower neck. Brown adipocytes have rich nerve and blood supply. They are tasked with thermogenesis; cold temperature and stimulation by sympathetic nerves induce UCP1 leading to heat generation.[2] In rodents, it participates in adaptation to cold as well as to ingestion of very low carbohydrate in diet.[4,5]

Brown adipose tissue was inversely correlated with body mass index, suggesting a potential role in the cause of insulin resistance.[6] This led to interest in brown adipocytes due to its promise as a potential drug target for human obesity via its thermogenetic ability.[7]

It has been hypothesized that the modern pandemic of obesity could be a result of reduction of basal metabolism and ineffective thermogenesis of the brown adipose tissue.[8] Studies in monozygotic twins showed that genetic factors influencing basal metabolic role play a role in the development of obesity. Of the three components of energy expenditure, differences in adaptive thermogenesis could be responsible for individual variations in daily expenditure of energy.

Nonshivering thermogenesis, mediated by brown adipose tissue, could have provided the role of thermogenesis in localized regions via ancient UCP1. The thermogenic properties of UCP1 evolved as early as the Cretaceous period in eutherian mammals, which allowed a stable body temperature through higher metabolic rates. These animals were able to hunt for food at dusk and night when the other predators were inactive. Evolution of brown adipose tissue aided their survival in a variety of environments.

During evolution of modern humans, about 2 million years ago, adaptation to the hot and arid sub-Saharan conditions would have been established.[9] Exposure to cold could have been responsible for the selection of genes that are involved in nonshivering thermogenesis in brown adipose tissue. In support of this, a variant form of the gene beta-3 adrenergic receptor (ADRB3) has been found to exist in high frequencies in nonhuman primates. The ADRB3, found on the surface of brown adipose tissue, stimulates lipolysis and activates nonshivering thermogenesis. Only humans have the energy wasting variant of the ADRB3, which promotes both lipolysis and nonshivering thermogenesis.

Migration of early humans out of Africa could have resulted in the selection of cold-adaptive genes, although current evidence for advantages of such genes is scant. However, Greenlandic Inuits continue to harbor thermogenesis by brown adipose tissue, suggesting an adaptive response.

Interestingly, south Asians, who are not exposed to extreme cold climates, have reduced nonshivering thermogenesis brown adipose tissue volume, which has an impact on basal metabolism and expenditure of energy.[10] Ethnic groups of Africa and south Asia demonstrate reduced activity of brown adipose tissue and basal metabolic rates, making them susceptible to obesity. However, it must be borne in mind that genetics alone cannot explain the differences in obesity among different ethnic groups. Cultural and socioeconomic factors undoubtedly play a significant role. Besides, another confounding factor is that people in cold regions are hardly ever exposed to the cold, as they mostly stay in temperature-regulated environments.[8]

Beige or brown adipocytes, the third category of adipocytes, are multilocular and express UCP1. They are a specific kind of brown-like adipocytes capable of thermogenesis. Beige adipocytes arise as white adipocytes, mainly from Myf5 progenitor cells.[1] They are found in the subcutaneous white fat tissue and in small quantities in visceral fat. Activation of beige adipocytes or beiging of white adipose tissue primarily results from exposure to cold or by beta-3 adrenoceptor agonist that mimics the effect of cold stress. Beige adipocytes were also shown to develop from $Sca1^+$ progenitor cells by the stimulation of bone morphogenetic protein-7 (BMP-7).[11]

Current interest in beige fat is mainly for two main reasons: Firstly, it provides insights into how environmental changes alter cell fate development and maintenance; secondly, its potential as a target for obesity and metabolic disorders in the adult.[12] Adult humans have inducible beige-like thermogenic adipocytes, which can regulate energy homeostasis. Beige adipocyte transformation is believed to be a transient regulatory event, operating through UCP1-independent mechanism.[12] These could involve the SERCA2-RyR2 signaling pathway.

There are intriguing possibilities for the role of beige adipocytes in addition to thermogenesis; there was an inverse correlation with adipose tissue fibrosis in white adipose tissue found subcutaneously. Secretions from beige adipocytes, called "batokines," could control the systemic metabolism of glucose.[13]

REGULATION OF BEIGE ADIPOCYTE PLASTICITY

The $UCP1^+$ beige adipocyte formation from white adipose tissue can occur in two ways. One, stimuli such as cold, excess nutrition, or physical exercise, which produce beige adipocytes via $PDGFRa^+$ or $PDGFRb^+$ or $MyoD^+$ progenitors in white adipose tissue. The second is via transdifferentiation of existing white adipose tissue cells. Sympathetic drive is the major driver for the formation of beige adipocytes. Other stimuli include immune cells, thyroid hormones, natriuretic peptides, interleukin-6 (IL-6), irisin, and metabolites such as lactate and succinate.[14]

BROWN ADIPOSE TISSUE AS A TARGET FOR TREATING OBESITY

Thermogenesis by brown adipose tissue results from high expression of UCP1 protein found in the inner membrane of mitochondria; activated UCP1 protein leads to dissipation of electrochemical gradient that develops during fatty acid synthesis across the mitochondrial membrane. Various substrates are taken up by brown adipose tissue such as glucose, nonesterified fatty acids, dietary fatty acids, and glutamate.[15]

THERMOGENESIS AND ADIPOCYTES

A rich network of transcription factors is responsible for activation of thermogenic fat. Key interactions occur among peroxisome proliferator-activated receptor gamma (PPAR-γ), PRDM16, and peroxisome proliferator-activated receptor gamma coactivator 1-alpha (PGC1-α).[16] PPARs play a central role in regulating fat storage along with influencing insulin resistance.[17] Chronic activation of PPAR-γ by the thiazolidinedione group of drugs during development of adipocytes leads to their increased ability for thermogenesis. Rosiglitazone, a PPAR agonist, upregulated gene transcripts that encode mitochondrial proteins, resulting in increased mitochondrial mass and structure. This led to increased consumption of oxygen and enhanced oxidation of palmitate.[18] While the use of rosiglitazone in the management of T2DM has been restricted due to its adverse cardiovascular effects, the mechanisms by which thermogenesis is promoted are being studied.

Posttranslational changes in PPAR-γ have been suggested to play a role in upregulating thermogenic program during differentiation of adipocytes. They drive the transcription of PRDM16 as well as work alongside it. PRDM16, a transcriptional cocomponent, has a key role in the regulation of brown fat cell fat and beige fat cell function.[16] It works in part by forming a complex with CCAAT/enhancer-binding protein and can, thus, be influenced by miRNAs that regulate C/EBPbeta.

The transcriptional factor PGC1-α, interacting with many nuclear receptors, has a pivotal role in the mitochondrial oxidative metabolism and biogenesis.[19]

Targeting thermogenesis at the level of brown adipose tissue has been a beguiling path in treating obesity. Early efforts failed in the translation of animal studies in humans because maximal activation of brown adipose thermogenesis occurred at maximal exposure to cold, which does not happen in humans who mostly stay in thermally controlled environments. Second, energy expenditure is inversely proportional to body size, a comparison that is unfavorable for humans compared to mice.[20]

Early manipulations using compounds for medicinal use did not meet with success either. Dinitrophenol was tried in the 1930s, but this and others were beset with serious side effects, some even leading to death, probably due to their actions on nonbrown adipose tissues. In the search for other "physiological" activators, hormones such as catecholamines and thyroid hormones also result in significant adverse effects. Search for selective ADRB3 agonist had initial drawbacks such as poor oral bioavailability, until the repurposing of mirabegron, a beta-3 adrenoceptor agonist, approved for use in overactive bladder. Other target molecules under investigation other than thiazolidinediones include regulators of fibroblast growth factor 21 (FGF21), natriuretic peptides, chenodeoxycholic acid, glucocorticoids, and cyclooxygenase, without much current success.[16,20]

ROLE OF ADRENERGIC SYSTEM IN ADIPOCYTE THERMOGENESIS

Selective activation of ADRB3 can occur via cold stress, leptin, or emotional stress; brown adipose tissue is the most densely innervated by sympathetic nerves. An alternative path of activation is by direct action on the adrenergic receptor.[21] Norepinephrine, released from the sympathetic nerves, binds to the ADRB3 on brown adipocytes, which, in turn, activating protein kinase A, which induces intracellular lipolysis.[22] UCP1, the mitochondrial membrane protein, uncouples respiratory chain of oxidative phosphorylation leading to generation of heat. Prolonged by beta-3 adrenergic nerves stimulation is required for sustained thermogenesis.

However, there is evidence for UCP1-independent thermogenesis, although the sites have not been clearly determined. Matrix-assisted transplantation of beige cells was shown to have a positive influence on insulin sensitivity, suggesting a potential role for FGF21 and IL-6 in mediating the beneficial effects.[21]

Though their role in energy store and thermogenesis is well established, one must carefully assess many variables involved in the regulation of adrenoceptors in adipocyte function.[23] Interestingly, a recent study showed that activation of downstream insulin effectors may not be necessary for the acute responses of beta-3 adrenoceptor agonists on thermogenesis.[24] Similarly, Fan et al. suggested that dietary *n*-3 polyunsaturated fatty acids could play a role in rejuvenating white adipose tissue—browning with aging.[25]

TARGETING THERMOGENESIS AS A THERAPEUTIC OPTION

Viewed broadly, a number of approaches can theoretically target thermogenesis, besides exposure to cold, activating the sympathetic nerves, and the use of beta-3 adrenoceptor agonists. Modulators of G protein-coupled receptors (GPCRs) ion channels and signaling pathway modulators such as adenosine receptor agonists, cannabinoid receptor type 1 (CB1) targets such as rimonabant, melatonin, nicotine, phosphodiesterase inhibitors, β-aminoisobutyric acid (BAIBA), and irisin; growth factors and cytokines such as BMP-7, BMP-4, FGF21, follistatin, and IL-6, besides food components.[22,26]

The initial results obtained in rodent models to enhance thermogenesis could not be translated in humans because of the issue of thermoneutrality and not conducting studies at lower temperatures.[27,28]

SLOW MARCH TO MIRABEGRON: THE BETA-3 ADRENOCEPTOR AGONIST

Given that beta-3 adrenoceptor activation has a role in beiging of white fat, efforts to develop beta-3 adrenoceptor agonists have long been in the pipeline. The impetus was provided by their efficacy in rodent models of obesity and T2DM. They increased the oxidation of fatty acids and lowered the concentration of metabolites of fatty acids, which activate protein kinase C isozymes, which, in turn, phosphorylating serine residues of insulin receptor substrate 1; they could also play a role in inflammation.[29]

Yet none of them could come into clinical practice because some of the compounds had little lipolytic effect in human adipocytes either due to poor expression of beta-3 adrenoceptor agonist in human white adipocytes or the compounds effective in the rodents had little effect in human receptors. Besides, human lipolysis, white adipocytes were chiefly mediated by classical beta-3 adrenoceptors. A few agents, which showed selective activity for the human receptor, were not effective orally.

Yet others, which were orally effective and highly selective agonists of the human beta-3 adrenoceptors to raise energy expenditure over 24 hours, failed because of toxicity, particularly of the cardiovascular system.[29]

Besides, rodents have a larger surface-area-to-volume ratio compared to humans and are, thus, more exposed to ambient temperature. Also, human sympathomimetic agents raise expenditure of energy by only up to 30%; the beta-3 adrenoceptor agonists even lesser <10%.[30] Finally, the amount of brown adipose tissue that is activated by drugs would be too small to be clinically significant.[29]

Mirabegron is a highly selective agonist of the beta-3 adrenoceptor agonist, approved for the treatment of overactive bladder.[31] The drug is orally effective when given in a dose of 25–50 mg/day; it has a half-life of 50 hours, being primarily metabolized by CYP3A4 and excreted through feces and urine.[32]

MIRABEGRON: EFFECTS ON ADIPOSE TISSUE BEIGING, COMPONENTS OF METABOLIC SYNDROME

Finlin et al. studied the effects of local ice application or administration of mirabegron in lean and obese subjects.[33] They assessed the ability of white adipose tissue from the subcutaneous tissue to beige following the exposure to cold and to administration of beta-3 adrenoceptor agonist mirabegron. UCP1 and TMEM26 protein expression was assessed. Biopsies were taken at day 0 and on day 10 after 30-minute treatment a day with an ice pack; they were obtained from the leg to which ice was applied and from the contralateral leg to assess the effect of response to activating sympathetic nervous system. Interestingly, expression of UCP1 and TMEM26 was increased to a similar extent in the subcutaneous white adipose tissue of the cold-treated leg as well as the contralateral leg, suggesting that the response was mediated by the sympathetic nervous system.[33]

To assess, if increased UCP1 protein has functional consequences in the mitochondria, mitochondria from abdominal subcutaneous white adipose tissue were studied in 11 lean subjects: Before and after repeated cold exposure for 10 days to one side of the thigh and the abdomen. On analysis of bioenergetics, it was found that cold increased UCP1 and TMEM26 protein staining.

Following the administration of mirabegron for 10 weeks, there was an upregulation of UCP1, TMEM26 and CIDEA, and hormone-sensitive lipase (HSL) serine phosphorylation in obese, insulin-resistant individuals. Compared to exposure of ice for 10 days, mirabegron induced nearly 1.5-fold greater expression of UCP1 and beige adipocyte markers.[33] It remains to be seen whether treatment with beta-3 adrenoceptor agonist for a longer duration or when combined with diet and other drugs could be effective on PGC1-α expression and further beiging.[33]

Two recent studies showed the effect of chronic mirabegron treatment on human brown fat, high-density lipoprotein cholesterol (HDL-C), insulin sensitivity, and glucose homeostasis.[34,35]

O'Mara et al. report the effect of mirabegron (100 mg/day for 4 weeks) on 14 healthy young women. The dose was higher than the maximum approved dose of 50 mg/day in order to stimulate the brown adipose tissue to a greater extent. At the end of the study period, mirabegron increased brown adipose tissue activity as assessed by [^{18}F]fluoro-2-deoxy-D-glucose (^{18}FDG) positron emission tomography (PET)/computed tomography (CT).[34] It was particularly effective in those who had little brown adipose tissue before treatment. This occurred without accompanying changes in body weight, fat mass, fat-free mass, or self-reported food intake.

There were no changes in the duration of sleep or of sleep efficiency. To address the concern about potential cardiovascular toxicity following overstimulation by beta 3 adrenoceptor agonists, cardiac stimulation was observed from day 1 and was found to be higher on day 28. The potential mechanisms could involve myocardial oxygen consumption.[34]

Plasma metabolite responses to mirabegron showed three patterns: (1) Most showed no effect; (2) Acute increase in nonesterified fatty acids and beta-hydroxybutyrate on day 28, likely due to beta-3 adrenoceptor agonist stimulation; and (3) Specific changes that could potentially mediate improvement of metabolic health: Elevated fasting levels of HDL-C, apolipoprotein A1, ApoE, bile acids, and adiponectin, along with reduced ApoB100/ApoA1 ratio.[34] Earlier studies showed that beta-3 adrenoceptor agonists improved glucose tolerance, insulin sensitivity, and pancreatic beta-cell secretion of insulin.

Therefore, chronic treatment with mirabegron increased metabolism of brown adipose tissue, similar to the effect of cold exposure. This occurred in the perirenal fat depots, which express high levels of beta-3 adrenoceptors. Considering the improvement in glucose and insulin metabolism without alterations in fasting glucose or insulin levels, the effects are similar to those of mild exercise. The mechanism of improved glucose metabolism is speculative and could involve higher adiponectin acting via skeletal muscle and liver, increased incretin glucose-dependent insulinotropic polypeptide (GIP), or directly by the pancreatic beta-cells.[34]

Finlin et al. studied the effect of mirabegron on glucose metabolism in obese, insulin-resistant humans.[35] Up to 13 overweight adults were given a daily dose of 50 mg mirabegron at 12 weeks. At baseline and at the end of the study, the following parameters were assessed: Oral glucose tolerance test, body composition by dual-energy X-ray absorptiometry scan, resting metabolic rate, euglycemic clamp, subcutaneous white adipose tissue and vastus lateralis biopsies, and PET-CT scans under cold stimulation for quantification of brown adipose tissue.

Mirabegron treatment improved overall glucose tolerance and lowered glycosylated hemoglobin, without changes in body composition, resting energy expenditure, or plasma lipid levels. There were no side effects reported; blood pressure and pulse rate did not alter with treatment. Mirabegron increased both the disposition index and insulinogenic index, showing an improvement in pancreatic beta-cell function. Overall, improved glucose tolerance resulted from both increased in beta-cell function and improved insulin sensitivity.[35]

With mirabegron, there was increased expression of beige adipose markers such as UCP1, transmembrane protein 26, and cell death-inducing DFFA-like effector in white adipocytes in the subcutaneous tissue. The beige fat was increased with mirabegron.

Mirabegron slightly reduced triglyceride levels, but did not have any effect on adiponectin, tumor necrosis factor-alpha (TNF-α), monoattractant protein 1, and lipotoxic lipids such as ceramide. It appeared that reduced muscle triglycerides were due to release of a factor from the adipocytes that led to induction of PGC-1α mRNA in muscle.[35]

To understand the effect of mirabegron on adipose tissue, gene expression was studied in white adipose tissue from subcutaneous tissue. Among a panel of 160 genes involved in the function of adipocytes, in angiogenesis, and in fibrosis, alterations in mRNA were found in fatty acid-binding protein, FGF21, and retinol-binding protein 4, involved in metabolic homeostasis and in inducing adipose tissue inflammation.[35]

CONCLUSION

White adipocytes can be transformed to thermogenic beige adipocytes through activation of the sympathetic nervous activation. Pharmacological agents such as mirabegron can target thermogenesis via activating the sympathetic nerves. Preliminary evidence indicates that mirabegron improved the homeostasis of glucose among insulin-resistant obese persons by enhancing insulin sensitivity and beta-cell function. It is interesting that the beneficial effects occurred without weight loss or the activation of brown adipose tissue. It is yet to be known if longer duration of treatment can have a sustained improvement in beta-cell function to delay the onset of diabetes and if it would have a beneficial effect in T2DM.[35] An accompanying commentary on the two studies concluded that "the potential therapeutic utility of beta-3 adrenoceptor agonists for metabolic disorders is down, but it is not yet out".[36]

REFERENCES

1. Luo L, Liu M. Adipose tissue in control of metabolism. J Endocrinol. 2016;231:R77-99.
2. Hafidi ME, Chontal MB, Muñoz FS, Carbó R. Adipogenesis: a necessary but harmful strategy. Int J Mol Sci. 2019;20:3657.
3. Engin A. Fatty acid turnover in obesity. Adv Exp Med Biol. 2017;960:135-60.
4. Cannon B, NedergaardIkeda J. Nonshivering thermogenesis and its adequate measurement in metabolic studies. J Exp Biol. 2011;214:242-53.
5. Kennedy AR, Pissios P, Out H, Xue B, Asakura K, Furukawa N, et al. A high-fat, ketogenic diet induces a unique metabolic state in mice. Am J Physiol Endocrinol Metab. 2007;292:E1724-39.
6. Cypess, AM, Lehman S, Williams G, Tal I, Rodman D, Allison B, et al. Identification and Importance of Brown Adipose Tissue in Adult Humans. N Engl J Med. 2009;360:1509-17.
7. Maretich P, Kajimura S. The common and distinct features of brown and beige adipocytes. Trends Endocrinol Metab. 2018;29:191-200.
8. Sellayah D. The impact of early human migration on brown adipose tissue evolution and its relevance to the modern obesity pandemic. J Endocr Soc. 2019;3:372-86.
9. Williams BA, Kay RF, Kirk EC. New perspectives on anthropoid origins. Proc Natl Acad Sci. 2010;107:4797-804.
10. Bakker LEH, Boon MR, van der Linden RAD, Bouda LPA, van Klinken JB, Smith F, et al. Brown adipose tissue volume in healthy lean south Asian adults compared with white Caucasians: a prospective, case-controlled observational study. Lancet Diabetes Endocrinol. 2014;2:210-7.
11. Schultz TJ, Huang TL, Tran TT, Zhang H, Townsend KL, Shadrach JL, et al. Identification of inducible brown adipocyte progenitors residing in skeletal muscle and white fat. Proc Natl Acad Sci. 2011;108:143-8.
12. Ikeda K, Maretich P, Kajimura S. The common and distinct features of brown and beige adipocytes. Trends Endocrinol Metab. 2018;29:191-200.
13. Hasegawa Y, Ikeda K, Chen Y, Alba DL, Stifler D, Shinoda K, et al. Repression of Adipose Tissue Fibrosis through a PRDM16-GTF2IRD1 Complex Improves Systemic Glucose Homeostasis. Cell Metab. 2018;27:180-94.e6.
14. Paulo E, Wang B. Towards a better understanding of beige adipocyte plasticity. Cells. 2019;8:1552.
15. Carpentier AC, Blondin DP, Virtanen KA, Richard D, Haman F, Turcotte EE. Brown adipose tissue energy metabolism in humans. Front Endocrinol. 2018;9:447.
16. Emont MP, Kim DI, Wu J. Development, activation, and therapeutic potential of thermogenic adipocytes. Biochim Biophys Acta Mol Cell Biol Lipids. 2019;1864:13-9.

17. Sridhar GR. Peroxisome proliferator-activated receptors as molecular targets for drug therapy. J Assoc Physicians India. 2003;51:49-52.
18. Fritch LW, Nicoloro S, Chouinard M, Lazar MA, Chui PC, Leszyk J, et al. Mitochondrial remodelling in adipose tissue associated with obesity and treatment with rosiglitazone. J Clin Invest. 2004;114:1281-9.
19. Handschin C, Spiegelman BM. Peroxisome proliferator-activated receptor gamma coactivator 1 coactivators, energy homeostasis and metabolism. Endocr Rev. 2006;27:728-35.
20. Rosen ED, Spiegelman BM. What do we talk about when we talk about fat. Cell. 2014;156:20-44.
21. Ramseyer VD, Granneman JG. Adrenergic regulation of cellular plasticity in brown, beige/brite and white adipose tissues. Adipocyte. 2016;5:119-21.
22. Pan R, Zhu X, Maretich P, Chan Y. Combating obesity with thermogenic fat: current challenges and advancements. Front Endocrinol. 2020;11:185.
23. Evans BA, Merlin J, Bengtsson T, Hutchinson DS. Adrenoceptors in white, brown and brite adipocytes. Br J Pharmacol. 2019;176:2416-32.
24. Olsen JM, Aslund A, Bokhari MH, Hutchinson DS, Bengtsson T. Acute B-adrenoceptor mediated glucose clearance in brown adipose tissue; a distinct pathway independent of functional insulin signalling. Mol Metab. 2019;30:240-9.
25. Fan R, Koehler K, Chung S. Adaptive thermogenesis by dietary n-3 polyunsaturated fatty acids: emerging evidence and mechanisms. Biochim Biophys Acta Mol Cell Biol Lipids. 2019;1864:59-70.
26. Merlin J, Evans BA, Dehvari N, Sato M, Bengtsso T, Hutchinson DS. Could burning fat start with a brite spark? Pharmacological and nutritional ways to promote thermogenesis. Mol Nutr Food Res. 2016;60:18-42.
27. Reitman ML. Of mice and men—environmental temperature, body temperature, and treatment of obesity. FEBS Lett. 2018;592:2098-107.
28. Perez MB, Zagmutt S, Vazquez MCS, Serra D, Mera P, Herrero L. Impact of adaptive thermogenesis in mice on the treatment of obesity. Cells. 2020;9:316.
29. Arch JRS. Challenges in B3-adrenoceptor agonist drug development. Ther Adv Endocrinol Metab. 2011;2:59-64.
30. Van Baak MA, Hul GB, Toubro S, Astrup A, Gottesdiener KM, DeSmet M, et al. Acute effect of L-796508, a novel B3-adrenergic receptor agonist, on energy expenditure in obese men. Clin Pharmacol Ther. 2002;71:272-9.
31. Warren K, Burden H, Abrams P. Mirabegronin overactive bladder patients: efficacy review and update on drug safety. Ther Adv Drug Saf. 2016;7:204-16.
32. Dehvari N, da Silver Junior ED, Bengtsson T, Hutchinson DS. Mirabegron: potential off target effects and uses beyond the bladder. Br J Pharmacol. 2018;175:4072-82.
33. Finlin BS, Memetimin H, Confides AL, Kasza I, Zhu B, Vekaria HJ, et al. Human adipose beiging in response to cold and mirabegron. JCI Insight. 2018;3:e121510.
34. O'Mara AE, Johnson JW, Linderman JD, Brychta RJ, McGehee S, Fletcher LA, et al. Chronic mirabegron treatment increases human brown fat, HDL cholesterol, and insulin sensitivity. J Clin Invest. 2020;130:2209-19.
35. Finlin BS, Memetimin H, Zhu B, Confides AL, Vekaria HJ, El Khouli RH, et al. The B3-adrenergic receptor agonist mirabegron improves glucose homeostasis in obese humans. J Clin Invest. 2020;130: 2319-31.
36. Flier JS. Might B3-adrenergic receptor agonists be useful in disorders of glucose homeostasis? J Clin Invest. 2020;130:2180-2.

CHAPTER 17

Is Fasting the New Feasting?

Sanjana Narasimhadevera SN, G Lakshmi, GR Sridhar

ABSTRACT

Until recently, in evolutionary terms, human activity was synchronized with the day–night cycle. Eating was generally restricted to daylight hours. In the preceding century and more, it was possible to override the body's natural rhythm of eating and sleeping. Sleep was abridged and the hours when food was ingested expanded. This asynergy has been a factor in the rising prevalence of obesity, insulin resistance, diabetes mellitus, (DM) and coronary artery disease. Efforts to lose weight by approaching the energy supply-expenditure binary have been ineffective. Recent evidence has shown that modifying the time window when food is eaten during the 24-hour period can address the problem. Calorie restriction is equally effective, but is difficult to follow in the long-term. The concepts of intermittent fasting and time-restricted eating are more practical to implement, particularly the latter. When food ingestion is restricted to <12 hours, human studies have shown improvements in body weight, insulin resistance, glycemic control, and lipid profile. These were initially established in animal models where a strict restriction could be implemented. However, evidence in humans is showing that similar results can be obtained. More evidence is needed for the time when it should be started, the time window for fasting in different groups of individuals, safety, and sustained efficacy.

Keywords: *Calorie restriction, Intermittent fasting, Time-restricted eating, Insulin resistance, Circadian rhythm, Metabolism.*

INTRODUCTION

Feasting traditionally happens at a time of celebration, when dietary prudence is temporarily forgotten. As the saying goes, too much of anything is bad; so is it with feasts. Our bodies did not evolve for continual feasts without fasts. The results are evident: Epidemic of obesity and its attendant ill-effects.

Current efforts at managing the epidemic have been unfruitful. Realizing that genetic causes play little if any modifiable role, attempts were made to recalibrate the energy equation: To reduce the intake of energy by psychological, physical, or pharmacological means, or ineffectual ways to increase the energy as heat. Judging from the results, neither offers hope for success. There is exciting evidence that not just the kind of eating, but the time of eating could help in tackling obesity, insulin resistance, and diabetes.

BACKGROUND

When one considers eating patterns, both evolutionary and cultural forces come into play. During evolution, food intake was characterized by intermittent consumption of energy, be it carnivorous animals or hunter-gatherer communities. This could have favored a biological response that supported the ability to function during long periods when there was no food.[1] Behavioral adaptations consisted of higher cognitive abilities of humans to acquire food. Advent of agricultural revolution nearly 10,000 years ago ensured constant rather than intermittent availability of food. Eating patterns were adapted to the new conditions. As the balance between food access and physical activity led to greater food consumption and lower physical activity, lifestyle diseases such as obesity and type 2 diabetes mellitus (T2DM) became frequent.

To enable anticipation of rhythms of daylight and darkness, circadian rhythms evolved; this extended to availability of food as well. When there was no artificial light, humans tended to find the scarce food chiefly in daytime, interspersed with long hours of fasting overnight. Modern lifestyle disturbed the natural rhythm by making food available on demand and abridged the night hours by artificial light.[1]

These circadian rhythms are regulated by internal clocks which enable activities at appropriate times. Several core clock genes have been identified which participate in a transcriptional-translational feedback loop.[2] These control energy metabolism by regulating the expression of enzymes involved in different biological processes.

Because of the differing times at which food was available, people developed strategies to deal with these circumstances, such as seasonal fasting.[3] Fasting is defined as the "ability to meet the body's requirements .. for nutrients .." using the body's energy stores. Daily exogenous calories are restricted below 500 kcal. Done properly, fasting is not tiresome, as part of a multimodal approach including mind-body-medicine techniques with or without spiritual components, fasting is not tiresome. It enhances vitality without hunger.[3]

Normal fasting-feeding circadian rhythms dampen with age; initial evidence from animal studies showed that the rhythms can be restored to prevent or even reverse chronic diseases.[4] On the contrary, epidemiological studies have shown that erratic eating patterns increase the risk of disease in humans. The purpose of time-regulated eating is to enable the proper timing of external cues with regulated eating patterns to sustain a robust circadian clock.[4]

The relation between circadian clocks and metabolism is reciprocal. Disturbances can also occur by genetic and behavioral factors.[5] The central clock situated in the suprachiasmatic nucleus (SCN) of the brain controls a hierarchical interconnected peripheral clock network. Environmental cues are conveyed to the central clock which in turn operates through peripheral clocks situated in all cells of the body. Metabolism of glucose, lipids, and amino acids is regulated by controlling expression of genes responsible for enzymes regulating their pathways.[5]

Fasting, which can be practiced for prevention or treatment, is associated with adaptations in the body's responses: Because there is little carbohydrates available, fats are used to generate energy; when incomplete, it results in ketogenesis. Ketone bodies can be used by muscles of the heart and skeletal muscles, and by the brain. The initial enhanced protein catabolism soon ceases so that proteins are spared. Nitrogen is excreted as urea and as glutamine, thereby sparing energy. Kidneys use glutamine as substrate for gluconeogenesis, forming ammonia, which in turn neutralize keto acids and uric acids in the kidneys.[3]

ARCHITECTURE AND REGULATION OF THE CIRCADIAN CLOCK APPARATUS

Existence of daily rhythms was recognized long back in history. A French scientist, Jean-Jacques d'Ortous de Mairan, in the 18th century, while studying plant behavior, identified the existence of a central clock for such rhythms. However, it was not until the early 1970s that the field of circadian biology took off.[6] The foundation was laid by an unlikely duo of Seymour Benzer and Ronald J Konopka. Benzer was a doctorate in physics, who veered to the study of biology, where he began with a study of bacteriophages and later shifted to behavioral biology. The work (his only publication in the field) of circadian biology[7] was done with his postdoctoral student, Ronald J Konopka. The publication in PNAS (Proceedings of the National Academy of Sciences of the United States of America), which was described as being far ahead of its time, was a result of luck and rigorous science.[6] Science progresses and is recognized in inscrutable ways. The Nobel Prize for discovering the molecular mechanisms regulating circadian rhythms was awarded to Hall, Rosbash, and Young in 2017. Their work had as the foundation the 1971 PNAS paper.[7]

The central core clock, entrained by light and dark cycles, while also being regulated by nutrient availability, both anticipates and adapts to demands of the environment to enhance the fitness of organisms.[8] Each mammalian cell contains a molecular clock with autoregulatory transcription-translational feedback loop. It is reset every day by the central clock located in the SCN. The clock system also influences the numerous metabolic rhythms acting through bioenergetic programs located in different tissues. This interaction is important in relation to evolution and its influence on circadian networks.[8] However, rapid changes in environment and lifestyle in the recent past outpaced the ability of the clock machinery to adapt. These are partly responsible for a surge of noncommunicable diseases such as obesity, diabetes, cardiovascular disorders, depression, and cancers. Understanding these interactions allows therapeutic strategies to deal with these diseases. Are there ways to match clock activities with modern times? The concept of time-restricted eating seeks to match the two.

From a bird's eye view, the cues from the environment consist of light and food, which influence the clock regulator in the brain and the peripheral tissues through hormones and autonomic innervation. The central clock in turn regulates sleep, wakefulness, and feeding and fasting. The peripheral clocks, acting through the complex hormonal networks, affect metabolic pathways including adipose tissue, insulin sensitivity, immune system, cardiorenal function, and food absorption among others.[9]

Nutrient sensors form a communication between the circadian clock and energy metabolism. They entrain the clocks so that when there is an asynchrony between the metabolic tissues and the central clock, metabolic dyshomeostasis results.[5] Restricted feeding can re-entrain the phase to feeding rhythm. Along with nutrient excess and voluntary abridgment of sleep, shift work is an important contributor to the loss of synchrony with the circadian clock. This involves disruption of timing of both eating and sleeping, leading to obesity and hypertriglyceridemia, which are components of the insulin resistance syndrome.[5] Shift work operates through many pathways: Altered eating patterns, changes in hormones such as melatonin and stress resulting from sleep disturbances.[10]

Disruption of the intrinsic circadian rhythms has far-reaching adverse effects, leading to cardiometabolic diseases mediated in the brain through metabolic pathways; the involved organs include the heart, adipose tissue, muscle, liver, pancreas, and the gut. Alignment of the cycles of sleeping-awakening and feeding-fasting is a promising way to prevent and to ameliorate diseases in these diverse organs.[9]

Individual chronotype refers to the "manifestation of a person's underlying circadian rhythm,"[11] which can be identified by questionnaires about sleep habits. People can be categorized into early chronotypes and late chronotypes.[5] Those with later chronotype slept later and woke up later than early chronotype; each hour of delay in mid-sleep time led to glycosylated hemoglobin elevation of 2.5% of original value.[12]

Chrononutrition refers to time of eating in consonance with the daily rhythm of the body.[13] Periodic fasting and limiting the hours of the day during which food is taken can postpone or prevent the development of metabolic disorders such as obesity and diabetes mellitus (DM). The underlying reason for the beneficial effects lies with conserved responses of cells acting to enhance intrinsic defense mechanisms against metabolic and oxidative stress.[13] Clock regulation is affected by quality and timing of diet such as high fat intake, skipping breakfast, and eating at nighttime. Time-restricted regular eating leads to synchronous amplified rhythm, whereas irregular feeding blunts the synchrony leading to attenuated rhythms and metabolic disorders.[2]

Most evidence in the early stages is derived from animal studies carried out under controlled conditions. Similar beneficial effects were shown in humans with time-related feeding.[14]

TYPES OF CALORIE RESTRICTION

Total calorie restriction is effective in achieving weight loss, but it is difficult to maintain in the long run; alternatives such as intermittent fasting proved to be equally effective. Intermittent fasting entails normal or reduced energy intake during nonfasting periods. In contrast, *intermittent energy restriction* consists of marked energy restriction for 24 hours or more, alternating with normal eating. A number of protocols are available such as time-restricted fasting for 14–18 hours a day, early time-restricted fasting for 18 years, weekly 24-hour fasting.[15]

Sustained chronic energy restriction refers to usual meal frequency, but with reduction of energy by 40%. In *intermittent fasting,* unchanged meal timing is practiced with one or more days of fasting. *Time-restricted feeding* entails consumption of food which is restricted to a set period in the day, with or without total energy restriction.[13] The last appears to be a practical method of chrononutrition in the current obesogenic environments.

TIME-RESTRICTED FEEDING IN PREVENTION AND TREATMENT OF DISEASE

Beneficial effects of time-restricted feeding operate through modifying stress and rhythmic variability along with peripheral tissue metabolic entrainment.[16] Time-restricted feeding regulates metabolism that is disturbed as a result of obesogenic diets by synchronizing fasting/feeding times with light-entrained circadian clock. The precise mechanisms are yet to be worked out.[17]

Early humans had a diurnal rhythm of food intake, with most being consumed in the natural period of wakefulness. These are synergistic with the molecular circadian clock to match physiological anabolic and catabolic metabolism rhythms. Animal studies showed that when eating patterns were disturbed, the normal circadian oscillatory rhythms are disturbed, leading to diet-induced obesity and related abnormalities. These were prevented when given time-restricted feeding.[18]

In human trials, daily eating periods ranged from 4 to 11 hours. Even though these trials were of a short duration lasting between 4 days and 12 weeks conducted, on relatively small numbers, they were well-tolerated and effective in obese subjects, with metabolic benefits as well.[19] In addition, hunger and a desire to eat was reduced; there was lowering of blood pressure, markers of oxidative stress, and improved sleep. Improvements in glucose and lipid levels were also noted.[19] Broadly, eating over an extended time results in higher risk of obesity, liver disease, cardiac and metabolic abnormalities, poor sleep, and impaired quality of life. Time-restricted feeding reverses all these changes, when food is consistently eaten within a daily window of 12 hours or less.[20]

Benefits, Risks, and Feasibility of Time-restricted Eating

Overall, intermittent fasting is effective for losing weight and improving glycemic control in subjects with T2DM. It has similar effects as calorie restriction, but needs close monitoring for sustainable benefits.[15] There are few adverse events other than the logical ones such as hypoglycemic episodes in subjects taking hypoglycemic agents; others include muscle wasting, gout, postural hypotension, cardiac arrhythmias, and menstrual disturbances. Therefore, it is essential to prescribe intermittent fasting diets under the supervision of an experienced nutritionist.[15] As a general rule, subjects on sulfonylureas or insulin must reduce their dose by 50% on fasting days; additional modifications may be necessary based on self-blood glucose monitoring. Long-term compliance could be an issue: Jospe et al. reported that of 250 overweight adults started on the intervention, only 54% remained at the end of 12 months in the absence of intensive dietary guidance.[21]

PATHWAYS FOR BENEFICIAL EFFECTS OF INTERMITTENT FASTING

Beneficial effects of intermittent fasting and calorie restriction go beyond weight loss or reduced production of free radicals. Improvements in glucose regulation, enhanced stress resistance, and suppression of inflammation result from evolutionarily conserved adaptive integrated cellular responses.[22] During periods of fasting, cells activate mechanisms to enhance inbuilt defenses against stress due to metabolic processes; during feeding, cells are engaged in growth and plasticity of specific tissues.[22]

Caloric restriction along with intermittent fasting activates a "metabolic switch," brought about by changes in a number of signaling pathways.[15] The changes may be considered in three areas following intermittent fasting: (1) Reduced adenosine triphosphate (ATP), elevated adenosine monophosphate (AMP), which lead to increased adenosine monophosphate-activated protein kinase (AMPK) resulting in suppressed anabolic actions and enhanced catabolism, cognition, autophagy, and mitochondrial function, (2) decreased amino acids and glucose lead to lower mammalian target of rapamycin (mTOR), which in turn results in reduced protein synthesis, increased autophagy, longevity, and mitochondrial biogenesis, and (3) lower availability of carbohydrates results in liver glycogen stores and increased release of fatty acids along with hepatic β oxidation; the latter results in higher levels of ketones and autophagy. Alongside increased NAD^+ deacetylase activity of sirtuins results in lowered oxidative stress and increased autophagy. All three lead to what is called "metabolic switch" ultimately resulting in increased health span and longevity in animals.[15] The benefits from metabolic switch are not divorced from that of weight loss.[22]

At the level of the hypothalamic nuclei which control energy balance, local inflammation may lead to positive energy balance resulting in metabolic syndrome. Fasting lowers the levels of insulin and leptin, while increasing ghrelin levels. These were shown to reverse components of the metabolic syndrome in animal models. Altered gut microbiota may also play a protective role.[23] In addition, fasting can trigger an adaptive stress response, leading to increased ability to cope with more severe stress. Advancing knowledge about the mechanisms of benefits of intermittent fasting brings forth a new set of questions, such as determining at which age in the life cycle the interventions should be started to reap the beneficial effects.[24]

Timing of food alone can exert beneficial effects independent of type of food. However, further molecular studies are needed to understand the mechanism of benefits accruing from intermittent fasting.[19]

RELIGIOUS FASTING

Fasting is incorporated in many religious practices: Muslims during Ramadan, Christians, Hindus, Jews, and Buddhists on specific days of the week.[23] This serves multiple purposes in spirituality and religion, in preserving health and in postponing aging. However, it may be associated with health risks, especially in subjects with diabetes mellitus who are on glucose-lowering medications. Clinicians must be knowledgeable about how to deal with metabolic fluctuations during these episodic fasts.

Types and Benefits of Religious Fasting

Religious fasting can be continuous or intermittent. Each is further categorized in terms of dietetic rules involving macro- and micronutrients, time and duration of fast, physical behavior and activity, and finally mental aspects of prayer and meditation.[25]

Broadly, religious fasting could be beneficial for health, although nuances must be worked out such as different types of fasts, in different age groups and with coexisting diseases.[25]

Ramadan Fasting

Muslims who observe Ramadan fast are generally restricted from eating, drinking, smoking, or engagement in sensual activities between dawn and sunset during the Holy month, viz. the ninth lunar month of the Islamic calendar.[26] People often wake early to have breakfast before dawn; energy intake is restricted to evening, nighttime, and very early morning.[27] Because of religion and spirituality influencing treatment of diabetes mellitus,[28] faith-based dietary practices could promote health following Ramadan for 12 weeks.[27]

Subjects with diabetes should not fast in the following situations: Poor glycemic control, those who are noncompliant to treatment or who have unstable cardiac conditions, who have problems in alertness, brittle diabetes, and pregnant women.[26] Potential risks include hypo- and hyperglycemia, diabetic ketoacidosis, dehydration, and thrombosis,[29] especially when Ramadan falls during the summer months in tropical climates.

People who wish to undertake Ramadan fast must be evaluated by their physician beforehand. Given a choice, simple once a day regimen of antidiabetes medicines must be prescribed. Written advice is preferable to oral instructions. Patients and their family must be aware of potential problems and how to deal with them. Importantly, fasting should not be interspersed with feasting, viz. avoid high fat, sweetmeats, and fast foods.[26]

Emergence of technologies such as continuous glucose monitoring during fasts could help in recognizing and treating hypoglycemia and hyperglycemia, although cost is a constraint.[30] The following recommendations can be made about the choice of antidiabetes medications during Ramadan fast: Despite limited data, metformin, acarbose, and thiazolidinedione group of drugs appears to be safe. Sulfonylureas, with the exception of gliclazide sustained release, carry a higher risk of hypoglycemia, and must be used carefully if at all, with adjustment in dosing and timing. The incretin group and sodium-glucose cotransporter-2 (SGLT2) inhibitor appear to be safe with little risk of hypoglycemia, when used alone, i.e., without sulfonylureas or insulin. Insulin regimes must be tailored to each patient who undertakes fast during Ramadan.[31]

Indirect benefits of following Ramadan fast in subjects with diabetes include an opportunity to engage patients about management to improve control in the short-term. Hopefully this would help them realize that the metabolic gains are sustainable by strict dietary and behavioral practices.[32]

Subjects with T1DM are a vulnerable group. They can still fast during Ramadan, with careful education about diet, adjustment of insulin dose, and support from the family and physician in the event of emergencies. Self-monitoring of glucose is imperative, with regulated dietary intake. When hypoglycemia either symptomatic or asymptomatic (<70 mg/dL) develops, fast should be immediately broken irrespective of the time of day.[33]

COVID-19 infection gave rise to special issues in adults who undertook Ramadan fast: Specific precautions included social distancing, hand hygiene, hand wash, and monitoring of blood glucose. Identification of COVID symptoms must be taken into consideration. Patients must be assured they can "pray, share and care, from a safe distance" [RSSDI (Research Society for the Study of Diabetes in India) guidelines for management of diabetes during Ramadan 2020].

Despite the existence of a plethora of guidelines, it is essential to individualize structured education for the patients and their family before and during Ramadan,[34] without which principles cannot be translated to practice.

Other Kinds of Religious Fasting

Orthodox Christian fasting occurs for 180–200 days every year, besides four periods of continuous fasting from 14 to 40 days. Meat, fish, dairy products, and alcohol are prohibited. Buddhism fasting avoids all animal products with the exception of milk.[25] Despite the many studies on the health effects of religious fasting, further investigations are necessary to unravel the interactions between orthodox fasting and health.[35]

India has many traditions of fasting (and feasting). Women observe Karva Chauth and Guru Purnima annually; monthly fasts on Ekadashi, Purnima, and Pradosha. During Navaratri, fasts are longer (9 days). The type of fast may differ, e.g., "nirahara" (without food), "phalahara" (fruit and milk are allowed), and "alpahara" (broken rice is allowed).[36]

In all these varied kinds of fasting, the principles of prefast counseling, monitoring during the fast, and postfast counseling to avoid feasting are essential components for the safe practice of rituals.

CONCLUSION

Studies originally carried out in animal models have been replicated in human beings. Epidemiological, clinical, and short-term controlled studies showed that time-restricted eating can improve obesity, insulin resistance, dysglycemia, and dyslipidemia. This is an exciting addition to lifestyle methods that attempt to address the energy intake-expenditure paradigm. Biochemical basis for its effectiveness is being established. Further well-designed trials over longer periods should lead to the widespread applicability of time-restricted feeding as a management option.

REFERENCES

1. Mattson MP, Allison DB, Fontana L, Harvie M, Longo VD, Malaisse WJ, et al. Meal frequency and timing in health and disease. Proc Natl Acad Sci U S A. 2014;111(47):16647-53.
2. Oike H, Oishi K, Kobori M. Nutrients, clock genes, and chrononutrition. Curr Nutr Rep. 2014;3(3):204-12.
3. Boschmann M, Michalsen A. Fasting therapy - old and new perspectives. Forsch Komplementmed. 2013;20(6):410-11.
4. Manoogian ENC, Panda S. Circadian rhythms, time-restricted feeding, and healthy aging. Ageing Res Rev. 2017;39:59-67.
5. Bae SA, Fang MZ, Rustgi V, Zarbl H, Androulakis IP. At the interface of lifestyle, behavior, and circadian rhythms: metabolic implications. Front Nutr. 2019;6:132.
6. Hardcastle M. Cracking the clock: Ronald J. Konopka and Seymour Benzer. Proc Natl Acad Sci U S A. 2021;118(39):e2115546118.
7. Konopka RJ, Benzer S. Clock mutants of Drosophila melanogaster. Proc Natl Acad Sci U S A. 1971;68(9):2112-6.
8. Gerhart-Hines Z, Lazar MA. Circadian metabolism in the light of evolution. Endocr Rev. 2015;36(3):289-304.
9. Maury E, Ramsey KM, Bass J. Circadian rhythms and metabolic syndrome: from experimental genetics to human disease. Circ Res. 2010;106(3):447-62.
10. Sridhar GR, Sanjana NS. Sleep, circadian dysrhythmia, obesity and diabetes. World J Diabetes. 2016;7(19):515-22.
11. Wittmann M, Dinich J, Merrow M, Roenneberg T. Social jetlag: misalignment of biological and social time. Chronobiol Int. 2006;23(1-2):497-509.
12. Sridhar GR, Gumpeny L. Sleep, obesity and diabetes: the circadian rhythm. In: Sridhar GR. Advances in Diabetes: Novel insights. New Delhi: The Health Sciences Publisher; 2016. pp. 197-207.
13. Hawley JA, Sassone-Corsi P, Zierath JR. Chrono-nutrition for the prevention and treatment of obesity and type 2 diabetes: from mice to men. Diabetologia. 2020;63(11):2253-9.
14. Summa KC, Turek FW. Chronobiology and obesity: Interactions between circadian rhythms and energy regulation. Adv Nutr. 2014;5(3):312S-9S.
15. Rajpal A, Ismail-Beigi F. Intermittent fasting and 'metabolic switch': Effects on Chrono-nutrition for the prevention and treatment obesity and type 2 diabetes: from mice to men, metabolic syndrome, prediabetes and type 2 diabetes. Diabetes Obes Metab. 2020;22(9):1496-510.
16. Sunderram J, Sofou S, Kamisoglu K, Karantza V, Androulakis IP. Time-restricted feeding and the realignment of biological rhythms: translational opportunities and challenges. J Transl Med. 2014;12:79.
17. Zarrinpar A, Chaix A, Panda S. Daily eating patterns and their impact on health and disease. Trends Endocrinol Metab. 2016;27(2):69-83.
18. Melkani GC, Panda S. Time-restricted feeding for prevention and treatment of cardiometabolic disorders. J Physiol. 2017;595(12):3691-700.
19. Schuppelius B, Peters B, Ottawa A, Pivovarova-Ramich O. Time restricted eating: A dietary strategy to prevent and treat metabolic disturbances. Front Endocrinol (Lausanne). 2021;12:683140.
20. Manoogian EN, Chow LS, Taub PR, Laferrère B, Panda S. Time-restricted eating for the prevention and management of metabolic diseases. Endocr Rev. 2021:bnab027.
21. Jospe MR, Roy M, Brown RC, Haszard JJ, Meredith-Jones K, Fangupo LJ, et al. Intermittent fasting, Paleolithic, or Mediterranean diets in the real world: exploratory secondary analyses of a weight-loss trial that included choice of diet and exercise. Am J Clin Nutr. 2020;111(3):503-14.
22. de Cabo R, Mattson MP. Effects of intermittent fasting on health, aging, and disease. N Engl J Med. 2019;381(26):2541-51.
23. Longo VD, Mattson MP. Fasting: molecular mechanisms and clinical applications. Cell Metab. 2014;19(2):181-92.
24. Helfand SL, de Cabo R. Evidence that overnight fasting could extend healthy lifespan. Nature. 2021;598(7880):265-6.

25. Persynaki A, Karras S, Pichard C. Unraveling the metabolic health benefits of fasting related to religious beliefs: A narrative review. Nutrition. 2017;35:14-20.
26. Akbani MF, Saleem M, Gadit WU, Ahmed M, Basit A, Malik RA. Fasting and feasting safely during Ramadan in the patient with diabetes. Pract Diab Int. 2005;22(3):100-4.
27. Hoddy KK, Marlatt KL, Çetinkaya H, Ravussin E. Intermittent fasting and metabolic health: From religious fast to time-restricted feeding. Obesity. 2020;28(S1):S29-37.
28. Sridhar GR. Diabetes, religion and spirituality. Intl J Diab Dev Cntrs. 2013;33:5-7.
29. Al-Arouj M, Assaad-Khalil S, Buse J, Fahdil I, Fahmy M, Hafez S, et al. Recommendations for management of diabetes during Ramadan: update 2010. Diabetes Care. 2010;33(8):1895-902.
30. Ibrahim M, Davies MJ, Ahmad E, Annabi FA, Eckel RH, Ba-Essa EM, et al. Recommendations for management of diabetes during Ramadan: update 2020, applying the principles of the ADA/EASD consensus. BMJ Open Diabetes Res Care. 2020;8(1):e001248.
31. Loh HH, Kamaruddin NA. Treatment options for patients with type 2 diabetes mellitus during the fasting month of Ramadan. Ann Acad Med Singap. 2020;49(7):468-76.
32. Ahmed SH, Chowdhury TA, Hussain S, Syed A, Karamat A, Helmy A, et al. Ramadan and diabetes: A narrative review and practice update. Diabetes Ther. 2020;11(11):2477-520.
33. Deeb A, Elbarbary N, Smart CE, Beshyah SA, Habeb A, Kalra S, et al. ISPAD Clinical Practice Consensus Guidelines: Fasting during Ramadan by young people with diabetes. Pediatr Diabetes. 2020;21(1): 5-17.
34. Yaqub F. Diabetes and fasting during Ramadan: a need for guidelines. Lancet Diabetes Endocrinol. 2014;2:454
35. Koufakis T, Karras SN, Antonopoulou V, Angeloudi F, Zebekakis P, Kotsa K. Effects of Orthodox religious fasting on human health: a systematic review. Eur J Nutr. 2017;56(8):2439-55.
36. Saboo B, Joshi S, Shah SN, Tiwaskar M, Vishwanathan V, Bhandari S, et al. Management of diabetes during fasting and feasting in India. J Assoc Physicians India. 2019;67(9):70-7.

CHAPTER 18

Drugs that Wear Different Hats: Sodium-glucose Cotransporter-2 Inhibitors

G Lakshmi, Sanjana Narasimhadevera SN, GR Sridhar

ABSTRACT

The sodium-glucose cotransporter 2 inhibitors (SGLT2i) belong to a different class of antidiabetes agents. They were first isolated from the root bark of the apple tree and used in treating malaria. Advances in technology led to the development of orally effective agents in the SGLT2i class that could be used in clinical practice. While their primary effectiveness in glycemic control is established, unexpected benefits were observed such as cardiorenal protection. Large multicentric global clinical trials confirmed their protective effects. Not only are they being used in diabetes, but nephrologists and cardiologists are beginning to use them for preventing or delaying heart failure and renal failure even in subjects without diabetes.

Keywords: *Adiposity, Cardiorenal, Glucosuria, Heart failure, Ketoacidosis, Renal failure, Renal tubule.*

INTRODUCTION

Plasma glucose levels are maintained in a narrow range by a balance between the rate of formation and metabolism. Glucose formation and utilization is regulated by hormones such as insulin, gut peptides, and glucagon. While it goes to the kidneys in large amounts, most of it is normally filtered by the proximal renal tubules so that little is excreted in the urine.

The drugs commonly used in treating diabetes focused on insulin: Its formation, secretion, action, and when all else failed by replacement. Still there was scope and need for improvement.

The ideal antidiabetes agent must have all or most of the following attributes: Not only lowering glucose levels, but also addressing the underlying pathological processes leading to diabetes; further value would be added if the agent can reduce nonglycemic risk factors that result in vascular disease. Over the past 10 years or so, regulatory agent requirements needed that newer antidiabetes agents must undergo cardiovascular outcome trials, and demonstrate that they do not cause adverse cardiovascular events. Therefore, a search was made for drugs that act on targets other than pancreatic β cells and tissue insulin resistance.[1]

With the focus primarily directed on various aspects of insulin metabolism, the role of kidney in glucose metabolism has for long remained a footnote in the management of dysglycemia. Yet, as long back as the early 1930s, Himsworth remarked that "the concentration of the sugar reabsorbed is determined by the sugar content of the blood in the peritubular capillaries," i.e., he recognized a parallel relationship between glucose levels in the blood and the urine.[2] Preceding the publication of Himsworth, Hjarne reported 19 persons in a Swedish family who had inherited glucosuria across generations. It was a rare, apparently benign condition characterized by persistent glucosuria in spite of having normal blood glucose levels.[3] An animal study showed that a chemical, derived from apple tree bark, phlorizin, induced glucosuria in dogs by blocking glucose reabsorption at the level of the renal tubules.[4] Putting all these together, it was evident that glucose was reabsorbed by the renal tubule, which depended on the presence of an "inherited factor," which could in turn be inhibited. The question remained: What was the "factor"?[1]

HISTORICAL ASPECTS

Nearly a 150 years ago in 1886, von Mering identified the glucose-lowering properties of phlorizin through its glucosuric effects.[5] In the early to mid-20th century, it was demonstrated that glucose is normally filtered in the glomerulus and almost fully reabsorbed in the proximal renal tubule. The need for active transport across the tubule was established in the 1960s, with glucose and sodium being cotransported.[6] The cotransporter responsible for the transport of glucose and sodium was recognized as sodium-glucose cotransporter (SGLT); when it was inhibited, both glucose and sodium were excreted in urine. In retrospect, phlorizin was shown to be a competitive inhibitor of this transport. Injecting phlorizin to diabetic animals lowered their plasma glucose. For clinical use, orally effective agents were developed because phlorizin needed to be injected and was associated with adverse effects. A number of sodium-glucose cotransporter 2 inhibitors (SGLT2i) oral analogs were synthesized for use in the treatment of diabetes mellitus.[7]

SODIUM GLUCOSE TRANSPORTER (FIG. 1 AND TABLE 1)

Glucose reabsorption across the renal tubules depends on membrane-associated transport proteins. Sodium-dependent glucose transporter types 1 and 2, the most extensively studied among the family of 6, are located on the

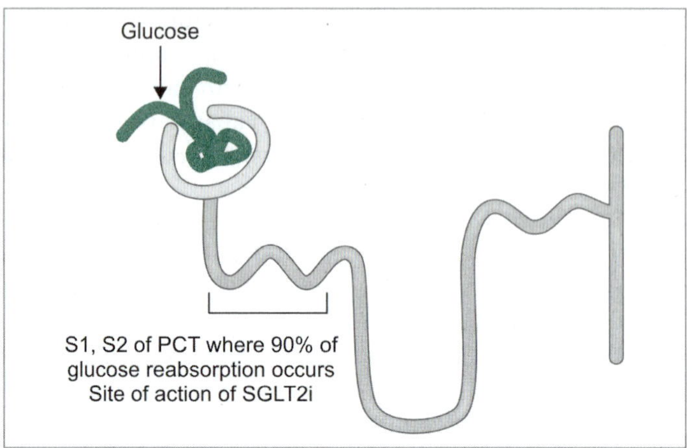

(PCT: proximal convoluted tubule; SGLT2i: sodium glucose-cotransporter 2 inhibitor)

FIG. 1: Sodium-glucose cotransporter.

TABLE 1 Types of SGLTs.

Types of SGLT	Major sites	Functions: Transport of–
SGLT1	Small intestine, trachea, heart, and kidney (Segment 3 of PCT)	Sodium, glucose, and galactose
SGLT2	Kidney (Segments 1 and 2 of PCT)	Sodium and glucose
SGLT3	Small intestine, thyroid, lung, liver, testis, and uterus	Sodium
SGLT4	Small intestine, stomach, lung, liver, and kidney	Glucose and mannose
SGLT5	Kidney	Unknown
SGLT6	Small intestine, spinal cord, brain, and kidney	Glucose and myo-inositol

(PCT: proximal convoluted tubule; SGLT: sodium-glucose cotransporter)

apical or luminal membrane. They serve as secondary active transporters,[8] bringing sodium and glucose into the cell.

Sodium-dependent glucose transporters have 15 exons and 580–718 amino acids. They act by a coordinated closing and opening of internal and external gates. SGLT1 and SGLT2, localized to the brush border membrane, have specific locations; SGLT1 is located in distal part of proximal renal tubule (segment 3) which reabsorbs 10% of glucose and SGLT2 in segments 1 and 2 of proximal renal tubule which reabsorbs 90%. Since the bulk of glucose is reabsorbed by SGLT2 which is located in the proximal tubules, inhibitors of SGLT2 were developed for the management of diabetes.

MECHANISM OF ACTION OF SODIUM-GLUCOSE COTRANSPORTER 2 INHIBITORS

The clinical effects of SGLT2 inhibitors depend on reduction of glucose reabsorption in the proximal tubule. They shift the renal threshold for glucose excretion from about 180 to 50 mg/dL. By lowering the levels of glucose via an insulin-independent mechanism, through inducing osmotic diuresis and loss of calories in the urine. They have favorable effects in type 2 diabetes mellitus (T2DM). These drugs do not go intracellularly, but inhibit SGLT2 from the extracellular surface of the tubular lumen.[8]

SODIUM-GLUCOSE COTRANSPORTER 2 INHIBITOR IN CLINICAL USE

Dapagliflozin was the first drug in the class to be approved by the European Medicines Agency in 2012, followed a year later by canagliflozin, which was approved by Food and Drug Administration. A number of other agents such as empagliflozin were shortly approved based on favorable effects not only on glycemic control, but also by inducing weight loss and cardiorenal benefits. Recently, a dual SGLT1 and SGLT2 inhibitor, sotagliflozin, has been developed and shown to improve postprandial glucose control.[9]

Canagliflozin, dapagliflozin, and empagliflozin have good oral bioavailability (60–80%) and their absorption is unaffected by food. They reach peak plasma levels 1–2 hours after ingestion. With a half-life of 12 hours, they are given as once daily dosing. Inactive metabolites are excreted by the kidney, with virtually none of the parent drugs being excreted.

CLINICAL STUDIES AND TRIALS OF SODIUM-GLUCOSE COTRANSPORTER 2 INHIBITOR DRUGS

Dapagliflozin, the first clinically approved SGLT2i drug (BMS-512148; BMS-512148), underwent global clinical trials for efficacy and safety in the early 2000s.[10,11] In randomized, double-blind trials among subjects with poorly controlled T2DM, dapagliflozin as monotherapy in drug-naive patients, or as add-on to metformin, glimepiride, pioglitazone, or insulin-based therapy, significantly reduced both glycosylated hemoglobin and fasting plasma glucose levels compared with placebo.[11] It was associated with weight loss and glycemic control was sustained for up to 2 years.

Cardiac Outcome Trials

The results of SGLT2i outcome trials on cardiovascular safety revealed that they are not only safe, but they slow the progression and improve the outcomes of heart failure and renal failure.

Dapagliflozin and Cardiovascular Outcomes in T2DM

In this large randomized double-blind trial, 17,160 subjects with T2DM having established cardiovascular disease ($n = 6{,}974$) or multiple risk factors ($n = 10{,}186$) were assigned to dapagliflozin 10 mg a day or to placebo. The treating physician used or continued all other agents for managing diabetes mellitus. The primary end points were major cardiovascular events (cardiovascular disease, myocardial infarction, ischemic stroke, and heart failure). Dapagliflozin group showed a lower risk of coronary artery disease and heart failure (4.9% compared to 5.8% in control group)[12]; similarly, the major cardiovascular events were also favorable with dapagliflozin: i.e., estimated glomerular filtration rate, end-stage renal disease, death due to renal or cardiovascular causes (4.3 vs. 5.6% in controls). All-cause mortality, another secondary end point tended to be lower with dapagliflozin (6.2 vs. 6.6%). However diabetic ketoacidosis occurred more often with dapagliflozin compared to placebo.[12]

Dapagliflozin in Patients with Heart Failure and Reduced Ejection Fraction

In the DAPA-HF trial, subjects with or without diabetes having heart failure and reduced ejection fraction were recruited: Inclusion criteria were New York Heart Association (NYHA) class II-IV dyspnea, left ventricular ejection fraction (LVEF) ≤40%, NT-proBNP (N-terminal-proB-type natriuretic peptide) ≥600 pg/mL as a biochemical marker. Following a 14-day run in period, either placebo ($n = 2{,}371$) or dapagliflozin 10 mg once a day ($n = 2{,}373$) were given. Dapagliflozin lowered the risk of cardiovascular deaths and hospitalization or urgent hospital visit due to heart failure in both groups, i.e., in those with diabetes and even in those without diabetes.[13]

Effect of Dapagliflozin on Left Ventricular Hypertrophy in People with T2DM

Sixty-six subjects with T2DM and left ventricular hypertrophy with controlled blood pressure received dapagliflozin 10 mg a day or placebo for 12 months. The active drug group showed significant reduction of left ventricular mass compared to control. It was associated with reduced body weight, systolic blood pressure, body fat, and insulin resistance.[14] Dapagliflozin can therefore contribute to cardiac protection by reverse remodeling and changes in left ventricular structure.[14]

Effect of Dapagliflozin on Worsening Heart Failure and Cardiovascular Death in Patients with Heart Failure with and without Diabetes

In this exploratory analysis of global trials, the effects of dapagliflozin on heart failure with reduced ejection fraction (HFrEF) were studied in subjects with and without diabetes. All but 2 of 4,744 patients who were recruited completed the trial. In those without diabetes, the primary outcome occurred in 13.2% in the dapagliflozin group and 17.7% in the placebo group. In patients with diabetes, the primary outcome was seen in 20% in the dapagliflozin group and 25.5% in the placebo group.[15] This exploratory analysis showed that addition of dapagliflozin to recommended therapy reduced the risk of worsening heart failure or cardiovascular death. The risk reduction was independent of diabetes status.

A post-hoc analysis of DAPA-HF (Dapagliflozin in Patients with Heart Failure and Reduced Ejection Fraction) trial showed that the beneficial effects of dapagliflozin in heart failure were seen despite the heterogeneous background treatments for heart failure.[16]

Dapagliflozin and Cardiovascular Outcomes in Patients with T2DM and Previous Myocardial Infarction (DECLARE-TIMI 58 Trial Subanalysis)

In view of increased baseline risk among patients with prior myocardial infarction, it was hypothesized that SGLT2i treatment may provide greater benefit in this subgroup. A subanalysis of the DECLARE-TIMI 58 (Dapagliflozin and Cardiovascular Outcomes in Type 2 Diabetes) trial showed that among those with previous myocardial infarction, dapagliflozin reduced the relative risk of major cardiovascular events by 16% and the absolute risk by 2.6%.[17] In contrast, there was no effect among subjects without prior cardiovascular event. Benefit was greater within 2 years of the last event. Further studies are needed to confirm these exploratory findings.

TRIALS ON RENAL OUTCOMES

Dapagliflozin on Clinical Outcomes in Patients with Chronic Kidney Disease, with and without Cardiovascular Disease

In the DAPA-CKD trial (Dapagliflozin on Clinical Outcomes in Patients with Chronic Kidney Disease, with and without Cardiovascular Disease), 4,304 subjects with chronic kidney disease were randomly assigned to two groups: Dapagliflozin 10 mg/day or placebo. The primary end point was a composite of sustained decline in estimated glomerular filtration rate (eGFR), end-stage renal disease or death due to renal failure or cardiovascular disease. Dapagliflozin reduced the risk of primary composite outcome, with low adverse effects. The beneficial effect was observed in those with and without T2DM, independent of the coexistence of cardiovascular disease.[18]

Canagliflozin and Cardiovascular and Renal Events in T2DM (CANVAS Program)

The CANVAS Program (Canagliflozin and Cardiovascular and Renal Events in Type 2 Diabetes) integrated data from two trials comprising 10,142 participants with T2DM carrying high risk of cardiovascular disease. Participants were randomly assigned to canagliflozin or placebo. They were followed for a mean duration of 188.2 weeks. The primary outcome was a composite of death from cardiovascular causes, nonfatal myocardial infarction, or nonfatal stroke. With participants having mean duration of diabetes for 13.5 years, 6% had a history of cardiovascular disease. The rate of the primary outcome was lower with canagliflozin compared to placebo.[19] Adverse effects were not different from those reported earlier, except for an increase in the risk of amputation at the level of the toe or the metatarsal.

Canagliflozin for Primary and Secondary Prevention of Cardiovascular Events [CANVAS Program (Canagliflozin Cardiovascular Assessment Study)]

In the CANVAS Program, the primary end-point was taken as a composite of cardiovascular death, nonfatal myocardial infarction, or nonfatal stroke. Secondary outcomes were heart failure hospitalization and a renal composite. Participants in the primary prevention group (n = 3,486; 34%) were younger, more often female and had diabetes for a longer period compared with secondary prevention participants. Canagliflozin improved cardiovascular and renal outcomes. There was no statistically significant heterogeneity of the treatment response between the primary and secondary prevention groups.[20] Further studies are needed to obtain better insights.

Adverse Outcomes with Canagliflozin

A retrospective analysis was made from nine placebo and active controlled studies in which canagliflozin given in doses of 100 mg and 300 mg a day (n = 10,194) from the CANVAS (n = 4,327) and another eight non-CANVAS studies (n = 5,867). The pooled results from non-CANVAS studies showed a similar fracture risk in both groups (viz. canagliflozin and placebo). However, in the CANVAS, fracture incidence was higher in canagliflozin group (2.7%) compared to placebo (1.9%).[21] The cause for the divergent results between the two groups could not be satisfactorily answered, although a potential link to volume-depleted adverse reactions leading to falls in CANVAS was suggested. A further analysis published in 2019 concluded that the differences could be due to a chance occurrence.[22] In addition, ketoacidosis is a recognized adverse effect, which must be identified and treated.

Empagliflozin, Cardiovascular Outcomes, and Mortality in T2DM

Similar to other agents in the group, empagliflozin showed improved glycemic control both as monotherapy and in combination regimens.[23] In the EMPA-REG OUTCOME study, empagliflozin was given in an oral dose of 10 or 25 mg. As a measure of primary composite outcome, deaths from cardiovascular causes, nonfatal myocardial infarction, or nonfatal stroke were considered. When empagliflozin was added to standard therapy in T2DM at high risk for cardiovascular events, it lowered the rate of the primary composite cardiovascular outcome and of death from any cause.[24] It was postulated that the beneficial effects could be mediated by additive cardioprotective effects through the activation of nonclassic renin-angiotensin-aldosterone system (RAAS) pathways.[25]

Empagliflozin was also shown to lower blood pressure in subjects with T2DM having hypertension. Among 825 individuals who participated in a double-blind randomized study, empagliflozin was administered in a dose of 10 or 25 mg once daily or placebo for 12 weeks. Study drug showed a significant, meaningful reduction of blood pressure and glycosylated hemoglobin.[26] It was well tolerated without significant adverse effects.

Cardiovascular and Renal Outcomes with Empagliflozin in Heart Failure

In a double-blind study, subjects ($n = 3{,}730$) with class II, III, or IV heart failure and an ejection fraction lower than 40% were given empagliflozin 10 mg/day or placebo. Other medications for heart failure were continued. At a median of 16 months, a primary outcome event (composite of cardiovascular death or hospitalization for heart failure which worsened), occurred in 19.4% of empagliflozin group and 24.7% in placebo. The annual rate of reduction in eGFR was slower in the empagliflozin group, associated with increased risk of uncomplicated genital tract infections.[27] Beneficial effects were observed even in nondiabetic individuals. The proposed beneficial effects on progression of atherosclerosis were due to modulation of lipid profiles and activity of the sympathetic nervous system.[28]

Dual Sodium-glucose Transporter Inhibitor, Sotagliflozin

While the first three drugs had their principal action on inhibiting SGLT2 receptors of the proximal renal tubule, sotagliflozin is a dual inhibitor, viz. of both SGLT2 and SGLT1 receptors. It was shown to be useful in the treatment of type 1 diabetes mellitus (T1DM) as well as T2DM.[9] It induces glucosuria like other SGLT2i drugs; in addition, it delays glucose absorption from the intestine by inhibiting SGLG2, improving postprandial glycemic swings. It is effective as monotherapy and in combination with other antidiabetic agents. Similar to SGLT2i, sotagliflozin improves glycosylated hemoglobin, lowers body weight and blood pressure.[9] SOLOIST-WHF trial was a multicenter, double-blind trial on patients with T2DM recently hospitalized due to worsening heart failure. They were randomized to receive sotagliflozin or placebo. The primary end point was the deaths due to cardiovascular causes, hospitalizations, and urgent visits for treatment of heart failure. Even though the trial (n = 1,222; 608 to sotagliflozin) was prematurely terminated early because the sponsor withdrew their funding of the drug, compared to placebo when begun before or shortly after discharge, led to lower total number of cardiovascular deaths and hospitalizations and urgent visits for heart failure.[29]

OVERVIEW OF SODIUM-GLUCOSE COTRANSPORTER 2 INHIBITORS ON CARDIOVASCULAR RISK

Considered as a class, SGLT2i drugs have extraglycemic benefits by modulating blood pressure, body weight, truncal obesity, hyperinsulinemia, stiffness of arteries, albuminuria, uric acid levels, and oxidative stress.[30] The basis of these putative pathways led to large international multicentric clinical trials which showed the cardiorenal benefit of a variety of SGLT2i, in addition to improving glycemic control. Novel insights were obtained such as their greater cardiovascular protective effect among those with lower eGFR and greater degree albuminuria.[31] Inhibition of SGLT2 in the proximal renal tubule has effects other than on plasma volume homeostasis: It has beneficial effects on adiposity and energy metabolism globally.[32]

A systematic review and meta-analysis on SGLT2i for the prevention of kidney failure in T2DM was published based on data from empagliflozin (EMPA-REG OUTCOME), canagliflozin (CANVAS program, CREDENCE), and dapagliflozin (DECLARE T1M1 58) (n = 38,723 subjects). It was concluded that they substantially reduced the incidence of dialysis, renal transplantation, or death due to chronic renal disease, and gave the strongest yet evidence for their routine use in patients with renal failure.[33]

A meta-analysis on cardiovascular outcomes trials with SGLT2i (n = 34,322 subjects) showed moderate benefits on atherosclerotic major adverse cardiovascular events; these were limited to those having established atherosclerotic cardiovascular disease. But they substantially reduce heart failure needing hospitalization and progression of renal disease.[34]

DO ALL SODIUM-GLUCOSE COTRANSPORTER 2 INHIBITORS HAVE SIMILAR CARDIORENAL BENEFITS?

In general, all three commonly used agents in the SGLT2i class, viz. empagliflozin, dapagliflozin, and canagliflozin, have biologically plausible class effects on cardiac and renal outcomes. It depends on the baseline glomerular filtration rate and degree of albuminuria.[35]

A recent systematic review and network meta-analysis of randomized controlled trials (RCTs) on comparative efficacy of SGLT2i drugs on cardiovascular outcomes in T2DM was published. 64 trials were included (n = 74,874 subjects) with the primary end point being all-cause mortality. It provided comparative cardiovascular benefits of different agents among subjects with T2DM. Empagliflozin, canagliflozin, and dapagliflozin reduced all-cause mortality in comparison with placebo. However, among the three, empagliflozin seemed more effective than the others.[36] The differences could, however, be attributed to trial populations heterogeneity. But there was no difference among the three agents on reduction of heart failure. They were attributed to reduction of circulating volume, natriuresis, lowering of blood pressure, modification of renal-renin-angiotensin axis, and reduced arterial stiffness.[36]

CONCLUSION

A relatively new group of antidiabetic agents, SGLT2i, have been shown to improve glycemic control as well as cardiorenal outcomes even in those without diabetes mellitus, although the real-world applicability of the benefits must be established.[37] A case has been made for initiation of SGLT2i early in the course of the disease,[38] and even in those without diabetes.[39] In the words of Eugene Braunwald, SGLT2i can be called the "statins of the 21st century."[6]

REFERENCES

1. Marshall SM. The bark giving diabetes therapy some bite: the SGLT inhibitors. Diabetologia. 2018;61(10):2075-8.
2. Himsworth HP. The relation of glycosuria to glycaemia and the determination of the renal threshold for glucose. Biochem J. 1931;25(4):1128-46.
3. Hjärne U. Study of orthoglycaemic glycosuria with particular reference to its hereditability. Acta Med Scand. 1927;67(1):422-571.
4. Poulsson LT. On the mechanism of sugar elimination in phlorrhizin glycosuria. A contribution to the filtration-reabsorption theory on kidney function. J Physiol. 1930;69(4):411-22.
5. Von Moring J. Über künstlichen Diabetes; Centralblatt für die medizinische Wissenschaft. 1886;22: 31-5.
6. Braunwald E. SGLT2 inhibitors: the statins of the 21st century. Eur Heart J. 2021:ehab765.
7. Adachi T, Yasuda K, Okamoto Y, Shihara N, Oku A, Ueta K, et al. T-1095, a renal Na+-glucose transporter inhibitor, improves hyperglycemia in streptozotocin-induced diabetic rats. Metabolism. 2000;49(8): 990-5

8. Gallo LA, Wright EM, Vallon V. Probing SGLT2 as a therapeutic target for diabetes: basic physiology and consequences. Diab Vasc Dis Res. 2015;12(2):78-89.
9. Cefalo CMA, Cinti F, Moffa S, Impronta F, Sorice GP, Mezza T, et al. Sotagliflozin, the first dual SGLT inhibitor: current outlook and perspectives. Cardiovasc Diabetol. 2019;18(1):20.
10. Dapagliflozin: BMS 512148; BMS-512148. Drugs R D. 2010;10(1):47-54.
11. Albarrán OG, Ampudia-Blasco FJ. Dapagliflozina, el primer inhibidor SGLT 2 en el tratamiento de la diabetes tipo 2. Med Clin (Barc). 2013;141 Suppl 2:36-43.
12. Wiviott SD, Raz I, Bonaca MP; DECLARE–TIMI 58 Investigators. Dapagliflozin and cardiovascular outcomes in type 2 diabetes. N Engl J Med. 2019;380(4):347-57.
13. McMurray JJV, Solomon SD, Inzucchi SE, Køber L, Kosiborod MN, Martinez FA, et al. Dapagliflozin in patients with heart failure and reduced ejection fraction. N Engl J Med. 2019;381(21):1995-2008.
14. Brown AJM, Gandy S, McCrimmon R, Houston JG, Struthers AD, Lang CC. A randomized controlled trial of dapagliflozin on left ventricular hypertrophy in people with type two diabetes: the DAPA-LVH trial. Eur Heart J. 2020;41(36):3421-32.
15. Petrie MC, Verma S, Docherty KF, Inzucchi SE, Anand I, Belohlávek J, et al. Effect of dapagliflozin on worsening heart failure and cardiovascular death in patients with heart failure with and without diabetes. JAMA. 2020;323(14):1353-68.
16. Docherty KF, Jhund PS, Inzucchi SE, Køber L, Kosiborod MN, Martinez FA, et al. Effects of dapagliflozin in DAPA-HF according to background heart failure therapy. Eur Heart J. 2020;41(25):2379-92.
17. Furtado RHM, Bonaca MP, Raz I, Zelniker TA, Mosenzon O, Cahn A, et al. Dapagliflozin and cardiovascular outcomes in patients with type 2 diabetes mellitus and previous myocardial infarction. Circulation. 2019;139(22):2516-27.
18. McMurray JJV, Wheeler DC, Stefánsson BV, Jongs N, Postmus D, Correa-Rotter R, et al. Effect of dapagliflozin on clinical outcomes in patients with chronic kidney disease, with and without cardiovascular disease. Circulation. 2021;143(5):438-48.
19. Neal B, Perkovic V, Mahaffey KW, de Zeeuw D, Fulcher G, Erondu N, et al. Canagliflozin and cardiovascular and renal events in type 2 diabetes. N Engl J Med. 2017;377(21):644-57.
20. Mahaffey KW, Neal B, Perkovic V, de Zeeuw D, Fulcher G, Erondu N, et al. Canagliflozin for primary and secondary prevention of cardiovascular events: results from the CANVAS Program (Canagliflozin Cardiovascular Assessment Study). Circulation. 2018;137(4):323-34.
21. Watts NB, Bilezikian JP, Usiskin K, Edwards R, Desai M, Law G, et al. Effects of canagliflozin on fracture risk in patients with type 2 diabetes mellitus. J Clin Endocrinol Metab. 2016;101(1):157-66.
22. Zhou Z, Jardine M, Perkovic V, Matthews DR, Mahaffey KW, de Zeeuw D, et al. Canagliflozin and fracture risk in individuals with type 2 diabetes: results from the CANVAS Program. Diabetologia. 2019;62(10):1854-67.
23. Dailey GE. Empagliflozin: a new treatment option for patients with type 2 diabetes mellitus. Drugs Today (Barc). 2015;51(9):519-35.
24. Zinman B, Wanner C, Lachin JM, Fitchett D, Bluhmki E, Hantel S, et al. Empagliflozin, cardiovascular outcomes, and mortality in type 2 diabetes. N Engl J Med. 2015;373:2117-28.
25. Muskiet MH, van Raalte DH, van Bommel EJ, Smits MM, Tonneijck L. Understanding EMPA-REG OUTCOME. Lancet Diabetes Endocrinol. 2015;3(12):928-9.
26. Tikkanen I, Narko K, Zeller C, Green A, Salsali A, Broedl UC, et al. Empagliflozin reduces blood pressure in patients with type 2 diabetes and hypertension. Diabetes Care. 2015;38(3):420-8.
27. Packer M, Anker SD, Butler J, Filippatos G, Pocock SJ, Carson P, et al. Cardiovascular and renal outcomes with empagliflozin in heart failure. N Engl J Med. 2020;383(15):1413-24.
28. Liu Y, Xu J, Wu M, Xu B, Kang L. Empagliflozin protects against atherosclerosis progression by modulating lipid profiles and sympathetic activity. Lipids Health Dis. 2021;20(1):5.
29. Bhatt DL, Szarek M, Steg PG, Cannon CP, Leiter LA, McGuire DK, et al. Sotagliflozin in patients with diabetes and recent worsening heart failure. N Engl J Med. 2021;384:117-28.
30. Inzucchi SE, Zinman B, Wanner C, Ferrari R, Fitchett D, Hantel S, et al. SGLT-2 inhibitors and cardiovascular risk: proposed pathways and review of ongoing outcome trials. Diab Vasc Dis Res. 2015;12(2):90-100.

31. Chun KJ, Jung HH. SGLT2 inhibitors and kidney and cardiac outcomes according to estimated gfr and albuminuria levels: A meta-analysis of randomized controlled trials. Kidney Med. 202;3(5):732-44.
32. Thomas MC, Cherney DZI. The actions of SGLT2 inhibitors on metabolism, renal function and blood pressure. Diabetologia. 2018;61(10):2098-07.
33. Neuen BL, Young T, Heerspink HJL, Neal B, Perkovic V, Billot L, et al. SGLT2 inhibitors for the prevention of kidney failure in patients with type 2 diabetes: a systematic review and meta-analysis. Lancet Diabetes Endocrinol. 2019;7(11):845-54.
34. Zelniker TA, Wiviott SD, Raz I, Im K, Goodrich EL, Bonaca MP, et al. SGLT2 inhibitors for primary and secondary prevention of cardiovascular and renal outcomes in type 2 diabetes: a systematic review and meta-analysis of cardiovascular outcome trials. Lancet. 2019;393(10166):31-9.
35. Kluger AY, Tecson KM, Lee AY, Lerma EV, Rangaswami J, Lepor NE, et al. Class effects of SGLT2 inhibitors on cardiorenal outcomes. Cardiovasc Diabetol. 2019;18(1):99.
36. Täger T, Atar D, Agewall S, Katus HA, Grundtvig M, Cleland JGF, et al. Comparative efficacy of sodium-glucose cotransporter-2 inhibitors (SGLT2i) for cardiovascular outcomes in type 2 diabetes: a systematic review and network meta-analysis of randomised controlled trials. Heart Fail Rev. 2021;26(6):1421-35.
37. Shao SC, Lin YH, Chang KC, Chan YY, Hung MJ, Yang YHK, et al. Sodium glucose co-transporter 2 inhibitors and cardiovascular event protections: how applicable are clinical trials and observational studies to real-world patients? BMJ Open Diabetes Res Care. 2019;7(1):e000742.
38. Handelsman Y. Rationale for the early use of sodium-glucose cotransporter-2 inhibitors in patients with type 2 diabetes. Adv Ther. 2019;36(10):2567-86.
39. Khunti K. SGLT2 inhibitors in people with and without T2DM. Nature Rev Endocrinol. 2021;17(2):75-6.

CHAPTER 19

Damned If You Do, Damned If You Do Not: Corticosteroids in COVID-19

GR Sridhar, G Lakshmi

ABSTRACT

The coronavirus disease 2019 (COVID-19) pandemic struck suddenly with a force that left health systems across the world in despair. While it was identified as a respiratory virus primarily involving the lungs, it became clear that the disease severity and outcomes were due to an abnormal immune response called "cytokine storm." Management directed against the virus by antivirals and specific cytokine blockers was ineffective in altering the outcome of the disease. It was realized that agents were needed to combat the abnormal immune reaction leading to cytokine storm. Among the various choices, corticosteroids were the most easily available and affordable. An early trial showed that use of dexamethasone improved the outcome of admitted subjects with COVID-19 infection. When it was realized that this group of anti-inflammatory agents could alter the outcome of the disease, it quickly became the principal drug in management. The dose to suppress the cytokine overproduction was arrived at by clinical trial and error, learning as one went along the way. It is well known that the use of corticosteroids is associated with adverse metabolic outcomes of which hyperglycemia is most prominent; in addition, hyperglycemia was identified to be a marker for adverse outcomes. The situation was like being stuck between Scylla and Charybdis: Do not administer corticosteroids and run the risk of losing the patient or give corticosteroids and face the problem of hyperglycemia. This made management of hyperglycemia a critical component in COVID-19 treatment.

Keywords: *Immune suppression, Cytokines, Storm, Glucocorticoids, Insulin resistance, Insulin, RECOVERY study.*

INTRODUCTION

Coronavirus disease 2019 (COVID-19) infection due to severe acute respiratory syndrome coronavirus 2 (SARS-CoV-2) virus started as a localized infection and rapidly spread worldwide causing widespread death and destruction. Being a novel infection, there were no immediate pharmacological agents to combat it; management became a process of learning on the job. It soon became evident that the phase of viral infection of cells was not cause of deaths; rather, it was the uncontrolled inflammatory response termed the "cytokine storm," which led to systemic damage. It was realized that the phase of viral infection was usually asymptomatic rendering the role of antiviral agents of limited use. Focus was shifted to extinguishing the inflammatory phase. Of the anti-inflammatory agents, corticosteroid group of agents were the most readily available and widely used. Initiated tentatively, their use became widespread after the publication of the first major study, the RECOVERY (Randomized Evaluation of COVID-19 Therapy) trial in February 2021.[1] While the known adverse effects of corticosteroids are well recognized,[2] in this desperate situation, they were utilized, considering the alternative outcome of near certain death.

Until alternatives to corticosteroids are shown to be effective or their derivatives without significant adverse effects are available, one must use the current group of agents judiciously, while trying to minimize, if possible, and treat, if necessary, the adverse metabolic effects.

BACKGROUND

What began in December 2019 as pneumonia of unknown cause in Wuhan, China was initially linked to the seafood wholesale market. The pathogen causing the pneumonia was identified as a beta-coronavirus, an enveloped ribonucleic acid (RNA) virus that was previously unknown.[3] The virus infection spread rapidly[4] until it was declared a global pandemic. Currently, the World Health Organization (WHO) has recorded 186,411,011 confirmed cases and 4,031,725 confirmed deaths.[5] The Johns Hopkins University of Medicine Coronavirus Resource Center reported 30,874,376 cases and 408,764 deaths in India.[6]

Malhotra et al. published the epidemiological profile and risk factors for SARS-CoV-2 infection from a large testing center located in north India using a retrospective record review method.[7] Between 6 April 2020 and 31 December 2020, among 125,600 participants who underwent reverse transcription-polymerase chain reaction (RT-PCR), the mean age was 33.1 years [standard deviation (SD) = ±15.3)] with 66% being men. COVID-19 positivity was found in 7.6% ($n = 9,515$) with most being asymptomatic. SARS-CoV-2 test positivity was more with increasing age in men, in those with history of international travel, and who were symptomatic.[7]

PATHOGENESIS OF CORONAVIRUS DISEASE 2019

To enter the cell, SARS-CoV-2 binds to the angiotensin-converting enzyme 2 (ACE2), which is expressed in cells of the respiratory tract, vascular endothelium, and macrophages.[8] Additionally, the spike protein of SARS-CoV-2 is primed by protease enzymes such as cellular transmembrane serine protease 2 (TMPRSS2). Viral entry to the cell occurs, if the two are coexpressed.[9] After first invasion of the superficial epithelium of the nasal cavity, the virus multiplies and spreads to other cells.[10]

Viral multiplication in the respiratory passageways leads to viremia and could lead to clinical worsening with the involvement of organs. The stage of COVID-19 storm is caused chiefly by immune-mediated injury that is induced by the virus.[8] The clinical course of infection may be considered as stages of viremia, acute pneumonia, and cytokine storm or recovery. Insights into the pathogenesis provide an opportunity to target interventions[11] with a potential window of opportunity existing between the first and second stages of infection.[8]

CLINICAL COURSE OF CORONAVIRUS DISEASE 2019 INFECTION

The course of COVID-19 can be arbitrarily grouped into phases as alluded to above: Initially, the disease shows mild-to-moderate symptoms similar to that seen in influenza; an asymptomatic phase preceding this consists of viral replication. By the time, patients present with symptoms and viral invasion of cells has already occurred, when antiviral drugs are no longer ineffective. Most individuals recover, while a minority proceeds to the next phase, where radiological changes in the lungs are seen. Even from here, only a minority proceeds to the stage of hyperinflammation and systemic sepsis requiring intensive care; mortality is high among those in the third stage.[12]

THERAPEUTIC INTERVENTIONS IN CORONAVIRUS DISEASE 2019

The virus and the body response can be logically targeted at many levels: Antivirals block viral entry via endosomes and by acting at the level of ACE2 receptor and serine proteases. Remdesivir, lopinavir, and ritonavir block the interaction with helicase, whereas favipiravir interferes with the genomic RNA transcription to mRNA.[12] Convalescent plasma acts at the level of quenching infection or sepsis. Tocilizumab blocks the release of the proinflammatory cytokines such as interleukin-6 (IL-6) and IL-1β.

Glucocorticoids inhibit interferon as well as production of proinflammatory cytokines.[13] They induce the expression of an inhibitor of nuclear factor-kappa B (NF-κB) and of the anti-inflammatory protein mitogen-activated protein (MAP) kinase phosphatase 1. In addition, they prevent recruitment of leukocytes by suppressing the synthesis of acute phase reactants and chemokines. Finally, they prevent the activation, proliferation, and immunoglobulin release by B cells.[13]

CLINICAL RESULTS OF CORONAVIRUS DISEASE 2019 THERAPEUTIC AGENTS

A number of agents were studied against COVID-19 including chloroquine hydroxychloroquine, lopinavir, favipiravir, ribavirin, remdesivir, and tocilizumab. None of them was shown to substantially improve the clinical outcomes, which makes the search for effective drugs a work in progress.[14] Cell-based therapies including stem cell therapy are being explored, but have not yet come into common clinical use.[15] Neutralizing monoclonal antibody may be considered on an outpatient basis early in the course particularly in those with are at high risk of progressive disease; convalescent plasma was used in high-risk patients early in the course of the disease.[16,17] Since the initial phase of infection is often asymptomatic antiviral medications and antibody-based methods have limited utility.

In the later stages when hyperinflammation and coagulopathy are the chief pathogenic factors, anti-inflammatory agents, immunomodulators, and anticoagulants, given alone or together, are the agents of choice.[17]

CORTICOSTEROIDS IN CORONAVIRUS DISEASE 2019

Considering the pivotal role of corticosteroids in the management of COVID-19, it may come as a surprise that indications for their use in previous critical settings such as septic shock or acute respiratory distress syndrome (ARDS) were inconclusive.[18] Not just their efficacy, but concerns about adverse reactions such as secondary infection and delirium held them back from widespread use.

Even in COVID-19 in the initial weeks, recommendations for use of corticosteroids were mixed in the absence of formal evidence; frontline workers, however, used them in critical conditions, citing their favorable outcomes in their experience.[19] While their use in COVID-19 had a rationale, evidence from randomized controlled trials was not available until the RECOVERY study published first as a preprint[20] and later in the New England Journal of Medicine in 2021.[1] The RECOVERY study was a controlled open-label trial to compare a range of treatments in subjects hospitalized with COVID-19. Patients were randomly assigned to dexamethasone given orally or intravenously in a dose of 6 mg once a day for up to 10 days. Comparator group consisted of those who received "usual care" without dexamethasone.[1] Dexamethasone group consisted of 2,104 patients and usual care consisted of 4,321 patients. Among the dexamethasone group, 482 patients (22.9%) died within 28 days of randomization in the usual care, 1,110 patients (25.7%) died within 28 days of randomization. When dexamethasone was given, mortality was lower than usual care in those who were receiving oxygen along or invasive mechanical ventilation. This was epochal in the management of critical COVID-19 infections with a commentary published in the Nature journal.[21]

This led to a change in the recommendations for corticosteroid use in COVID-19 including by the WHO.[22] However, based on the available evidence from RECOVERY study, the use was restricted to dexamethasone 6 mg only for critically ill patients.

Results of a retrospective analysis from Spain showed that when glucocorticoids were given in SARS-CoV-2 pneumonia, survival was higher than in controls.[23] A study by Han et al. reported that corticosteroids reduce the release of inflammatory mediators in patients with comorbid conditions and SARS-CoV-2 and may have a beneficial effect on outcomes.[24] The issue of delayed viral clearance by corticosteroids was addressed by Fu et al. who showed in mild cases of COVID-19, when given in low doses, corticosteroids do not affect the final clearance of viral nucleic acid nor do they lead to adverse clinical outcomes.[25] The issue of viral clearance, however, is still under debate,[26] although there is evidence for corticosteroids not adversely affecting clearance.[27,28]

PLACE OF CORTICOSTEROID THERAPY IN CORONAVIRUS DISEASE 2019

To provide context to treatment options, network meta-analysis and living systemic review methods are being utilized. Unlike traditional reviews, which are limited to a specific time, living network meta-analysis allows a "complete, updated, and broad view of evidence".[29] Thereby, it provides knowledge about different treatments that have not been compared in head-to-head trials. Siemieniuk et al. analyzing 196 trials where 76,767 patients were enrolled, concluded that compared with standard care, corticosteroids reduce death, mechanical ventilation, and increase the number of days free from mechanical ventilation.[29]

The second edition of a living systematic review with meta-analyses and trial sequential analyses (the LIVING Project) published in 2021 reported that corticosteroids might reduce the risk of death, serious adverse events, and mechanical ventilation, but cautioned that the quality of evidence is of "very low certainty".[30]

When and in what dose must corticosteroids be started?

While results from the RECOVERY trial led to the widespread use of corticosteroids in COVID-19, the indications were circumscribed by the narrow parameters used in the trial, viz., inpatients admitted in intensive care unit (ICU) requiring assisted respiratory support.[22] An understanding of the pathogenesis of COVID-19 course reveals that inflammatory markers presage the progress to cytokine storm, which requires admission and critical care. Logically, corticosteroids in the earlier stages could prevent the progression to the late critical stages. Recent studies have indicated that immune interventions can be chosen based on the disease presentation and trajectory.[31] Although there are no documented studies to prove or disprove this approach, clinical evidence suggests that it may be the logical approach, considering the lack of established markers for progress, and the lack of access to such investigations in much of the world where COVID-19 is prevalent.[32] (Suresh Anne 2021, personal communication).

DYSGLYCEMIA WITH CORTICOSTEROID USE IN SURGICAL STRESS

Studies in postoperative patients showed that dexamethasone increases plasma glucose level in nondiabetic individuals and even more so among individuals with diabetes.[33] In an international study assessing the effect of dexamethasone on surgical site infection, 8,725 participants were included in the modified intention-to-treat population, 4,372 participants were in the dexamethasone group and 4,353 participants were in the placebo group, and 13.2% (576 participants in the dexamethasone group and 572 participants in the placebo group) had diabetes mellitus. Hyperglycemic events were low, although they were higher in those without diabetes in the dexamethasone group (22 of 3,787; 0.6%) compared to the control group (6 of 3,776; 0.2%).[34] There was no significant difference in wound site infection between the two. Clinical studies in healthy individuals showed that glucocorticoids might elevate fasting plasma glucose, worsen insulin resistance assessed by homeostatic model assessment (HOMA), and could contribute to insulin resistance.[35]

Dysglycemia is an acknowledged adverse effect of corticosteroid use. Yet, considering the limited efficacy of available agents in treatment,[36] they form the bulwark of drugs for managing COVID-19 infection.

DIABETES AND CORONAVIRUS DISEASE 2019

Comorbid conditions such as obesity, diabetes, and coronary artery disease in the elderly were associated with susceptibility to COVID-19 infection and with adverse clinical outcomes.[37,38] Specifically, older age, male gender, preexisting diabetes, and hypertension were risk factors for severe infection and death.[39] In a population study of persons with diabetes from Scotland, risks of fatal or critical unit-treated COVID-19 were higher compared to background population.[40]

The CORONADO (Coronavirus SARS-CoV-2 and Diabetes Outcomes) is a nationwide multicenter observational study conducted in France, where 1,317 participants with diabetes and confirmed COVID-19 were admitted to 53 French hospitals between 10th and 31st March, 2020. While there was no association between elevated glycated hemoglobin (HbA1c) and the primary outcome or death on day 7, it was observed that body mass index was positively and independently associated with the primary outcomes.[41]

Updated results from the nationwide CORONADO study showed that clinical factors associated with poorer outcomes include history of microvascular disease, use of anticoagulants, and dyspnea at admission.[42]

A modeling study on the mortality from COVID-19 in India showed that compared to England, mortality is increased by uncontrolled diabetes and reduced by obesity.[43] The difference was attributed to the difference in population structure between the two nations.

In a recent literature synthesis, it was reported that in a longitudinal study of >6,000 persons, need for hospitalization due to COVID-19 infection was more common in those with diabetes mellitus.[44]

Additionally, the pandemic resulted in social disruption leading to poor identification and management of diabetes.[44]

Diabetes is associated with comorbidities, which could also adversely impact the course of COVID-19 infection.[45] Obesity, associated with diabetes, causes immune dysfunction, an increase of proinflammatory cytokines, and overactivation of complement storm. In addition, it is associated with disturbances in lung mechanics and physiology.[45]

A study from Mexico showed that diabetes and obesity can be modeled to give prognostic information about the outcomes of COVID-19 infection.[46] It is simple to use, although further studies across different ethnic population groups are necessary before it comes into wider clinical use.[47]

In addition, built environment of cities and living spaces contribute to the spread of COVID-19 and other respiratory virus infections.[48] It also contributes to the quality of life and adjustment to living with physical restrictions that are accompaniments of quelling the spread of COVID-19 infection.[49]

MANAGEMENT OF DIABETES IN CORONAVIRUS DISEASE 2019

It is evident that hyperglycemia may be precipitated or unmasked by the infection itself apart from the use of corticosteroids employed in the management.[50] Diabetes is associated with poorer outcomes, while being difficult to manage, especially with high doses of glucocorticoids. COVID-19 being a new condition, evidence-based therapy has been a work in progress, even for glucocorticoid-induced hyperglycemia. A review of managing diabetes in hospitalized patients without reference to COVID suggested that use of chronic high-dose corticosteroids is associated with hyperglycemia in the afternoon and evening for which multiple dose insulin was advised. In those without known diabetes, a single morning dose of intermediate-acting insulin is effective.[51]

Early in the course of pandemic, practical recommendations for managing diabetes in subjects with COVID-19 were published by a group of clinicians.[52] The management recommendations consisted in preventing COVID-19 infections in subjects with diabetes and to monitor inpatients for hyperglycemia and management when it is identified. The recommended aims in outpatient subjects were a plasma glucose concentration between 72 and 144 mg/dL and an HbA1c of 7%. Inpatient target plasma glucose levels were between 72 and 180 mg/dL.[52]

On the choice of specific agents, one must carefully monitor renal function with metformin and with sodium-glucose cotransporter-2 (SGLT-2) inhibitors; the institution of the latter is best avoided in the phase of respiratory illness. Adequate fluid intake should be especially ensured with glucagon-like peptide-1 (GLP-1) receptor agonists. Dipeptidyl peptidase-4 (DPP-4) inhibitors are safe and can be continued. Insulin must not be stopped; its dose is adjusted by careful monitoring.[52]

In view of patients with COVID-19 and diabetes being at greater risk for severe infections, poorer prognosis, and higher mortality, glycemic control should be aggressive, often employing insulin. One must decide on insulin use depending on the severity of infection; intense monitoring of glycemic excursions is a critical part of insulin therapy.[53]

The Concise Advice on Inpatient Diabetes (COVID:Diabetes) guidelines given by Diabetes UK on managing dexamethasone-induced hyperglycemia was recently published in Diabetic Medicine.[54] The salient recommendations include the initiation of rapid-acting analog insulin when capillary blood glucose exceeds 216 mg/dL. The dose of insulin is calculated based on the weight of the patient. Higher doses are usually recommended because of associated insulin resistance in COVID-19. For maintenance, neutral protamine Hagedorn (NPH) insulin, rather than long-acting insulin analogs, is recommended because of greater flexibility in adjusting the dose. After the acute phase, those with steroid-induced hyperglycemia must undergo a yearly assessment of HbA1c.[54]

INDIAN GUIDELINES

The Endocrine Society of India has published a position statement on the diagnosis and management of steroid-related hyperglycemia in COVID-19.[55] *Four classes* have been recognized: (1) COVID-19-induced diabetes, (2) Preexisting diabetes, (3) COVID-19 treatment-related hyperglycemia, and (4) Stress hyperglycemia. Steroids induce postprandial elevation of plasma glucose and reliance on fasting samples may underestimate the prevalence of hyperglycemia. Among the risk factors, dose of corticosteroids and duration are important; others include elderly age, central obesity, and family history of diabetes.

Insulin is the recommended drug of choice for hyperglycemia in hospitalized patients with COVID-19. Indications include premeal glucose level of >180 mg/dL and postmeal glucose level of >250 mg/dL.[55] Other indications are hyperglycemic emergencies and irregular intake of food.

Insulin infusion is recommended in emergencies (e.g., diabetic ketoacidosis), sepsis, severely ill, failure of basal-bolus insulin regimen, and irregular food intake.

Insulin infusion can be initiated at a dose of 0.05–0.1 units/kg/h with regular plasma glucose monitoring. Expected fall of capillary blood glucose is 50–70 mg/dL hourly. If it lies outside the range, the infusion rate must be appropriately stepped up or down. Hypokalemia is a recognized accompaniment of both COVID-19 infection and insulin therapy, which must be identified and corrected.

Once glycemia is stable, the frequency of capillary glucose monitoring can be extended from 1 to 2 hours to every 4 hours.

Less emergent situations in hospital can be managed with basal insulin regimens. A single dose of NPH insulin (0.27 units/kg) can be given in the morning along with the morning dose of oral prednisolone based on evidence from non-COVID-19 inpatients.[56]

At discharge, patients and their attendants must be educated about tapering of steroid dose, monitoring of glucose levels, measures to control, if they rise, and to present for medical attention, if required. In addition, one must identify and manage other potential adverse effects with corticosteroid use such as adrenal suppression, hypertension, gastritis, and, rarely, mucormycosis infection.

CONCLUSION

Coronavirus disease 2019 gave no time for considered and proper evidence-based treatment. Since most adverse outcomes resulting from unbridled inflammatory response leading to cytokine storm, immunosuppressants were identified to alter the course of the disease. Corticosteroids were the widely available and used agents that made a difference in the outcome. The RECOVERY study placed dexamethasone in a fixed dose and duration as a treatment standard. Depending on the clinical condition and pathogenesis of the disease, the use of corticosteroids has been expanded with the possibility of potential adverse metabolic actions. Hyperglycemia is the most significant result of both corticosteroid use and of COVID-19 infection itself. It is also a harbinger of poorer outcomes, if left uncontrolled, which must be identified and treated assiduously. Being commonly used in hospital and ICU settings, insulin is the drug of choice to manage hyperglycemia, although recent evidence questions its role in the ultimate outcome.[57] Despite its potential drawbacks, metformin has been suggested to have a favorable effect in COVID-19.[58] It must be recognized that the course and management of COVID-19 are evolving and evidence-based protocols are being developed. Yet, for now, based on the knowledge of pathogenesis and clinical experience, the effective drugs such as corticosteroids must be judiciously used until better options are available.

REFERENCES

1. RECOVERY Collaborative Group, Horby P, Lim WS, Emberson JR, Mafham M, Bell JL, et al. Dexamethasone in Hospitalized Patients with Covid-19. N Engl J Med. 2021;384:693-704.
2. Rhen T, Cidlowski JA. Anti-inflammatory action of glucocorticoids—new mechanisms for old drugs. N Engl J Med. 2005;353:1711-23.
3. Zhu N, Zhang D, Wang W, Li X, Yang B, Song J, et al. A Novel Coronavirus from Patients with Pneumonia in China, 2019. N Engl J Med. 2020;382:727-33.
4. Wang D, Hu B, Hu C, Zhu F, Liu X, Zhang J, et al. Clinical Characteristics of 138 Hospitalized Patients With 2019 Novel Coronavirus-Infected Pneumonia in Wuhan, China. JAMA. 2020;323:1061-9.
5. World Health Organization (WHO). (2021). Coronavirus disease (COVID-19) pandemic. [online] Available from https://www.who.int/emergencies/diseases/novel-coronavirus-2019. [Last accessed on August, 2021].
6. John Hopkins University and Medicine. (2021). Coronavirus resource center. [online] Available from https://coronavirus.jhu.edu/map.html. [Last accessed on August, 2021].
7. Malhotra S, Rahi M, Das P, Chaturvedi R, Chhibber-Goel J, Anvikar A, et al. Epidemiological profiles and associated risk factors of SARS-CoV-2 positive patients based on a high-throughput testing facility in India. Open Biol. 2021;11:200288.
8. Cao W, Li T. COVID-19: towards understanding of pathogenesis. Cell Res. 2020;30:367-9.
9. Gupta A, Madhavan MV, Sehgal K, Nair N, Mahajan S, Sehrawat TS, et al. Extrapulmonary manifestations of COVID-19. Nat Med. 2020;26:1017-32.
10. Osuchowski MF, Winkler MS, Skirecki T, Cajander S, Shankar-Hari M, Lachmann G, et al. The COVID 19 puzzle: deciphering pathophysiology and phenotypes of a new disease entity. Lancet Respir Med. 2021;9:622-42.
11. Domingo P, Mur I, Pomar V, Corominas H, Casademont J, de Benito N. The four horsemen of a viral Apocalypse: The pathogenesis of SARS-CoV-2 infection (COVID-19). EBioMedicine. 2020;58:102887.
12. Santos WGD. Natural history of COVID-19 and current knowledge on treatment therapeutic options. Biomed Pharmacother. 2020;129:110493.
13. Annane D. Corticosteroids for COVID-19. J Intensive Med. 2021;1:14-25.
14. Giovane RA, Rezai S, Cleland E, Henderson CE. Current pharmacological modalities for management of novel coronavirus disease 2019 (COVID-19) and the rationale for their utilization: a review. Rev Med Virol. 2020;30:e2136.
15. Mirtaleb MS, Mirtaleb AH, Nosrati H, Heshmatnia J, Falak R, Emameh RZ. Potential therapeutic agents to COVID-19: An update review on antiviral therapy, immunotherapy, and cell therapy. Biomed Pharmacother. 2021;138:111518.
16. Shang L, Lye DC, Cao B. Contemporary narrative review of treatment options for COVID-19. Respirology. 2021;26:745-67.
17. Gandhi RT, Lynch JB, Del Rio C. Mild or moderate COVID-19. N Engl J Med. 2020;383:1757-66.
18. Prescott HC, Rice TW. Corticosteroids in COVID-19 ARDS: Evidence and Hope during the Pandemic. JAMA. 2020;324:1292-5.
19. Yang R, Yu Y. Glucocorticoids are double-edged sword in the treatment of COVID-19 and cancers. Int J Biol Sci. 2021;17:1530-7.
20. Horby P, Lim WS, Emberson J, Mafham M, Bell J, Linsell L, et al. Effect of Dexamethasone in Hospitalized Patients with COVID-19—Preliminary Report. medRxiv. 2020.
21. Ledford H. Coronavirus breakthrough: dexamethasone is first drug shown to save lives. Nature. 2020;582:469.
22. World Health Organization (WHO). (2020). Corticosteroids for COVID-19: Living Guidance. [online] Available from https://www.who.int/publications-detail-redirect/WHO-2019-nCoV-Corticosteroids-2020.1. [Last accessed on August, 2021].
23. Fernández-Cruz A, Ruiz-Antorán B, Muñoz-Gómez A, Sancho-López A, Mills-Sánchez P, Centeno-Soto GA, et al. A Retrospective Controlled Cohort Study of the Impact of Glucocorticoid Treatment in SARS-CoV-2 Infection Mortality. Antimicrob Agents Chemother. 2020;64:e01168-20.

24. Han D, Peng C, Meng R, Yao J, Zhou Q, Xiao Y, et al. Estimating the release of inflammatory factors and use of glucocorticoid therapy for COVID-19 patients with comorbidities. Aging (Albany NY). 2020;12:22413-24.
25. Fu HY, Luo Y, Gao JP, Wang L, Li HJ, Li X, et al. Effects of Short-Term Low-Dose Glucocorticoids for Patients with Mild COVID-19. Biomed Res Int. 2020;2020:2854186.
26. Liu J, Zhang S, Dong X, Li Z, Xu Q, Feng H, et al. Corticosteroid treatment in severe COVID-19 patients with acute respiratory distress syndrome. J Clin Invest. 2020;130:6417-28.
27. Ji J, Zhang J, Shao Z, Xie Q, Zhong L, Liu Z. Glucocorticoid therapy does not delay viral clearance in COVID-19 patients. Crit Care. 2020;24:565.
28. Almas T, Ehtesham M, Khan AW, Khedro T, Hussain S, Kaneez M, et al. Safety and Efficacy of Low-Dose Corticosteroids in Patients With Non-severe Coronavirus Disease 2019: A Retrospective Cohort Study. Cureus. 2021;13:e12544.
29. Siemieniuk RA, Bartoszko JJ, Ge L, Zeraatkar D, Izcovich A, Kum E, et al. Drug treatments for covid-19: living systematic review and network meta-analysis. BMJ. 2020;370:m2980.
30. Juul S, Nielsen EE, Feinberg J, Siddiqui F, Jørgensen CK, Barot E, et al. Interventions for treatment of COVID-19: A living systematic review with meta-analyses and trial sequential analyses (The LIVING Project). PLoS One. 2021;16:e0248132.
31. Bolouri H, Speake C, Skibinski D, Long SA, Hocking AM, Campbell DJ, et al. The COVID-19 immune landscape is dynamically and reversibly correlated with disease severity. J Clin Invest. 2021;131:e143648.
32. Matthay MA, Wick KD. Corticosteroids, COVID-19 pneumonia, and acute respiratory distress syndrome. J Clin Invest. 2020;130:6218-21.
33. Polderman JA, Farhang-Razi V, Dieren SV, Kranke P, DeVries JH, Hollmann MW, et al. Adverse side effects of dexamethasone in surgical patients. Cochrane Database Syst Rev. 2018;11:CD011940.
34. Corcoran TB, Myles PS, Forbes AB, Cheng AC, Bach LA, O'Loughlin E, et al. Dexamethasone and Surgical-Site Infection. N Engl J Med. 2021;384:1731-41.
35. Zhou PZ, Zhu YM, Zou GH, Sun YX, Xiu XL, Huang X, et al. Relationship Between Glucocorticoids and Insulin Resistance in Healthy Individuals. Med Sci Monit. 2016;22:1887-94.
`36. Malhotra V, Basu S, Sharma N, Kumar S, Garg S, Dushyant K, et al. Outcomes among 10,314 hospitalized COVID-19 patients at a tertiary care government hospital in Delhi, India. J Med Virol. 2021;93:4553-8.
37. Chen N, Zhou M, Dong X, Qu J, Gong F, Han Y, et al. Epidemiological and clinical characteristics of 99 cases of 2019 novel coronavirus pneumonia in Wuhan, China: a descriptive study. Lancet. 2020;395:507-13.
38. Chen R, Liang W, Jiang M, Guan W, Zhan C, Wang T, et al. Risk Factors of Fatal Outcome in Hospitalized Subjects With Coronavirus Disease 2019 From a Nationwide Analysis in China. Chest. 2020;158:97-105.
39. Wolff D, Nee S, Hickey NS, Marschollek M. Risk factors for Covid-19 severity and fatality: a structured literature review. Infection. 2021;49:15-28.
40. McGurnaghan SJ, Weir A, Bishop J, Kennedy S, Blackbourn LAK, McAllister DA, et al. Risks of and risk factors for COVID-19 disease in people with diabetes: a cohort study of the total population of Scotland. Lancet Diabetes Endocrinol. 2021;9:82-93.
41. Cariou B, Hadjadj S, Wargny M, Pichelin M, Al-Salameh A, Allix I, et al. Phenotypic characteristics and prognosis of inpatients with COVID-19 and diabetes: the CORONADO study. Diabetologia. 2020;63:1500-15.
42. Wargny M, Potier L, Gourdy P, Pichelin M, Amadou C, Benhamou PY, et al. Predictors of hospital discharge and mortality in patients with diabetes and COVID-19: updated results from the nationwide CORONADO study. Diabetologia. 2021;64:778-94.
43. Novosad P, Jain R, Campion A, Asher S. COVID-19 mortality effects of underlying health conditions in India: a modelling study. BMJ Open. 2020;10:e043165.
44. Gregg EW, Sophiea MK, Weldegiorgis M. Diabetes and COVID-19: Population Impact 18 Months Into the Pandemic. Diabetes Care. 2021;44:1916-23.
45. Zhou Y, Chi J, Lv W, Wang Y. Obesity and diabetes as high-risk factors for severe coronavirus disease 2019 (Covid-19). Diabetes Metab Res Rev. 2021;37:e3377.

46. Bello-Chavolla OY, Bahena-López JP, Antonio-Villa NE, Vargas-Vázquez A, González-Díaz A, Márquez-Salinas A, et al. Predicting Mortality Due to SARS-CoV-2: A Mechanistic Score Relating Obesity and Diabetes to COVID-19 Outcomes in Mexico. J Clin Endocrinol Metab. 2020;105:dgaa346.
47. Muniyappa R, Wilkins KJ. Diabetes, Obesity, and Risk Prediction of Severe COVID-19. J Clin Endocrinol Metab. 2020;105:dgaa442.
48. Lai KY, Webster C, Kumari S, Sarkar C. The nature of cities and the Covid-19 pandemic. Curr Opin Environ Sustain. 2020;46:27-31.
49. Pasala SK, Gumpeny L, Kosuri M, Tippana S, Sridhar GR. Effect of lockdown on activities of daily living in the built environment and wellbeing. UCL Open Environ. 2021;2:5.
50. Montefusco L, Nasr MB, D'Addio F, Loretelli C, Rossi A, Pastore I, et al. Acute and long-term disruption of glycometabolic control after SARS-CoV-2 infection. Nat Metab. 2021;3:774-85.
51. Pasquel FJ, Lansang MC, Dhatariya K, Umpierrez GE. Management of diabetes and hyperglycaemia in the hospital. Lancet Diabetes Endocrinol. 2021;9:174-88.
52. Bornstein SR, Rubino F, Khunti K, Mingrone G, Hopkins D, Birkenfeld AL, et al. Practical recommendations for the management of diabetes in patients with COVID-19. Lancet Diabetes Endocrinol. 2020;8:546-50.
53. Jin S, Hu W. Severity of COVID-19 and Treatment Strategy for Patient With Diabetes. Front Endocrinol (Lausanne). 2021;12:602735.
54. Rayman G, Lumb AN, Kennon B, Cottrell C, Nagi D, Page E, et al. Dexamethasone therapy in COVID-19 patients: implications and guidance for the management of blood glucose in people with and without diabetes. Diabet Med. 2021;38:e14378.
55. Das S, Rastogi A, Harikumar KVS, Dutta D, Sahay R, Kalra S, et al. Diagnosis and Management Considerations in Steroid-Related Hyperglycemia in COVID-19: A Position Statement from the Endocrine Society of India. Indian J Endocrinol Metab. 2021;25:4-11.
56. Grommesh B, Lausch MJ, Vannelli AJ, Mullen DM, Bergenstal RM, Richter SA, et al. Hospital insulin protocol aims for glucose control in glucocorticoid-induced hyperglycemia. Endocr Pract. 2016;22:180-9.
57. Yang Y, Cai Z, Zhang J. Insulin Treatment May Increase Adverse Outcomes in Patients With COVID-19 and Diabetes: A Systematic Review and Meta-Analysis. Front Endocrinol (Lausanne). 2021;12:696087.
58. Ibrahim S, Lowe JR, Bramante CT, Shah S, Klatt NR, Sherwood N, et al. Metformin and Covid-19: Focused Review of Mechanisms and Current Literature Suggesting Benefit. Front Endocrinol (Lausanne). 2021;12:587801.

CHAPTER 20

Exercise-mimetic Medicines: Could They be a Reality?

GR Sridhar

ABSTRACT

There is ample evidence for the health benefits of physical activity; this is only matched by the lack of physical exercise in most populations. Since changing people's lifestyle behavior is proving to be cumbersome, efforts are made if chemical analogs of chemicals produced by skeletal muscle in response to exercise to bypass the necessity of exercising. A number of proteins and metabolites have been identified; some were used in early clinical trials, but they suffered from adverse effects and poor responses. It is possible that advances could overcome the problems that have been encountered. However, one must bear in mind that there is intense complexity in the number and interactions of released compounds; in addition, exercise has benefits unrelated to skeletal muscle secretory products. Yet, the concept of exercise-mimetic chemicals is beguiling and may find niche use, although they may not be a panacea of all ills.

Keywords: *Acute exercise, Cognition, Complexity, Exercise factors, Mitochondria, Myokines.*

INTRODUCTION

Physical exercise for health is a relatively recent construct. Earlier, activity was an integral part of living for survival. Over millennia energy as food is available without having to go foraging for it as in the past. It must be realized that this concept has been romanticized with little evidence that hunter-gatherer people were constantly in action to find food, interspersed by periods of fasting while in search of their next meal. Without good evidence, it is difficult to confirm or refute the hypothesis.

Studies on the now dwindling hunter-gatherer populations have provided interesting information, although the lifestyle of "hunter-gatherers" is no longer as isolated as it was in the past; yet they offer insights. Recently, Pontzer,

Wood, and Raichlen reviewed the lifestyle and health status of hunter-gatherer communities.[1] Hadza adults accumulate around 135 minutes of moderate-to-vigorous physical activity per day, which is maintained across the life span.[2] This was associated with good cardiovascular health, which supports the evolutionary model of physical activity and cardiovascular fitness with healthy diet habits contributing. Interestingly their daily energy expenditure was comparable to that of persons from the industrialized world.[1]

Why and how did the notion of lack of adequate physical exercise arise? The reasons are many, not all related to health and well-being. There are interesting traits related to social mores and to the concept of nationalism.[3,4]

CURRENT RECOMMENDATIONS OF PHYSICAL ACTIVITY FOR HEALTH

Despite these caveats, there has been a rise in lifestyle diseases accompanied by a rise of unhealthy food habits and lower levels of physical activity. National and global bodies have provided guidelines for physical exercise to promote health and prevent disease. Over the past >40 years, exercise guidelines have evolved from focusing on exercise, performance, and cardiac rehabilitation; from healthy adults and those with cardiovascular diseases to those with other chronic diseases and disability. The kind of exercises also shifted from aerobic to add muscle strengthening and balance. Similarly, guidelines about the intensity, frequency, duration, and volume were modified based on accumulating evidence.[5]

The World Health Organization guidelines for physical activity cover the age range 5 years and above.[6] For children 5–17 years of age, the recommendation for moderate-to-various intensity aerobic exercise across the week is at least an average 60 minutes every day. Muscle and bone strengthening exercises must be incorporated at least thrice a week. Adults between the ages of 18 and 64 years, including those with chronic conditions, are recommended to do regular physical activity: The duration is at least 150–300 minutes of vigorous aerobic activity throughout the week; and muscle-strengthening exercises involving all major muscle groups at least twice a week. Performing additional activity increases the benefits of exercise. For the elderly, aged 65 years and above, multicomponent physical activities are recommended; they must include physical balance and strength training for 3 or more days a week.

In addition, adults should minimize time spent in sitting, which can be offset by doing more than the recommended levels of physical activity.

ARE THESE BEING PUT IN PRACTICE?

Despite the availability of evidence that physical exercise has unequivocal health benefits, few people actually follow the advice. Nearly 20 years ago, we reported that just about one half of men and a far lower proportion of women with diabetes did regular physical exercise.[7] Exercise involves not just the desire and ability, but depends on a number of other social and family factors, that are more often a deterrent to going out for physical exercise.[8]

A recent study from Jamaica showed an equally disheartening pattern. Among subjects with diabetes, just about a third (38.7%) were "low active," another third (33.5%) moderately active, and a quarter (26%) were highly active.[9] The common barriers attributed were perceiving exercise as "hard work" causing tiredness and fatigue, particularly among the older age-group. Evidently, more needs to be done to break the barriers.

To decipher the barriers, Nagaraju et al. evaluated the stages of physical activity behavior change by a transtheoretical model approach.[10] To the stages of precontemplation, contemplation, preparation, action, and maintenance; a sixth phase was added, viz. reversal, when there can be a reversion to an earlier phase. When this model was applied to a cohort of 150 subjects, many were in the precontemplation (29%) and reversal phase (20%), with only 23% in the maintenance phase.

IS EXERCISE TRULY BENEFICIAL?

Given the many obstacles and the difficulties in overcoming them, the question arises whether exercise is truly beneficial. From an evolutionary perspective, genes were wired to hunter-gather lifestyle. Exercise selected the genome to optimize aerobic metabolism, conserve energy in food scarce times. What is the evidence for beneficial effects of exercise?

Epidemiological evidence shows that exercise is protective against cardiovascular risk factors. Athletes, who have high physical activity levels, live longer than nonathletic counterparts.[11] Exercise improves endothelial function as a protector against cardiovascular disease. It has been proven to lower glycosylated hemoglobin, a measure of average glycemic levels. Similarly, serum triglycerides and blood pressure are also lowered. Exercise has been called the "real polypill."[11]

Considering the unequivocal health benefits of physical exercise, and the roadblocks in inducing people to exercise, is there another way of offering the benefits without really doing physical exercise? To try to mimic the effects of exercise, the physiological and biochemical mediators of physical activity in the muscles, which are the main tissues involved in exercise, were studied. The aim was to develop chemical agents to mimic their effects without actually doing exercise.

THE CONCEPT OF EXERCISE MIMETICS

In response to exercise, adaptive changes occur in muscles; increased muscle oxidative capacity, mitochondrial density, and insulin sensitivity. Myokines must be differentiated from exercise factors. Myokines are proteins secreted by muscles which play a signaling role in an autocrine, paracrine, and endocrine manner. Exercise factors are produced by skeletal muscle in response to exercise and are released into the circulation; the latter consists of both proteins and metabolites.[12] There are overlaps between the two, but they cannot be used interchangeably. Over 100 myokines have been identified, but not all in humans.

Acute exercise releases interleukin 6 (IL-6), C–C motif chemokine ligand-2 (CCL-2), and chemokine (C-X3-C motif) ligand 1 (CX3CL1). Secreted protein acidic, rich in cysteine (SPARC) is released following both acute exercise and exercise training as shown by microarray studies carried out in mice. On the other hand, exercise training results in the release of myostatin, which results in muscle hypertrophy. Possible exercise factors are irisin, IL-8, and IL-15, whereas autocrine and paracrine factors include fibroblast growth factor 21 (FGF21), brain-derived neurotrophic factor (BDNF), and apelin.[12]

While a number of myokines have been identified, there is limited information about their function. Most of them appear to have principally local actions. The only well-established myokine is IL-6, while there are other promising exercise factors, "viz." SPARC, CCL-2, CX3CL1, and angiopoietin like 4 (ANGPTL4).

Effects in different exercise states are represented by the following evidence.[12] Acutely, IL-6 improves insulin sensitivity in skeletal muscle; chronically it reduces hepatic and adipocyte insulin sensitivity. CCL-2 acutely leads to local metabolic adaptation and repair and hypertrophy of skeletal muscle. Chronically it promotes insulin resistance and is important for the chronic low-grade adipose tissue inflammation. ANGPTL1 directs fatty acids bound with triglycerides to skeletal muscles which are active, away from inactive skeletal muscles. CX3CL1 is associated with β-cell dysfunction and type 2 diabetes mellitus (T2DM). SPARC improves glucose metabolism. Irisin improves glucose hemostasis and increases energy expenditure in adipose tissue.

WHAT ARE EXERCISE MIMETICS?

Exercise mimetics are defined as pharmacological agents that can produce the benefits of fitness such as mitochondrial remodeling effects, comprising increased mitochondrial oxidative phosphorylation and fatty acid metabolism.[13] Prototype exercise mimetics include GW501516 and AICAR. AICAR lowers blood glucose levels, reduces inflammation, and increases endurance. Adenosine monophosphate-activated protein kinase (AMPK) activators act as metabolic sensors that directly respond to exercise-induced energetic stress. Cpd14 is a synthetic small molecule; R419 activates AMPK more potently than metformin.

PPARδ ligands promise to have a role as exercise mimetic. GW501516, a synthetic PPARδ ligand when co-administered AICAR, can boost mitochondrial biogenesis and oxidative metabolism. Its use however is not legal, although safer agents can be developed.

Resveratrol is an SIRT1 activator which has exercise-mimicking effects in muscle. It activates muscle SIRT1 to increase PGC1a activity leading to triple action of ERRa, ERRd, and PPARd. Together there is induction of genes controlling mitochondrial biogenesis, fatty acid transport, and oxidative metabolism. It has weak exercise-mimicking benefits.

REV-ERBa ligands such as SR9009 and SR9011 are synthetic ligands of REV-ERBα. Acting at nuclear receptors, they affect circadian rhythm and energy metabolism, by selectively acting in the skeletal muscle. ERRγ is a target for exercise mimetics, which directly regulate mitochondrial oxidative genes.

Currently, exercise-mimetic chemicals have been tested only in animal models, which showed severe side effects. They act mainly by inhibiting mitochondrial adenosine triphosphate (ATP) production. Aside from other side effects, the risk of lactic acidosis is a major problem. AMPK activators cause cardiac and gastrointestinal (GI) disturbances. New-generation agents can overcome these limitations.

In addition, the potential for misuse exists. GW501516 and AICAR which were widely used by endurance athletes for improved performances have been listed under the category of banned agents by World Anti-Doping Agency.[13]

COMPLEXITY INVOLVED IN OUTCOMES OF EXERCISE

To identify the signaling molecules of human muscle following acute exercise, Hoffman et al. performed an integrated AMPK substrate prediction in human muscle and cells, with targeted validation of exercise-regulated AMPK substrates.[14] Since exercise is essential in regulating energy metabolism and whole-body insulin sensitivity, a global analysis of protein phosphorylation in human skeletal muscle biopsies was performed from untrained healthy males before and after a single high-intensity exercise bout. The aim was to explore the exercise signaling network. Altogether 1,004 unique exercise-regulated phosphosites on 562 proteins were identified.[14] This underscores the unexplored complexity of acute exercise signaling and reveals how exercise factors must be integrated to identify exercise mimetic agents.

IS EXERCISE ALL ABOUT MYOKINES AND EXERCISE FACTORS?

The beneficial outcomes of physical exercise are a composite of many effects and not just of biochemical products. Exercise has beneficial effects on the musculoskeletal and cardiorespiratory systems, in addition to body composition and metabolism. It also has positive effects on cognition and on psychological well-being.[15]

The health benefits of physical exercise comprise the following:

- Reduced abdominal obesity and help in weight control
- Increased coronary arterial blood flow and cardiorespiratory function
- Lowering the level of triglycerides, low-density lipoprotein (LDL) cholesterol, blood pressure, increasing high-density lipoprotein (HDL) cholesterol level; improvement of endothelial function, leading to improved glucose homeostasis and insulin sensitivity
- Improved psychological well-being, increased expression of neurotropic factors, improved memory, cognition and sleep, while reducing anxiety and depression[15]

It is evident that signaling pathways that mediate the diverse effects are not limited to a set of chemicals.

Therefore, no single agent can be expected to mimic the entire range of exercise-related benefits, it may be possible to target particular aspects of the exercise response.[16] This includes identifying the molecules that are altered with exercise, dubbed as "exercise responsome" to understand the many layers of control which can be simulated by pharmacological agents.[17] The degree of complexity is immense, involving the central nervous system, different body organs, down to the cellular and subcellular level. These are in turn modified by inherent genetic, epigenetic, and gender, as well as acquired traits including age, presence of disease, environmental influences, nutrition, and fitness level.[17]

CONCLUSION

Regular exercise is beneficial beyond reducing conventional cardiovascular risk factors; in some ways, it is even better than currently available agents, due to its preventive multisystem effects with little cost and few adverse effects.[11] The benefits result from an interplay of hundreds of genes involved in tissue maintenance and homeostasis; results from proteomics have shown that the effects can vary depending on the cell of their origin, whether at rest or exercising when they are secreted.

One must therefore be cautious in applying the reductionist paradigm when understanding and trying to regulate the effects of exercise.[18] Benefits of exercise beyond the skeletal muscle relate to improvement of endothelial function, remodeling of large arteries, improved autonomic balance, and psychological effects. In addition, exercise induces episodic physical shear stress which contributes to arterial health.

Given the enormous range of beneficial effects from exercise, the reductionist view of mimicking chemicals secreted by the skeletal muscle in response to exercise must be reconsidered. Following the excitement generated by an early study of exercise mimetic, Goodyear titled his commentary "The exercise pill – too good to be true"?[19] More than a decade later, the question still remains unanswered.

REFERENCES

1. Pontzer H, Wood BM, Raichlen DA. Hunter-gatherers as models in public health. Obes Rev. 2018;19 Suppl 1:24-35.
2. Raichlen DA, Pontzer H, Harris JA, Mabulla AZP, Marlowe FW, Snodgrass JJ, et al. Physical activity patterns and biomarkers of cardiovascular disease risk in hunter-gatherers. Am J Hum Biol. 2017;3(29):e22919.
3. Lieberman D. Are We Born to Rest or Run: In Exercised: The Science Of Physical Activity, Rest and Health. New York: Allen Lane; 2020; pp. 3-24.
4. McKenzie S. Getting Physical: The Rise of Fitness Culture in America. Kansas: University Press of Kansas; 2013.
5. Ding D, Mutrie N, Bauman A, Pratt M, Hallal PRC, Powell KE. Physical activity guidelines 2020: comprehensive and inclusive recommendations to activate populations. Lancet. 2020;396(10265): 1780-2.
6. Bull FC, Al-Ansari SS, Biddle S, Borodulin K, Buman MP, Cardon G, et al. World Health Organization 2020 guidelines on physical activity and sedentary behaviour. Br J Sports Med. 2020;54(24):1451-62.
7. Sridhar GR. Diabetes in India: Snapshot of a panorama. Curr Sci. 2002;83(7):791.
8. Sridhar GR, Madhu K, Veena S, Madhavi R, Sangeetha BS, Rani A. Living with diabetes: Indian experience. Diabetes Metab Syndr. 2007;1(3):181-7.
9. Gordon CD, Nelson GA. Physical activity correlates among persons with type 2 diabetes in Jamaica. Int J Diabetes Dev Ctries. 2019;39(2):108-14.
10. Nagaraju AS, Tondare D, Gopichandran V. What makes patients with diabetes adopt physical activity behaviors?—a trans-theoretical model approach. Int J Diabetes Dev Ctries. 2019;39:739-48.
11. Fiuza-Luces C, Garatachea N, Berge NA, Lucia A. Exercise is the real polypill. Physiology. 2013;28(5):-330-58.
12. Catoire M, Kersten S. The search for exercise factors in humans. FASEB J. 2015;29(5):1615-28.
13. Fan W, Evans RM. Exercise mimetics: Impact on health and performance. Cell Metab. 2017;25(2): 242-7.
14. Hoffman NJ, Parker BL, Chaudhuri R, Fisher-Wellman KH, Kleinert M, Humphrey SJ, et al. Global phosphoproteomic analysis of human skeletal muscle reveals a network of exercise-regulated kinases and AMPK substrates. Cell Metab. 2015;22(5):922-35.
15. Vina J, Sanchis-Gomar F, Martinez-Bello V, Gomez-Cabrera MC. Exercise acts as a drug; the pharmacological benefits of exercise. Br J Pharmacol. 2012;167(1):1-12.
16. Carey AL, Kingwell BA. Novel pharmacological approaches to combat obesity and insulin resistance: targeting skeletal muscle with 'exercise mimetics'. Diabetologia. 2009;52(10):2015-26.
17. Neufer PD, Bamman MM, Muoio DM, Bouchard C, Cooper DM, Goodpaster BH, et al. Understanding the cellular and molecular mechanisms of physical activity-induced health benefits. Cell Metab. 2015;22(1):4-11.
18. Hawley JA, Joyner MJ, Green DJ. Mimicking exercise: what matters most and where to next? J Physiol. 2021;599(3):791-802.
19. Goodyear LJ. The exercise pill--too good to be true? N Engl J Med. 2008;359(17):1842-4.

Index

Page numbers followed by *b* refer to box, *f* refer to figure, and *t* refer to table.

A

B

C

K

L

M

N

O

P

R

S

T

U

V

W

X